Case Based Reviews in
Pediatric Pulmonology

Case Based Reviews in
Pediatric Pulmonology

Editors

Kana Ram Jat MD FCCP MAMS
Assistant Professor
Department of Pediatrics
All India Institute of Medical Sciences
New Delhi, India

Jhuma Sankar MD
Assistant Professor
Department of Pediatrics
All India Institute of Medical Sciences
New Delhi, India

Rakesh Lodha MD
Additional Professor
Department of Pediatrics
All India Institute of Medical Sciences
New Delhi, India

Sushil K Kabra MD DNB
Professor
Department of Pediatrics
All India Institute of Medical Sciences
New Delhi, India

JAYPEE

JAYPEE BROTHERS MEDICAL PUBLISHERS
The Health Sciences Publisher
New Delhi | London

Jaypee Brothers Medical Publishers (P) Ltd

Headquarters
EMCA House
23/23-B, Ansari Road, Daryaganj
New Delhi 110 002, India
Landline: +91-11-23272143, +91-11-23272703
+91-11-23282021, +91-11-23245672
E-mail: jaypee@jaypeebrothers.com

Corporate Office
4838/24, Ansari Road, Daryaganj
New Delhi 110 002, India
Phone: +91-11-43574357
Fax: +91-11-43574314
E-mail: jaypee@jaypeebrothers.com

Overseas Office
J.P. Medical Ltd.
83, Victoria Street, London
SW1H 0HW (UK)
Phone: +44-20 3170 8910
E-mail: info@jpmedpub.com

EU GPSR Authorised Representative
Logos Europe, 9 rue Nicolas Poussin
17000, La Rochelle, France
Phone: +33 (0) 6 67 93 73 78
E-mail: contact@logoseurope.eu

Website: www.jaypeebrothers.com
Website: www.jaypeedigital.com

Inquiries for bulk sales may be solicited at: jaypee@jaypeebrothers.com

Case Based Reviews in Pediatric Pulmonology / Kana Ram Jat, Jhuma Sankar, Rakesh Lodha, Sushil K Kabra

First Edition: 2017, Reprint: 2026

ISBN: 978-93-85891-86-1

Printed in India

Contributors

EDITORS

Kana Ram Jat MD FCCP MAMS
Assistant Professor, Department of Pediatrics
All India Institute of Medical Sciences
New Delhi, India

Jhuma Sankar MD
Assistant Professor, Department of Pediatrics
All India Institute of Medical Sciences
New Delhi, India

Rakesh Lodha MD
Additional Professor, Department of Pediatrics
All India Institute of Medical Sciences
New Delhi, India

Sushil K Kabra MD DNB
Professor, Department of Pediatrics
All India Institute of Medical Sciences
New Delhi, India

CONTRIBUTING AUTHORS

Prahalad Kumar A MD FIAP
Professor
Department of Pediatric Medicine
Indira Gandhi Institute of Child Health
Bengaluru, Karnataka, India

Pooja Abbey MD DNB
Associate Professor
Department of Radio-Diagnosis
Lady Hardinge Medical College
New Delhi, India

Shalini Akunuri DCH DNB
Consultant
Department of PICU
Lotus Hospital for Women and Children
Visakhapatnam, Andhra Pradesh, India

Narendra K Bagri MD
Assistant Professor
Department of Pediatrics
All India Institute of Medical Sciences
New Delhi, India

Abdus S Bhat MD
Lecturer, Department of Pediatrics
Government Medical College and
Associated GB Pant Children Hospital
Srinagar, Jammu and Kashmir, India

Esra Caylan MD
Clinical Fellow, Department of Pediatric
Pulmonology, Maria Fareri Children's Hospital
at WMC and NYMC
VALHALLA, New York, United States

Arindam Choudhury MD MNAMS
Assistant Professor
Department of Cardiac Anesthesiology
All India Institute of Medical Sciences
New Delhi, India

Krishan Chugh MD MNAMS
Director and Head
Department of Pediatrics and Pediatric Intensive
Care Unit, Fortis Memorial Research Institute
Gurgaon, Haryana, India

Rashmi R Das MD FCCP FAPSR
Assistant Professor
Department of Pediatrics
All India Institute of Medical Sciences
Bhubaneswar, Odisha, India

Dhulika Dhingra MD
Assistant Professor
Department of Pediatrics
Chacha Nehru Bal Chikitsalya
New Delhi, India

Rakesh K Dogra DCH
Senior Specialist
Department of Pediatrics
Hindu Rao Hospital
North Delhi Municipal Corporation
New Delhi, India

Swati Dublish MD
Assistant Professor
Department of Pediatrics
Lady Hardinge Medical College
New Delhi, India

Fei Jamie Dy MD
Fellow, Department of Respiratory Medicine
Boston Children's Hospital
Boston, Massachusetts, United States

Sudhendra R Fattepur MD
Assistant Professor
Department of Pediatrics
Karnataka Institute of Medical Sciences
Hubli, Karnataka, India

Gautam Ghosh MD DCH DNB MNAMS FIAP FIMAAMS
Senior DNB Faculty
Department of Pediatrics
BR Singh Hospital for Medical Education and
Research
Kolkata, West Bengal, India

Jagdish P Goyal MD
Assistant Professor
Department of Pediatrics
All India Institute of Medical Sciences
Rishikesh, Uttarakhand, India

Mukesh K Gupta MD
Associate Professor and Head
Department of Pediatrics
Mahatma Gandhi Medical College and
Hospital
Jaipur, Rajasthan, India

Paramesh D H MD FAAP FAIP FIAMS FIAA FICAAI
Director
Department of Pediatric Pulmonology
Lakeside Center for Health Promotion
Bengaluru, Karnataka, India

Anupam Jaiswal MD
Consultant
Department of Pediatrics
Manipal Hospital
Bengaluru, Karnataka, India

Deo K Jha MD
Chief Medical Officer
Department of Pediatrics
Kasturba Hospital
New Delhi, India

Vidya K MD
Associate Professor
Department of Pathology
Vydehi Institute of Medical Sciences and Research Centre
Bengaluru, Karnataka, India

Subramanya N K MD
Professor
Department of Pediatrics
Vydehi Institute of Medical Sciences and Research Centre
Bengaluru, Karnataka, India

Salim A Khatib DNB DCH
Consultant
Department of Pediatrics
Columbia Asia Hospital
Bengaluru, Karnataka, India

Umakanth Khatwa MD
Director
Sleep Laboratory
Attending Pulmonary and Sleep Medicine
Boston Children's Sleep Center
Division of Respiratory Diseases
Boston Children's Hospital
Boston, Massachusetts, United States

Daisy Khera MD
Associate Professor
Department of Pediatrics
All India Institute of Medical Sciences
Jodhpur, Rajasthan, India

Indu Khoshla MD DCH RCPCH
Consultant and Director
Dr Indu's New Born and Childcare Centre
Mumbai, Maharashtra, India

Ilin Kinimi MD
Consultant
Department of Pediatrics
Manipal Hospital
Bengaluru, Karnataka, India

Sankaran Krishnan MD MPH FAAP
Associate Professor
Department of Pediatric Pulmonology
Maria Fareri Children's Hospital
at Westchester Medical Center and
New York Medical College
Valhalla, New York, United States

Ajay Kumar MD
Professor
Department of Pediatrics
Vardhman Mahavir Medical College and
Safdarjang Hospital
New Delhi, India

Prawin Kumar MD
Assistant Professor
Department of Pediatrics
All India Institute of Medical Sciences
Jodhpur, Rajasthan, India

Saptharishi Lalgudi Ganesan MD DM
Senior Resident
Department of Pediatrics
Postgraduate Institute of
Medical Education and Research
Chandigarh, India

Anirban Maitra DCH MRCP FRCPCH MMedSci CCT
Consultant
Royal Manchester Children's Hospital
Central Manchester University Hospitals
NHS Trust
Manchester, United Kingdom

Vivek Manchanda MS DNB MCh MBA
Associate Professor
Department of Pediatric Surgery
All India Institute of Medical Sciences
Jodhpur, Rajasthan, India

Poonam Mehta MD
Assistant Professor
Department of Pediatrics
Pt. B.D. Sharma Postgraduate Institute of
Medical Sciences
Rohtak, Haryana, India

Ramesh P Menon MD FAIMER
Assistant Professor
Department of Cardiothoracic and
Vascular Surgery, Pediatrics
All India Institute of Medical Sciences
New Delhi, India

Mudit Mittal MD
Senior Resident
Department of Pediatrics
All India Institute of Medical Sciences
Jodhpur, Rajasthan, India

Aparna Mukherjee MD PhD
Early Career Fellow, Wellcome Trust/DBT India
Alliance
Department of Pediatrics
All India Institute of Medical Sciences
New Delhi, India

Vishal Mukhija MD
Consultant
Dr Indu's New Born and Childcare Centre
Mumbai, Maharashtra, India

Shashidhara R Nagabhushana DCH DNB FIAP
Clinical Associate
Department of Pediatrics
Church of South India Hospital
Bengaluru, Karnataka, India

Devki Nandan MD
Professor and Head
Department of Pediatrics
Post Graduate Institute of Medical Education
and Research and Dr RML Hospital
New Delhi, India

Praveen Narsaria MD
Consultant
Department of Pediatrics
Nagarmal Modi Seva Sadan
Ranchi, Jharkhand, India

Varun Narwal MD FNBE
Consultant
Department of Pediatrics
Kainos Superspeciality Hospital
Rohtak, Haryana, India

Gowrishankar NC MD DCH DNB FIAP
Head, Pediatrics–Clinical Operations and Quality
Department of Pediatric Medicine
Dr Mehta's Children's Hospital
Chennai, Tamil Nadu, India

Ankit Parakh MD DNB MNAMS
Consultant
Department of Pediatrics
Dr. B.L. Kapur Memorial Hospital
New Delhi, India

Nandini Paul MSc
PhD Student
Department of Pediatrics
Postgraduate Institute of
Medical Education and Research
Chandigarh, India

Umar A Qureshi MD
Lecturer
Department of Pediatrics
Government Medical College and
Associated GB Pant Children Hospital
Srinagar, Jammu and Kashmir, India

Dinesh Raj MD
Associate Consultant
Department of Pediatrics
Holy Family Hospital
New Delhi, India

Vinod H Ratageri MD DCEH
Associate Professor
Department of Pediatrics
Karnataka Institute of Medical Sciences
Hubli, Karnataka, India

Santosh K Rathia MD
Assistant Professor
Department of Pediatrics
Pt Jawahar Lal Nehru Memorial Medical College
Raipur, Chhattisgarh, India

Anil K Sapare MD
Consultant
Department of Pediatrics
Narayana Hrudayalaya
Bengaluru, Karnataka, India

Rohit Sasidharan MD
Senior Resident
Department of Pediatrics
All India Institute of Medical Sciences
New Delhi, India

Julius X Scott MD
Chief
Department of Pediatric Hemato-Oncology
Sri Ramachandra University
Chennai, Tamil Nadu, India

Vineet Sehgal MD
Consultant
Department of Pediatrics
Max Healthcare
New Delhi, India

Bhagwan S Sharma MD
Senior Professor
Department of Pediatrics
Sawai ManSingh Medical College
Jaipur, Rajasthan, India

Meenu Singh MD
Professor
Department of Pediatrics
Postgraduate Institute of
Medical Education and Research
Chandigarh, India

Kamal K Singhal DCH MD
Assistant Professor
Department of Pediatrics
Kalawati Saran Chidlrens' Hospital
New Delhi, India

Tanu Singhal MD MSc
Consultant
Department of Pediatrics and
Infectious Disease
Kokilaben Dhirubhai Ambani Hospital and
Medical Research Institute
Mumbai, Maharashtra, India

Latha M Sneha MD
Assistant Professor
Department of Pediatric Hemato-Oncology
Sri Ramachandra University
Chennai, Tamil Nadu, India

Ravitanya Sodani MD
Senior Resident
Department of Pediatrics
Kalawati Saran Chidlrens' Hospital
New Delhi, India

Sivabalan X Somu MD DNB MNAMS FCCP FIAP
Consultant
Department of Pediatrics
Kanchi Kamakoti CHILDS Trust Hospital
Chennai, Tamil Nadu, India

Balasubramanian Sundaram MD DCH FRCPCH
Head, Department of Pediatrics
Kanchi Kamakoti CHILDS Trust Hospital and
CHILDS Trust Medical Research Foundation
Chennai, Tamil Nadu, India

Vikas Taneja DNB IDPCCM
Senior Consultant
Department of Pediatrics
Fortis Memorial Research Institute
Gurgaon, Haryana, India

Wonashi R Tsanglao MD
Senior Resident
Department of Pediatrics
Post Graduate Institute of
Medical Education
and Research and Dr RML Hospital
New Delhi, India

Pankaj C Vaidya MD
Associate Professor
Department of Pediatrics
Postgraduate Institute of
Medical Education and Research
Chandigarh, India

Ajoy M Varghese MS DNB
Professor
Department of ENT
Christian Medical College
Vellore, Tamil Nadu, India

Sneha D Varkki Dch DNB
Professor
Department of Pediatrics
Christian Medical College
Vellore, Tamil Nadu, India

Nishant Verma MD
Assistant Professor
Department of Pediatrics
King George's Medical University
Lucknow, Uttar Pradesh, India

Prabhakar M Veturi DCH MD
Pediatrician
Department of Pediatrics
Veturi Polyclinic and Diagnostic Centre
Bengaluru, Karnataka, India

Jasmeet K Wadhwa DCH DNB
Senior Consultant
Department of Pediatrics
Sri Balaji Action Medical Institute and
BLK Super Speciality Hospital
New Delhi, India

Preface

Respiratory diseases are a common cause of morbidity and mortality in children. Significant advances have occurred leading to better understanding of pediatric respiratory illnesses. Diagnostic tests have improved and with better treatment, outcome of acute as well as chronic illnesses has improved.

Basic principles of clinical medicine include, making a provisional diagnosis from history and clinical examination and confirming diagnosis by using available investigations judiciously.

In the first edition of this multi-author book, we have included cases of common respiratory illnesses and discussed them based on clinical findings to reach a diagnosis by using available investigations, where indicated. We have also discussed the principles of management and outcome of patients. The cases were selected considering the local epidemiological situation, sociodemographic background of patients, and available resources.

The basic aim of the book is to equip practicing pediatricians with necessary knowledge to consider and confirm various respiratory illnesses in children. We hope the book will achieve its objective.

Kana Ram Jat

Jhuma Sankar

Rakesh Lodha

Sushil K Kabra

Acknowledgments

We acknowledge the team of Jaypee Brothers Medical Publishers (P) Ltd., especially Miss Barkha Arora (Editorial co-ordinator) and Dr Neeraj Choudhary (Senior Acquisition Editor-Corporate) for their outstanding support in shaping the outlook of chapters as reader friendly. Gladden Savieo (Copy editors), Neha Bhatia (Development Editor), and Birendra Kumar (DTP operator) from his team have also put a lot of hard work and diligence during the creation of this book.

Contents

Section 3: Wheezing Disorders in Children

Section 4: Respiratory Tract Infections

Section 5: Suppurative Lung Diseases

Section 9: Miscellaneous Respiratory Disorders

PLATE 1

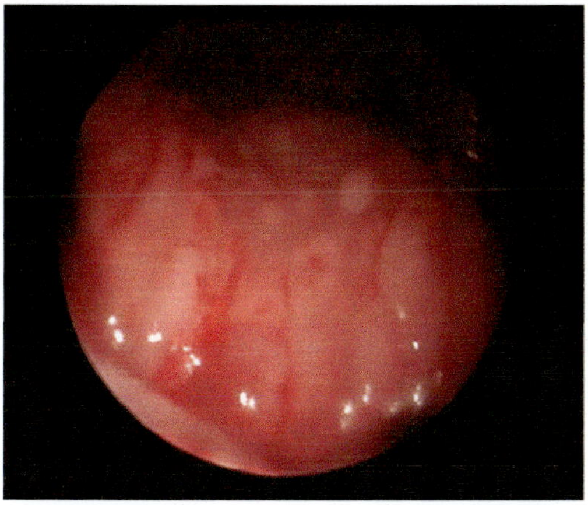

Figure 2: Posterior pharyngeal wall showing cobblestone appeareance *(Chapter 2)*

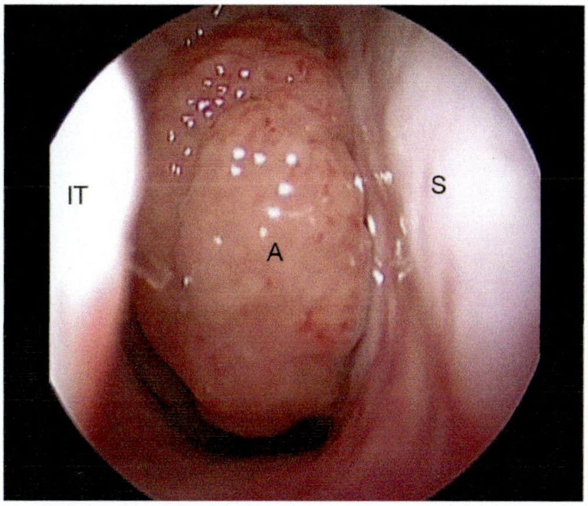

IT, inferior turbinate; S, septum; A, adenoids.

Figure 1: Nasal endoscopic images showing adenoid obstructing choana almost completely *(Chapter 6)*

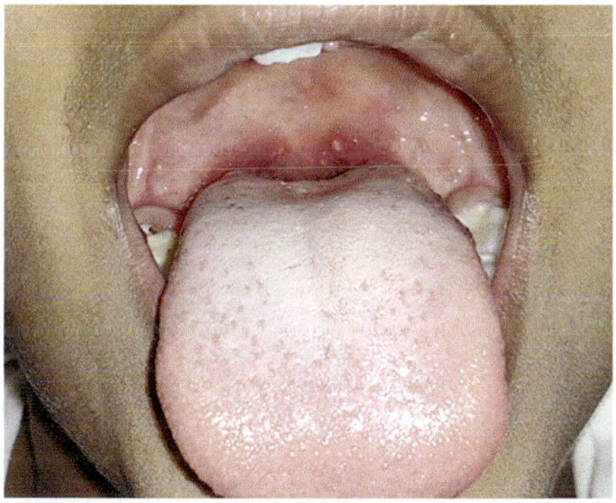

Figure 1: Throat examination showing small ulcers around the edges of faucial pillars *(Chapter 4)*.

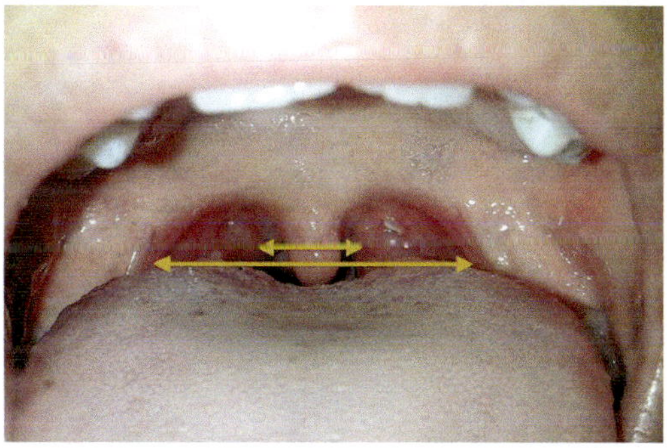

Figure 1: Bilateral tonsillar enlargement *(Chapter 7)*

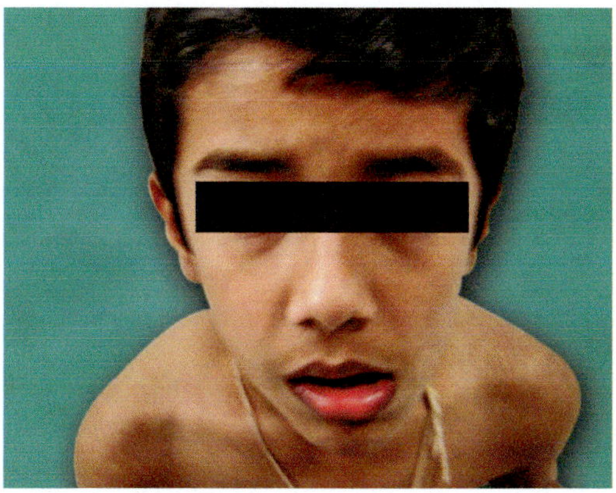

Figure 2: Scarlatiniform rash after partial improvement *(Chapter 4)*

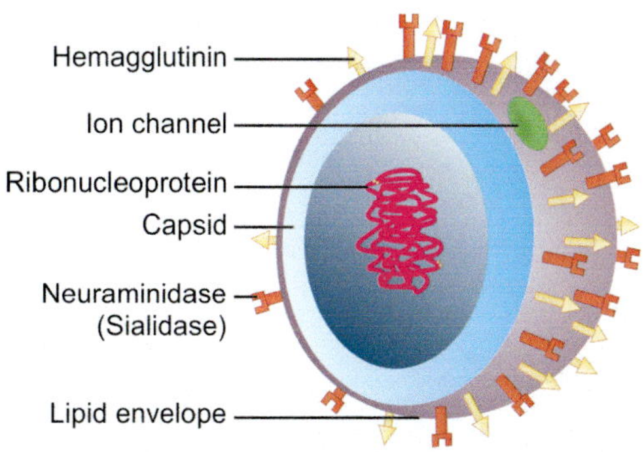

Figure 1: Influenza virus *(Chapter 18)*

PLATE 2

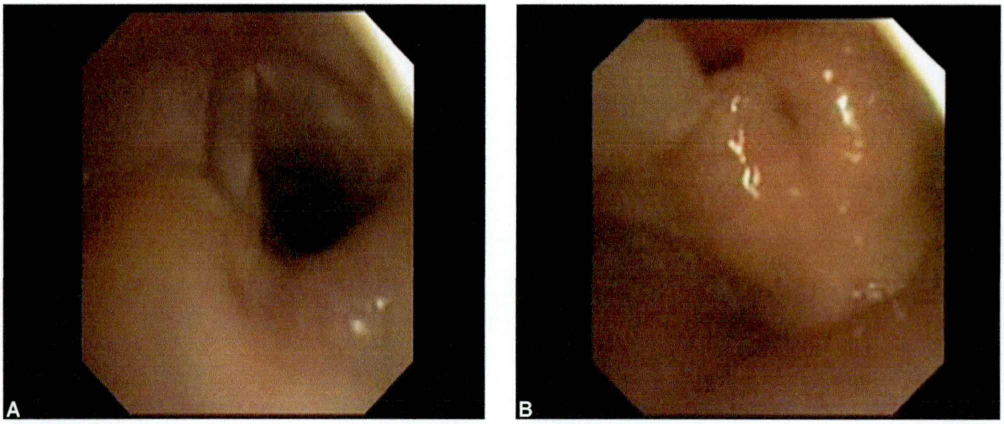

Figure 1: Fiber optic laryngoscopic view of child with laryngomalacia. **A,** during expiration and **B,** during inspiration *(Chapter 10)*

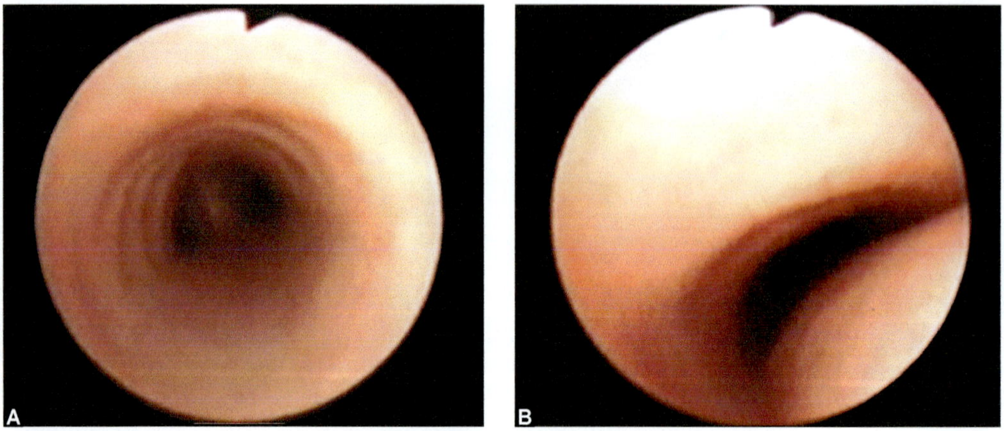

Figure 3: Bronchoscopic findings. **A,** in normal trachea and **B,** in tracheomalacia ***(Chapter 10)***

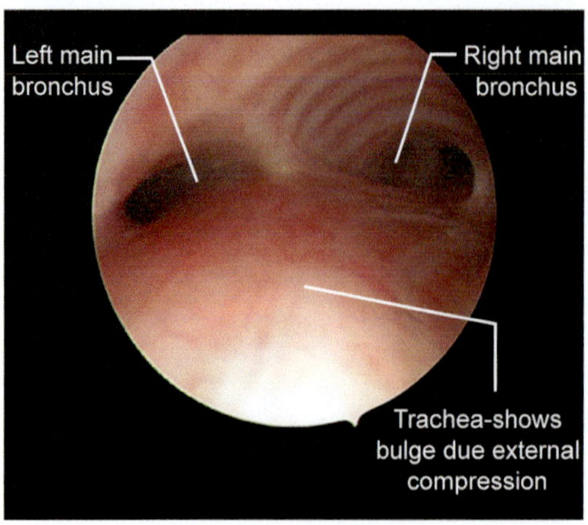

Figure 4: Bronchoscopic findings. Compression of left main bronchus ***(Chapter 10)***

Courtesy: Anilkumar Sapare, NH Hospital, Bengaluru.

PLATE 3

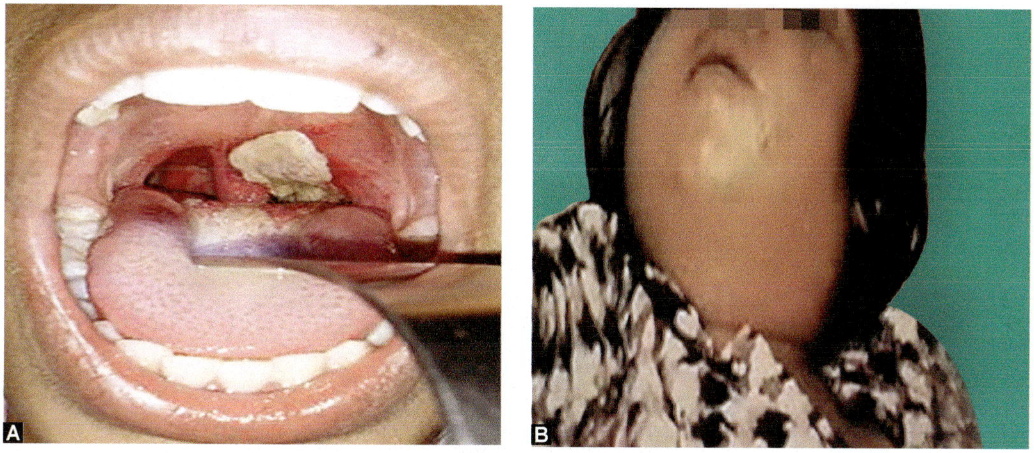

Figure 2: Tonsillar and pharyngeal diphtheria in two patients *(Chapter 19)*

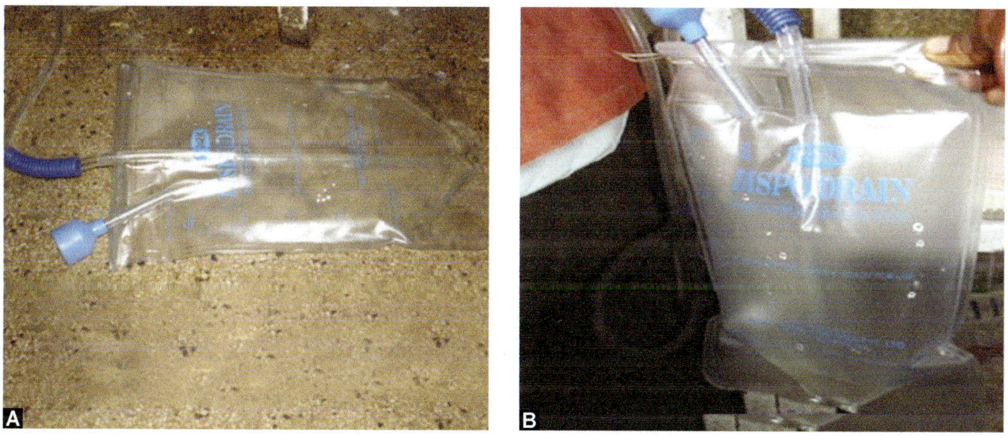

Figure 7: Pitfalls in intercostal drain management *(Chapter 38)*

1

SECTION

Disorders of Upper Respiratory Tract

CHAPTER

1

Common Cold

Deo K Jha

> **CASE 1**
>
> A 4-month-old female child was brought by her mother because the child had become irritable and was taking less feed since the last 48 hours. She had running nose since the last 24 hours and seems to have fever on touch. Her mother had cough, cold, and fever the previous week. On examination, her face was a bit red with red eyes and nasal discharge which was watery. Her vitals were stable with temperature of 100.4°F in axilla, no respiratory distress, and chest on auscultation was clear.

Q. What may be diagnostic possibilities here?

Diagnostic possibilities include common cold, influenza or swine flu, bronchiolitis, pneumonia, or allergic rhinitis. Let us explore all possibilities: *allergic rhinitis* is rare in this age group. It may be associated with other allergic conditions like allergic dermatitis, allergic conjunctivitis, or allergic airways disease and history should be of long time. There may be family history of atopy which we should ask the parents. In *pneumonia*, there should be high fever, with toxic look of baby with tachypnea which is a constant feature of pneumonia with or without chest retraction. On chest auscultation, one should get the finding of reduced intensity of breath sound or bronchial breath sound over affected area. There may be deep inspiratory crackles on auscultation. In *bronchiolitis*, there may be low- to high-grade fever, but if it is high grade at onset, it usually wanes over next 2–3 days. Child does not look toxic and respiratory distress may or may not be present. On auscultation of chest, there will be wheezes with or without early inspiratory crackles. In *influenza* or *swine flu*, the presentation will be more severe with continuous high-grade fever, vomiting, and loose motion and it is very difficult to feed the child. There may be history of proven swine flu in the family or in the society.

Looking on the case above, these possibilities are remote. So, it may be a case of our first possibility that is *common cold.*

Q. What is epidemiology of common cold?

The most common infective disease of human being is common cold. It is a great burden on society in terms of sufferings by children and number of working days lost by parents for caring of their children, despite enormous advancement in medical science in terms of preventive, diagnostic, and treatment facilities. It affects more infants and children than adults. Children <6 years of age may have one episode of common cold every month without any cause of concern. It is a self-limiting viral infection of upper respiratory tract. Symptoms vary depending upon the type of virus responsible for a particular infection. More than 50% of infections in children are caused by *Rhinoviruses* which have >100 serotypes. Other less common viruses responsible are adenovirus, respiratory syncytial virus (RSV), human metapneumovirus, influenza virus, and parainfluenza virus.

Seasonal patterns

Common cold is not caused by exposure to cold air or cold environment. It can occur in any season but occurs more commonly during fall and spring season irrespective of geographical locations. Any virus can infect children in any season, but the highest prevalence of some of the viruses has been seen in different seasons of the year as follows: *Rhinovirus*—early fall and late spring like in July-August and March-April; *parainfluenza virus*—late fall and late spring like in September-October and March-April; and *RSV* and *influenza virus*—mid winter throughout spring up to late spring like from December-April.

Mode of transmission

It is transmitted from person to person. When a child or adult suffering from common cold rubs his or her nose and then touches the hands of other person and then he or she touches his or her eyes or nose, the virus enters into that person because the virus remains alive on hands for about 2 hours. Common cold virus remains alive for about 24 hours on surfaces of toys, door handles, and table-tops and it can infect other person during this period. Common cold virus, particularly *Rhinovirus,* does not usually get transmitted by droplets but influenza virus can. Common cold is not usually transmitted by saliva.

Susceptibility

Mannose-binding lectin deficiency with impaired innate immunity in children makes them excessive susceptible to common cold. Asthmatic bronchial cells produce less β-interferon, which makes asthmatic children more susceptible to rhinovirus infection. There is variation in severity of common cold symptoms due to the polymorphism of cytokine genes, suggestive of genetic predisposition.

Pathogenesis

Viruses induce inflammation of nasal mucosa with or without mucosal lining of sinuses without damaging the epithelium. Kinin and cytokines are secreted by the epithelial lining after contact with viruses. Interleukin-8, which is secreted, attracts polymorphonuclear inflammatory cells. Inflammatory cells may block opening of sinuses or Eustachian tube with its complications. Prostsglandin and kinin which are released locally, cause vasodilatation; increased vascular permeability, and excessive secretion from exocrine glands. Stimulation of parasympathetic nerve endings along with these is responsible for symptoms.

CASE 2

An 18-month-old boy, who was completely well till 2 days back, was suddenly noticed with watery discharge through nose by his mother, which became yellowish the next day and then turned greenish after 2 days. He started sneezing many times a day with occasional cough 2–3 times a day. He started taking less feed and his forehead was warm to touch and her mother recorded temperature of 100.4°F. On examination, fever was confirmed to that extent and systemic examination was noncontributory.

Q. What are common clinical features of common cold?

The most common complaint in children suffering from common cold is nasal congestion which starts after 24–48 hours of exposures. Incubation period is 12–72 hours, but symptom has been noticed as early as 2 hours after contact. Fever of low grade 38°C or 100.4°F is common in first 3 days of illness. Nasal discharge may be watery, yellowish, or green. Other features are sore throat, cough, irritability, decrease in appetite with difficulty to feed the child, and difficulty in getting sleep which is disturbing for parents also. There may be watering from eyes with redness secondary to rubbing of eyes. There may be mild headache and loss of taste and loss of smell during the period. There may be hoarseness of voice in some children. There may be malaise with loss of interest in play and study.

Nasal mucosa may be swollen and edematous, and there may be nontender enlargement of cervical lymph nodes. Symptoms usually last for 7–10 days but may be prolonged to 14 days in some cases. Some times a second common cold virus infects the child during this prolonged period which gives confusion to physician that the first one is prolonging, but it should not be a cause of concern unless any sign of secondary bacterial infection is there.

Q. How we can diagnose common cold? What is the role of various investigations?

Diagnosis is primarily clinical. There is no role of investigations like hemogram, chest X-ray, throat swab and X-ray paranasal sinuses. There is no benefit of isolation of virus as antiviral agents are available for only few viruses.

> **CASE 3**
>
> A 5-year-old male child was noticed with watery discharge through the nose 5 days back by his mother when he returned from school. He was sneezing frequently for last the 3 days and on asking, he complained of some discomfort in his throat for the last 6 days. For the last 4 days he had temperature of >102°F. On examination his throat was congested, tonsil enlarged and congested, and there was tender anterior cervical lymph node enlargement. Systemic examination was noncontributory.

Q. When one should worry in common cold and what complications may be there?

The following features may be the cause of concern in a child with common cold—fever of 100.4°F in infants from birth up to 12 weeks of age; fever lasting >1 day (24 hours) in a child <2 years of age, fever lasting >2 days (48 hours) in a child >2 years of age, fever of 104°F and being repeated to such an extent in a child of any age, fever >101°F lasting for >3 days in any age of child, excessive sleepiness, pain abdomen, vomiting, impaired consciousness, very poor or no oral intake, severe headache, neck stiffness, ear pain, persistent cry, difficulty in breathing, and persistent cough.

Complications

Common colds are usually self-limiting but sometimes get complicated by the following: (1) acute otitis media, is the commonest complication; (2) asthma: children who are predisposed for asthma may get first episode of wheezing during common cold or the common cold may exacerbate the pre-existing asthma; (3) sinusitis: it should be suspected if the symptoms of common cold are prolonged for >10–14 days or if there is worsening of symptoms after initial improvement or the symptoms start with high-grade fever which prolong for >3 days; (4) secondary bacterial infection like bacterial tonsillopharyngitis as seen in case 3: and (5) pneumonia: child may be complicated by viral as well as secondary bacterial pneumonia which should be suspected if there is tachypnea, cough and high-grade fever.

Q. How to manage a child with common cold?

Market is flooded of formulations for common cold remedy with antihistaminics, antitussive cough syrups, decongestants, and expectorants. These are being used by parents very frequently. But no randomized controlled trials have shown benefit with these medications in children under the age of 6 years. Moreover, The Food and Drug Administration (FDA) has banned these medications for use in children below 2 years of age and further studies have indicated no benefit of these below 6 years of age. It has been seen in our experience that it gives only psychological benefits to the parents, so the use of these medications should be discouraged.

Symptomatic treatment in the form of paracetamol for fever and discomfort due to malaise should be given in the dose of 10–15 mg/kg body weight, which can be repeated 4–6 hourly if needed. Ibuprofen can be used in infants above 6 months of age in the dose of 7.5–10 mg/kg body weight, repeated every 6–8 hours if needed. Aspirin should not be used in children below 18 years of age due to fear of Reye syndrome. Symptoms due to nasal blockage should be taken care by instilling saline nasal drop into each nostril several times a day or it can be sprayed into the nostrils and secretions sucked out by bulb syringe. Nighttime cough may be treated by giving honey to children above 12 months of age. Symptoms of rhinorrhea may be decreased by 25–35% by giving first generation antihistaminics and anticholinergics. Child should be encouraged to take adequate fluid without forcing to take extra water intake.

Second generation nonsedative antihistaminics are not effective. There is no role of any antibiotics and its use may increase the resistance of antibiotics in society. Moreover, excessive irrational use of antibiotics to treat viral infections in children below 1 year of age may predispose the child to develop asthma after 6 years of age. Steam (warm humidified air) inhalation is not found to be effective for common cold and there is risk of burn in children and should not be used. Other preparations like zinc, vitamin C, and herbal product like *Echinacea* have no proven role, although being used with variable results.

Q. How common cold can be prevented? Is vaccine effective for common cold?

By the time we notice the symptoms of common cold in children, it might have infected several children because it is most infectious in initial 2–4 days. The most effective way of limiting the spread is by hand-washing for 15–30 seconds with soap water, without the need of any soap containing antibacterial. If water and sink is not available, hand rub containing alcohol as disinfectant can be used, it should be spread over both surfaces of hands until it dries. It is practically impossible to keep the infected person away from contact but they should be advised to cough or sneeze into tissues and wash hands frequently.

Vaccines to prevent common cold are not possible, seeing the large variation in antigenic type of virus.

LEARNING POINTS

- The most common cause of common cold is rhinovirus infection
- It is a self-limiting disease requiring only symptomatic treatment
- Some individuals are more susceptible and severity of symptoms varies among individuals
- It may be complicated by bacterial infection which should be detected and treated at the earliest
- There is no role of antibiotic in uncomplicated case, rather it may be harmful
- It may exacerbate asthma in children.

SUGGESTED READINGS

1. Cohen HA, Rozen J, Kristal H, Laks Y, Berkovitch M, Uziel Y, et al. Effect of honey on nocturnal cough and sleep quality: a double-blind, randomized, placebo-controlled study. Pediatrics. 2012;130(3):465-71.
2. Doyle WJ, Casselbrant ML, Li-Korotky HS, Doyle AP, Lo CY, Turner R, et al. The interleukin 6-174 C/C genotype predicts greater rhinovirus illness. J Infect Dis. 2010;201(2):199-206.
3. Heikkinen T, Järvinen A. The common cold. Lancet. 2003; 361(9351):51-9.
4. Martin ET, Fairchok MP, Stednick ZJ, Kuypers J, Englund JA. Epidemiology of multiple respiratory viruses in childcare attendees. J Infect Dis. 2013;207(6):982-9.
5. Van der Zalm MM, Uiterwaal CSPM, Wilbrink B, de Jong BM, Verheij TJ, Kimpen JL, et al. Respiratory pathogens in respiratory tract illnesses during the first year of life: a birth cohort study. Pediatr Infect Dis J. 2009;28:472-6.

CHAPTER

2

Allergic Rhinitis

Vineet Sehgal

CASE 1

An 8-year-old boy presented with complaints of:

- Constant cold for 3 years in the form of early morning sneezing and feeling of blocked nose
- He had intermittent cough for the past 6 months; cough was more on lying down
- The cold was disturbing his sleep, had lacrimation and would feel sleepy in school
- He had been given cold and cough syrups and nasal drops at night, intermittently

Family history of atopy was present.

Examination showed the following:

- Child had height and weight around 60th centile for age
- Dark under-eyes, gaping mouth (Fig. 1), with mouth breathing
- Inferior nasal turbinates hypertrophied, mucosa bluish in color
- Cobblestoned appearance of posterior pharyngeal wall (Fig. 2)
- Systemic examination was normal.

Q. What is diagnosis of the case?

It is allergic rhinitis (AR).

Q. What is AR?

Allergic rhinitis is a chronic inflammatory disease of nose induced by an immunoglobulin (Ig)E-mediated inflammation, after allergen exposure of mucus membrane of nose.

Four major cardinal symptoms of AR are:

1. Sneezing
2. Itching
3. Rhinorrhea (running nose)
4. Congestion (nasal obstruction or blocked nose).

Two or more of these symptoms present for >1 hour/day on most days are suggestive of AR. Other symptoms of AR may be:

- Lacrimation, itching eyes, conjunctivitis
- Feeling of ear fullness, otalgia
- Palatal pruritus, halitosis
- Headache, fatigue, sleep impairment
- Speech and cognitive impairment, depression.

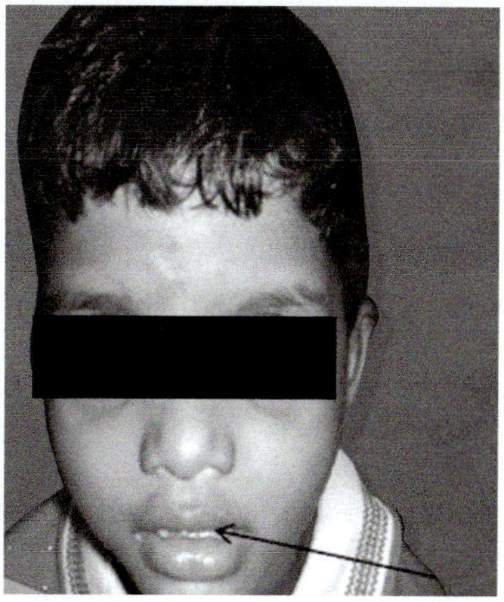

Figure 1: A child with allergic rhinitis showing gaping mouth (arrow head)

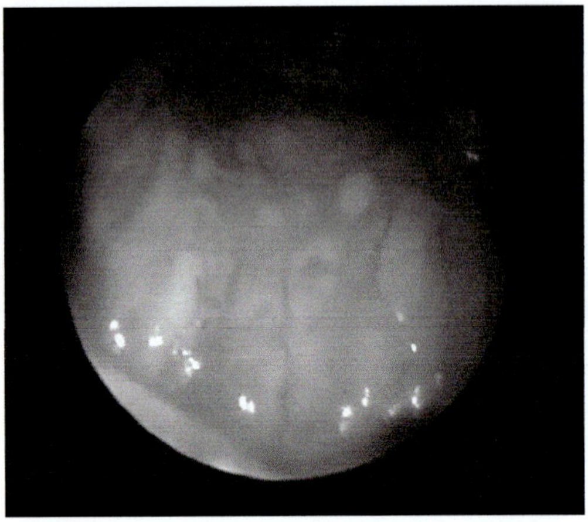

Figure 2: Posterior pharyngeal wall showing cobblestone appeareance *(For color version, see Plate 1)*

Q. What is the differential diagnosis?

Differential diagnosis of AR includes:

- Recurrent viral infections: usually febrile illnesses. More frequent in smaller children. Usually clustering of cases in contacts
- Vasomotor/occupational/hormonal/drug-induced/atrophic rhinitis
- Adenoidal hypertrophy/sinusitis, mouth breathing, snoring, disordered sleep, headaches
- Anatomic abnormalities like deviated nasal septum (DNS), polyps: usually unilateral symptoms
- Cystic fibrosis, mucociliary defects: will have other systemic symptoms
- Cerebrospinal fluid (CSF) rhinorrhea
- Foreign bodies, tumors, sarcoidosis.

Q. How AR can be diagnosed?

Diagnosis is entirely clinical. Investigations may be done to establish atopic sensitization in selected patients and these include blood counts, serum immunoglobulin E levels, Phadiatop and skin tests for allergy. Sometimes investigations may be needed to rule out alternate diagnosis or comorbidities if suggested on history and examination: X-ray soft tissue neck, X-ray paranasal sinuses, computed tomography (CT) scan for sinuses, sweat chloride, etc.

Q. How can AR be classified?

Earlier, AR used to be classified as seasonal or perennial, depending on persistence of symptoms. Indoor allergen sensitization was considered to be associated with perennial AR while aeroallergen sensitization was equated with seasonal AR. However, persistence of symptoms and intermittent exacerbations tend to overlap, making clear-cut delineation difficult. So ARIA (Allergic Rhinitis and it's impact on Asthma) group has proposed a functional classification, based on frequency of symptoms and their effect on quality of life. The classification is as under:

- Frequency:
  - Intermittent: if symptoms <4 days/week or for <4 consecutive weeks
  - Persistent: if symptoms >4 days/week and for >4 consecutive weeks
- Severity:
  - Mild: if normal sleep; no impairment of daily activities (including sport and leisure); normal work and school attendance; and no troublesome symptoms
  - Moderate-severe: if one or more of above mentioned is present
  - So, one can have a combination of intermittent and mild; intermittent and moderate-severe; persistent and mild; or persistent and moderate-severe.

CASE 1 *continued*

- On further detailed history taking, it was elicited that cough was more at night and early mornings. Climbing stairs and running precipitated paroxysmal cough. The cough would respond well to nebulized bronchodilators
- There was also history of snoring during sleep, more comfortable sleeping propped up and not getting up fresh in the morning.

Q. What are the possibilities now?

The boy had moderate-severe persistent and allergic rhinitis.

There is associated bronchial asthma and adenoid hypertrophy.

Q. What are comorbidities and complications associated with AR?

Allergic rhinitis may be associated or complicated by following conditions: asthma, sinusitis, allergic conjunctivitis, eczema, otitis media, adenoid hypertrophy, sleep-disordered breathing, speech impairment, and dentofacial anomalies.

Q. What is the management of AR?

The management strategies for AR are shown in table 1.

TABLE 1: Management strategies for allergic rhinitis and their action

Strategy	Action
Allergen control	Simple, effective, and essential means of controlling allergen exposure
Pharmacotherapy	
Antihistamines	Antagonize histamine action
Decongestants	Vasoconstriction
Corticosteroids	Anti-inflammatory action
Leukotriene receptor antagonists	Inhibition of early allergic response
Immunotherapy	Trigger induction of competing IgG antibodies
Surgery	Essentially to treat complications

Ig, immunoglobulin.

Treatment goals as outlined by ARIA include unimpaired sleep; ability to undertake normal daily activities, including work, school and leisure; no troublesome symptoms; and no or minimal side effects of the medications. Stepwise management of AR is shown in figure 3.

Allergen and irritant avoidance

Environmental control is basic treatment modality, whatever be the severity of AR. Common aeroallergens are dust mites, cockroach antigen, pollen, molds, and pet dander. Common irritants are dust, smoke, volatile organic compounds, mosquito coils, etc. These triggers should be eliminated or avoided by various measures, as much as possible.

Pharmacotherapy

Symptom wise efficacy of medicine class is shown in table 2.

Antihistamines

Oral second-generation antihistamines include cetirizine, levocetirizine, fexofenadine, loratadine and desloratadine. Doses of these drugs are shown in table 3. These are the first-line treatment for mild AR. They are effective for rhinorrhea, nasal pruritus, and sneezing, but less effective for nasal blockage. These may have possible additional anti-allergic and anti-

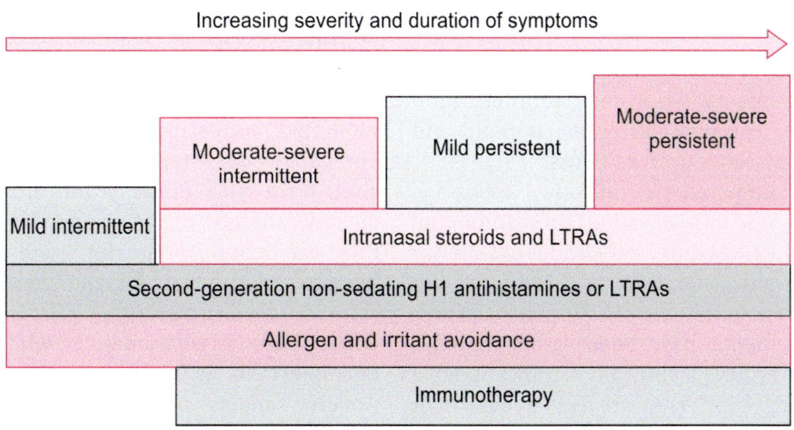

LTRAs, leukotriene receptor antagonists.

Figure 3: Stepwise management of allergic rhinitis based on severity

TABLE 2: Efficacy of various classes of drugs for allergic rhinitis symptoms

Characteristic	Nasal steroids	Oral antihistamine	Nasal antihistamine	Nasal decongestant	LTRA	Ipratropium bromide
Rhinorrhea	+++	++	++	--	+	++
Sneezing	+++	++	++	--	+	--
Itching	+++	++	++	--	+	--
Nose blockage	+++	+	+	+++	++	--
Eye symptoms	++	++	--	--	++	--

LTRA, leukotriene receptor antagonist.

TABLE 3: Doses of second-generation antihistamines for allergic rhinitis

Drug	Dose
Cetirizine	• 6–12 months: 2.5 mg OD • 12–24 months: 2.5 mg OD or BD • 2–5 years: 2.5 mg OD/BD or 5 mg OD • 6–11 years: 5 or 10 mg OD • >12 years: 5–10 mg OD
Levo-cetirizine	• 6 months–5 years: 1.25 mg OD • 6–11 years: 2.5 mg OD • >12 years: 5 mg OD
Fexo-fenadine	• 6 months–12 years: 30 mg BD • >12 years: 120–180 mg OD
Loratadine	• 1–2 years: 2.5 mg OD • 2–12 years: 5–10 mg OD • >12 years: 10 mg OD
Deslora-tadine	• 6–11 months: 1 mg OD • 12 months–5 years: 1.25 mg OD • 6–11 years: 2.5 mg OD • >12 years: 5 mg OD

BD, twice daily; OD, Once daily.

inflammatory effects. There are minimal or no sedative effects. Once daily administration is sufficient. The onset of action is rapid and duration of action is upto 24 hours.

Topical preparations include azelastine, olopatadine, and levocabastine. These intranasal antihistamines are equally efficacious or superior to oral second-generation antihistamines for treatment of intermittent AR. Systemic absorption occurs, hence have been associated with sedation. They have a clinically significant effect on nasal congestion. They are less effective than intranasal corticosteroids (INCS).

Intranasal corticosteroids

It is the most effective class of medicines for AR. Effect appears within 7–8 hours, while peak effect takes 2 weeks. Intranasal corticosteroids are effective in all symptoms of AR, including nasal obstruction. Intranasal corticosteroids are first-line pharmacotherapy for persistent AR. Comparing the available INCS, clinical response does not vary significantly between products irrespective of the differences in topical potency, lipid solubility, and binding affinity. They are overall safe to use. Adverse effects such as nasal irritation, epistaxis, septal perforation (extremely rare), hypothalamus-pituitary-adrenal axis suppression (inconsistent and not clinically significant), and suppressed growth (with beclomethasone) may be kept in mind. Available INCS with recommended dosages are shown in table 4.

Decongestants

These may be oral (pseudoephedrine, phenylephrine) or topical (xylometazoline, oxymetazoline). They reduce nasal congestion or obstruction, not much effect on histamine-mediated nasal symptoms, such as rhinorrhea. Topical decongestants can be considered for short-term and possibly for intermittent or episodic therapy of nasal congestion. However, they are inappropriate for regular daily use because of the risk for the development of rhinitis medicamentosa. Efficacy of oral decongestants is moderate while of nasal decongestants is high, in nasal obstruction. Adverse effects of oral decongestants may include insomnia, tachycardia, hyperkinesia,

TABLE 4: Intranasal corticosteroids and recommended doses and age group

Drug	Dosage	Lowest age group
Budesonide	• 6–11 years: 1 spray each nostril OD • >12 years: 2 sprays each nostril BD	6 years +
Fluticasone propionate	• 4–11 years: 1 spray each nostril OD • >12 years: 2 sprays each nostril OD	4 years +
Fluticasone furoate	• 2–11 years: 1 spray each nostril OD • >12 years: 2 sprays each nostril OD	2 years +
Mometasone furoate	• 2–11 years: 1 spray each nostril OD • >12 years: 2 sprays each nostril OD	2 years +

BD, twice daily; OD, once daily.

tremor, increased blood pressure, and stroke. Adverse effects of nasal decongestants include tachyphylaxis, rebound congestion, nasal hyperresponsiveness and rhinitis medicamentosa.

Leukotriene receptor antagonist (predominantly montelukast)

They are effective in improving asthma, AR symptom score by modulating inflammation. Less efficacious compared to nasal steroids. No data to suggest that combined leukotriene receptor antagonist (LTRA) + antihistamine or LTRA + INCS reduce symptoms more than either alone. May be used for simultaneous treatment of AR and asthma.

Dyspepsia (approximately 2%) and neuropsychiatric side effects have been reported.

Q. What is the role of immunotherapy in AR?

Desensitization or specific immunotherapy (SIT) is the only therapeutic option that modifies underlying cause of allergy and not just symptoms of allergy. It can be done by subcutaneous or sublingual route. It can be considered if there is a definite specific allergen

CASE 1 *continued*

- The boy was started on once daily combination of levocetirizine and montelukast. However, there was no improvement after 2 weeks of therapy
- On review of his environment, it was discovered that the roof of his bedroom had seepage with some mold sort of growth
- Parents were advised to get seepage fixed at earliest. For nasal obstruction, oral decongestants were given for 4–5 days. In view of moderate-severe persistent symptoms, he was also started on intranasal fluticasone furoate once at night
- On follow-up after 1 month, child was symptomatically much better.

trigger identified with inadequate response to environment control and appropriate pharmacotherapy, patient does not tolerate pharmacotherapy, has poor compliance or there are severe and persistent symptoms.

Q. What is the role of surgery in AR?

Although there is no surgical treatment for AR, it may be indicated in the management of comorbid conditions such as nasal obstruction due to severe nasal septal deviation, polyps, inferior turbinate hypertrophy or adenoidal hypertrophy, and refractory sinusitis and its complications.

LEARNING POINTS

- ☞ Environmental control/allergen avoidance is a crucial component of treatment
- ☞ There is no rationale of levocetirizine + montelukast combinations
- ☞ For symptoms of nasal block or obstruction, oral decongestants are better for short-term control
- ☞ Intranasal corticosteroids are preferred first-line controllers for moderate-severe or persistent symptoms.

SUGGESTED READINGS

1. ARCTM (Allergic rhinitis and co-morbidities module) of Indian Academy of Pediatrics.
2. Bousquet J, et al. Allergic rhinitis and its impact on asthma (ARIA) 2008 update (in collaboration with the World Health Organization, GA(2)LEN and AllerGen). Allergy. 2008 Apr;63 Suppl 86:8-160.

CHAPTER

3

Sinusitis

Devki Nandan, Wonashi R Tsanglao

CASE 1

A 5-year-old boy presented with persistent nasal discharge, with day-time non-spasmodic cough since 12 days. He had fever at the onset of illness that lasted around 2 days. He had been receiving symptomatic treatment, but had come back again due to persistence of symptoms.

Past medical history: None.

Family history: None.

Physical examination: Mucoid nasal discharge and congested middle turbinates. Postnasal drip was seen in the posterior pharynx.

Q. What are the diagnostic possibilities?

Persistent nasal discharge and cough for 10 days with history of fever in the beginning of illness and postnasal drip suggest a possibility of sinusitis.

Q. What are the clinical manifestations of sinusitis, and when to suspect sinusitis in children?

Acute bacterial sinusitis is a common complication of viral upper respiratory infection (URI) or allergic inflammation. Approximately 5–13% of viral upper respiratory tract infections (URTIs) are complicated by bacterial sinusitis. On an average, children have 5–10 episodes of viral URI in a calendar year. Presumptive diagnosis of acute bacterial sinusitis should be made when a child with an acute URI presents with one of the following:

- Persistent nasal discharge (any quality) and/or daytime cough of more than 10 days duration without improvement
- Worsening course or initial improvement followed by new onset of nasal discharge, daytime cough, or fever
- Severe onset, i.e., fever more than or equal to 39°C/102.2°F and purulent nasal discharge for at least three consecutive days.

In children, the most common manifestations of bacterial sinusitis are cough (80%) followed by nasal discharge (76%), and fever (63%). Bad breath, fatigue, headache, and decreased appetite, erythema and swelling of the nasal turbinates are not reliable. Percussion of the sinuses is not useful. Transillumination of the sinuses is also unreliable.

CASE 2

A 7-year-old girl, following an episode of URTI lasting for 7 days, presented with fever of 102°F, increasing nasal discharge, and headache since 3 days. She was initially given symptomatic treatment to which she responded well and her symptoms had subsided but had worsened since 3 days.

Past medical history: None.
Family history: None.
Physical examination: Febrile, with purulent nasal discharge. Right tympanic membrane was congested.

Q. What is the natural course of an uncomplicated viral URTI?

Viral URIs are usually characterized by either nasal symptoms or cough or both. Most often, the nasal discharge begins as clear and watery, that becomes thicker, but soon reverses to mucoid and resolves over a period of 5–7 days. However, resolving symptoms may persist in some patients after 10 days. Fever tends to occur early in the illness, often associated with headache and myalgias, which altogether typically disappears in the first 24–48 hours, and the respiratory symptoms become more prominent (Fig. 1).

Q. What are the predisposing conditions for acute bacterial sinusitis?

Conditions that predispose a child to development of bacterial sinusitis include following:

- *Interference with local defense mechanism:* Viral URIs (most common) and allergic rhinitis (2nd most common), causing inflammation and edema of the respiratory mucosa leading to obstruction of the ostium
- *Anatomic abnormalities:* Deviated nasal septum, concha bullosa (aerated middle turbinate causing blockade of ostiomeatal complex), Haller cells (infra-orbital cells causing narrowing of maxillary sinus ostium), and hypoplastic maxillary sinus
- *Defect in systemic defense mechanism:* Chiefly common variable disease, immunoglobulin (Ig) A and IgG subclass deficiency
- *Defect in mucociliary clearance:* Cystic fibrosis and primary ciliary dyskinesia
- *Others:* Bronchial asthma and gastro-esophageal reflux disease (GERD), inflammation of Eustachian tube orifices, or sinus ostia secondary to mucosal irritation.

Causes 2–4 are causes of recurrent acute bacterial sinusitis (RABS) or chronic sinusitis.

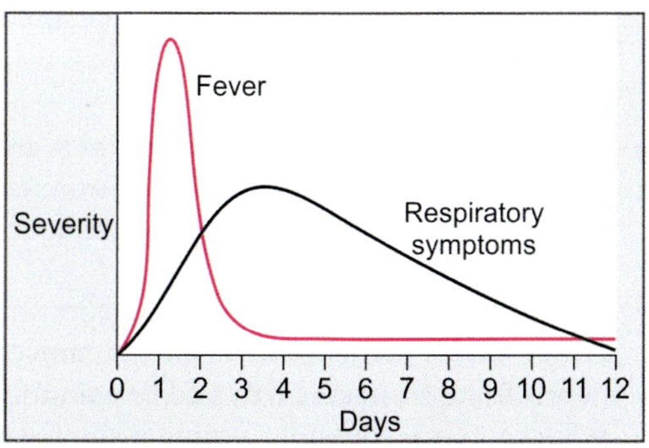

Figure 1: Natural course of uncomplicated viral upper respiratory infection

Q. How to make a diagnosis of acute sinusitis?

Acute bacterial sinusitis in children is diagnosed on the basis of clinical criteria. Non-resolving cough, cold for more than 10 days or recurrence of symptoms after initial relief in symptoms following a viral URTI indicates sinusitis. In young infants and children, there may be periorbital puffiness and in older children there may be tenderness on percussion of sinuses. Imaging for confirmation of diagnosis is not recommended routinely.

Q. When to consider imaging in acute bacterial sinusitis?

Imaging should be considered when complications of acute bacterial sinusitis are suspected. Complications are mainly orbital (ethmoid sinusitis) and intracranial (frontal sinusitis). Orbital complications include orbital cellulitis, orbital abscess, subperiosteal abscess, and cavernous sinus thrombosis. These are best visualized by contrast-enhanced computed tomography (CECT) scanning. These should be suspected when a child presents with swollen eyes, proptosis, or impaired function of the extra-ocular muscles. Intracranial complications include subdural empyema, epidural empyema, venous thrombosis, brain abscess, and meningitis. These should be suspected when a child presents with severe headache, vomiting, seizures, photophobia, or focal neurologic findings. Both magnetic resonance imaging (MRI) and CECT are complementary examinations when evaluating intracranial complications.

> **CASE 3**
>
> A 6-year-old boy presented with fever of 103°F, associated with purulent nasal discharge since 4 days.
>
> Past medical history: None.
>
> Family history: None.
>
> Physical examination: Febrile, toxic appearance, with purulent nasal discharge, and congested nasal mucosa. Tenderness was present over both maxillary sinuses. A diagnosis of acute bacterial sinusitis was made.

Q. How to treat acute bacterial sinusitis?

For severe onset and worsening course of acute bacterial sinusitis, antibiotic should be prescribed. For persistent illness, either prescribe an antibiotic or offer additional observation for 3 days, and prescribe antibiotic only if the child does not improve clinically or worsens at anytime. Pathogens involved in acute bacterial sinusitis are *Streptococcus pneumoniae (~30%),* and nontypeable *Haemophilus influenzae,* and *Moraxella catarrhalis (~20%). Staphylococcus aureus* is usually associated with infections of dental origin, and in orbital and intracranial complications.

Amoxicillin remains the drug of choice in uncomplicated acute bacterial sinusitis in situations where resistance is not suspected. Risk factors for amoxicillin resistance include age younger than 2 years; receipt of antibiotic therapy within the previous 30 days; and attendance at child care. The recommended dosage of amoxicillin is 45 mg/kg/day in two divided doses. Patients presenting with moderate to severe illness as well as those with risk factors for amoxicillin resistance may be treated with amoxicillin-clavulanate 80–90 mg/kg/day in two divided doses with a maximum of 2 g per dose. For children who are vomiting or not accepting orally, a single 50 mg/kg dose of ceftriaxone, intravenous (IV) or intramuscular (IM) may be given (all three major bacteria are susceptible to ceftriaxone in 95%–100% cases). Oral antibiotic can be commenced if improvement is observed at 24 hours; otherwise additional parenteral doses may be given. Patients who are allergic to penicillin or amoxicillin (both type I and non-type I) can be safely treated with cefdinir, cefuroxime, or cefpodoxime. Susceptibility of *S. pneumoniae* to these agents varies from 60% to 75%, *H. influenzae* is 85%–100% susceptible. Linezolid has excellent activity against all *S. pneumonia,* but lacks activity against *H. influenzae* and *M. catarrhalis.* Levofloxacin has a high level of activity against both *S. pneumoniae* and *H. influenzae.*

Recommended duration of treatment varies from 10–14 days, or for 7 days after the patient becomes free of signs and symptoms. Re-assessment should be done after 72 hours. If there is failure to improve or worsening in a confirmed case of acute bacterial sinusitis, change of antibiotic therapy may be considered.

Patients, who are acutely ill and appear toxic, can be considered for maxillary sinus aspiration to obtain sample for Gram stain, culture, and sensitivity. Alternatively, inpatient therapy can be initiated with IV ceftriaxone. Patient can be referred to an otolaryngologist if worsening is observed or fails to improve in 48 hours.

Q. What is the role of intranasal steroids, saline irrigation of nares and nasal decongestants?

- *Intranasal corticosteroids:* Currently there are no recommendations for the use of intranasal corticosteroids as adjuvant therapy in acute bacterial sinusitis in children
- *Saline irrigation*: Saline nasal irrigation or lavage (with hypertonic saline) removes debris from the nasal cavity and temporarily reduces tissue edema to promote drainage from the sinuses. However, there is only one study in children that showed greater

improvement in nasal airflow and quality of life and better rate of improvement, compared to placebo

- *Nasal decongestants:* The use of decongestants, antihistamines, and mucolytics has not been studied adequately in children and is not recommended for the treatment of acute uncomplicated bacterial sinusitis.

Q. What is recurrent acute bacterial sinusitis (RABS) and chronic sinusitis?

Recurrent acute bacterial sinusitis (RABS) is defined as episodes of acute bacterial sinusitis, lasting fewer than 30 days and separated by intervals of at least 10 days during which the patient is asymptomatic, or at least four episodes of acute bacterial sinusitis in a calendar year.

Chronic sinusitis is defined by duration of 90 or more days of daily respiratory symptoms such as cough, nasal discharge, or nasal obstruction.

Children presenting with RABS and chronic sinusitis should be worked up for allergic rhinitis, immunodeficiencies (particularly IgA and IgG deficiency), cystic fibrosis, gastroesophageal reflux disease, and primary ciliary dyskinesia. Anatomic abnormalities also should be ruled out.

The microbiology of RABS is similar to that of isolated episodes of acute bacterial sinusitis, and warrants the same treatment. The pathogenesis of chronic sinusitis is poorly understood and appears to be multifactorial; however, many of the conditions associated with RABS have also been implicated in chronic sinusitis and should be evaluated accordingly. The bacteriology of chronic sinusitis is different from that of acute sinusitis. The main pathogens include *S. aureus, Enterobacteriaceae* species and *Pseudomonas* species commonly. Less commonly implicated are *S. pneumoniae, H. influenzae,* and coagulase-negative staphylococcus.

Treatment of chronic rhinosinusitis includes administration of at least 4 weeks of broad-spectrum β-lactamase-resistant second-line antibiotic therapy. Failure of maximal medical therapy is an indication for surgical intervention which includes adenoidectomy and functional endoscopic sinus surgery. Excluding or maximally treating all associated conditions is essential.

LEARNING POINTS

- Acute bacterial sinusitis most often complicates viral upper respiratory infections and allergic rhinitis in children
- Diagnosis is on the basis of clinical criteria (persistent nasal discharge and/or cough of more than 10-days-duration, worsening course, or severe onset of more than 3-days-duration), and imaging is not recommended unless complications are strongly suspected
- Duration of treatment is 10–14 days, or for 7 days after resolution of signs and symptoms. Adjuvant therapies like intranasal corticosteroids and nasal decongestants are not recommended
- Recurrent acute bacterial sinusitis and chronic sinusitis should be further worked up for underlying cause(s).

SUGGESTED READINGS

1. Chow AW, Benninger MS, Brook I, Brozek JL, Goldstein EJ, Hicks LA, et al. Infectious Diseases Society of America. IDSA clinical practice guideline for acute bacterial rhinosinusitis in children and adults. Clin Infect Dis. 2012;54:e72-e112.
2. Desrosiers M, Evans GA, Keith PK, Wright ED, Kaplan A, Bouchard J, et al. Canadian clinical practice guidelines for acute and chronic rhinosinusitis. Allergy Asthma Clin Immunol. 201;7(1):2.
3. Shaikh N, Hoberman A, Kearney DH, Colborn DK, Kurs-Lasky M, Jeong JH, et al. Signs and symptoms that differentiate acute sinusitis from viral upper respiratory tract infection. Pediatr Infect Dis J. 2013;32:1061-5.
4. Wald ER, Applegate KE, Bordley C, Darrow DH, Glode MP, Marcy SM, et al. American Academy of Pediatrics. Clinical practice guideline for the diagnosis and management of acute bacterial sinusitis in children aged 1 to 18 years. Pediatrics. 2013;132: e262-80.
5. Wang YH, Yang CP, Ku MS, Sun HL, Lue KH. Efficacy of nasal irrigation in the treatment of acute sinusitis in children. Int J Pediatr Otorhinolaryngol. 2009;73(12):1696-701.

Chapter 4

Acute Tonsillopharyngitis

Shashidhara R Nagabhushana, Salim A Khatib, Prabhakar M Veturi

CASE 1

A toddler presented with history of fever, cough, and cold of 1 day duration. All symptoms started almost simultaneously. His elder sibling had similar problems 5 days ago and was improving. Two other members of the family had milder symptoms.

On examination, he was febrile, active but irritable, had watery rhinorrhea, dull-looking throat with small ulcers around the edges of faucial pillars (Fig. 1). There was dry cough, but no lymph nodes were palpable. Chest examination was normal.

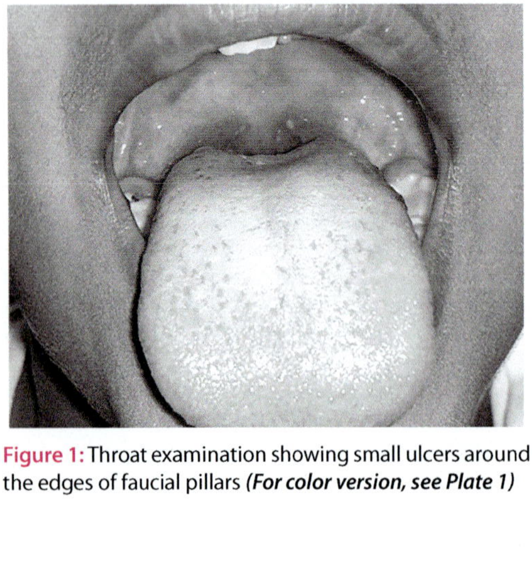

Figure 1: Throat examination showing small ulcers around the edges of faucial pillars *(For color version, see Plate 1)*

Q: What is the likely diagnosis?

Herpangina—viral tonsillopharyngitis. Although it is difficult to distinguish between viral and bacterial tonsillopharyngitis purely on clinical grounds, certain features are strongly associated with viral etiology. Presence of cough, rhinorrhea, watery red-eyes, diarrhea, and exanthema suggest viral etiology. In a younger child, tonsillopharyngitis is usually associated with viral infections. Conversely, presence of high fever, tonsillar exudates, palatal hemorrhages and tender anterior cervical adenitis in an older child (>5 years) and the absence of symptoms of coryza, rhinorrhea, and cough make the diagnosis of group A β-hemolytic streptococcal (GABHS) tonsillopharyngitis more likely. In general, viral infections tend to be more generalized with panmucositis, and bacterial infections more focal.

Group A streptococcal tonsillopharyngitis is suggested by presence of:
- Sudden onset of sore throat
- Age 5–15 years
- Fever
- Headache
- Nausea, vomiting, abdominal pain
- Tonsillopharyngeal inflammation
- Patchy tonsillopharyngeal exudates

- Palatal petechiae
- Anterior cervical adenitis (tender nodes)
- Winter and early spring presentation
- History of exposure to streptococcal pharyngitis
- Scarlatiniform rash.

Viral tonsillopharyngitis is suggested by presence of:

- Conjunctivitis
- Coryza
- Cough
- Diarrhea
- Hoarseness
- Discrete ulcerative stomatitis
- Viral exanthema.

Several clinical scoring systems and criteria-based diagnostic algorithms have been developed to aid this differentiation, but establishing or ruling out GABHS infection with certainty still depends on etiological diagnosis using microbiological tests.

Q. What is tonsillopharyngitis and how common it is?

- Acute tonsillopharyngitis is defined as an infection of the tonsils and pharynx. It is a common entity among children and adolescents
- Although viruses cause most acute tonsillopharyngitis, group A streptococcus (GABHS) causes 37% of acute tonsillopharyngitis in children older than 5 years
- Other bacterial causes of tonsillopharyngitis are group C streptococcus (5% of total), *Chlamydophila pneumoniae* (1%), *Mycoplasma pneumoniae* (1%), and anaerobic species (1%). Between viruses *Rhinovirus, Coronavirus* and *Adenovirus* account for more than 30% of the total cases, Epstein-Barr virus for 1%, and influenza and parainfluenza virus for about 4%.

Q: What are the probable etiologies of acute tonsillopharyngitis?

The etiologies of acute tonsillopharyngitis with associated clinical syndrome(s) are shown in table 1.

TABLE 1: Causative organisms of acute tonsillopharyngitis with associated clinical syndrome(s)

Organisms	Clinical syndrome(s)
Bacterial	
Group A streptococcus	Pharyngotonsillitis, scarlet fever
Group C and group G streptococcus	Pharyngotonsillitis
Arcanobacterium haemolyticum	Scarlatiniform rash, pharyngitis
Neisseria gonorrhoeae	Tonsillopharyngitis
Corynebacterium diphtheriae	Diphtheria
Mixed anaerobes	Vincent's angina
Fusobacterium necrophorum	Lemierre's syndrome, peritonsillar abscess
Francisella tularensis	Tularemia (oropharyngeal)
Yersinia pestis	Plague
Yersinia enterocolitica	Enterocolitis, pharyngitis
Viral	
Adenovirus	Pharyngoconjunctival fever
Herpes simplex virus 1 and 2	Gingivostomatitis
Coxsackievirus	Herpangina
Rhinovirus	Common cold
Coronavirus	Common cold
Influenza A and B	Influenza
Parainfluenza	Cold, croup
EBV	Infectious mononucleosis
Cytomegalovirus	CMV mononucleosis
HIV	Primary acute HIV Infection
Mycoplasma	
Mycoplasma pneumoniae	Pneumonitis, bronchitis
Chlamydia	
Chlamydophila pneumoniae	Bronchitis, pneumonia
Chlamydophila psittaci	Psittacosis

CMV, cytomegalovirus; EBV, Epstein-Barr virus; HIV, human immunodeficiency virus.

Several bacteria and viruses cause tonsillopharyngitis. Acute tonsillopharyngitis group A streptococcus is the commonest and most important bacterial pathogen. Other streptococci of group C and G, *Arcanobacterium haemolyticum*, *M. pneumonia,* anaerobic bacteria, etc. can cause tonsillopharyngitis. *Corynebacterium diphtheriae* causing membranous pharyngitis can be life-threatening but thankfully has become rare due to diptheria, pertussis, and tetanus toxoids (DPT) immunization. Viruses are by far the commonest cause of tonsillopharyngitis. Some viruses cause typical, clinically recognizable forms of pharyngitis, e.g., herpangina and hand-foot-mouth disease caused by Coxsackie viruses; pharyngoconjunctival fever by adenovirus, and typical gingivostomatitis by herpes simplex viruses. *Rhinoviruses* and adenoviruses account for approximately 20% each of all viral pharyngitis. Viral tonsillopharyngitis is self-limiting and resolves spontaneously, rarely leading to complications.

CASE 2

A 6-year-old boy presented with history of fever, throat pain for last 4 days. He had generalized rash, dysphagia, and decreased food intake for 2 days. There was no history of cough or nasal discharge.

On examination, he had bilateral tonsillar enlargement with exudates and congested pharynx and anterior cervical lymph nodes enlargement. The child had macular rash (scarlatiniform) (Fig. 2)

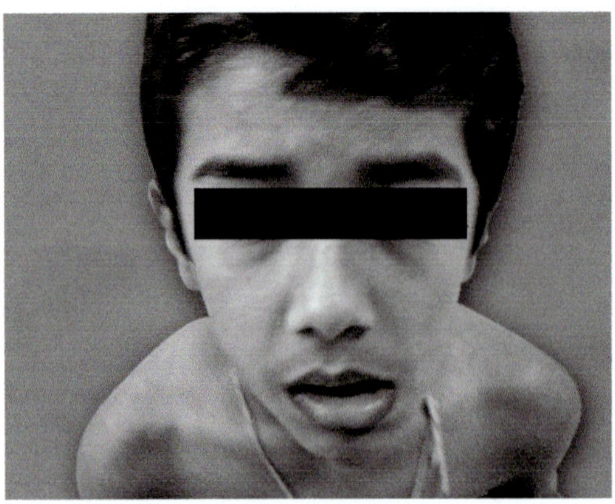

Figure 2: Scarlatiniform rash after partial improvement *(For color version, see Plate 1)*

Q: What is the likely diagnosis?

As mentioned above, absence of symptoms of coryza and presence of exudates and enlarged anterior cervical lymph nodes make the diagnosis of bacterial tonsillitis very likely. Although exanthematous rash generally tilts the diagnosis toward a viral etiology, typical rash of scarlet fever is the hallmark of GABHS tonsillopharyngitis. The rash appears 2–4 days after the onset of fever and has rough "sandpaper" like feel and fades with characteristic desquamation, especially in the palms and around the fingers.

Q: What is the importance of distinguishing GABHS tonsillopharyngitis from other etiologies?

Group A β-hemolytic streptococcus tonsillitis is associated with acute rheumatic fever and rheumatic heart disease as well as acute post-streptococcal glomerulonephritis. These potentially life-threatening complications can be avoided by adequate treatment and elimination of streptococcal throat carriage. In addition, acute suppurative complications, like peritonsillar abscess and systemic infections, make adequate treatment of GABHS infection essential.

CASE 3

A 4-year-old girl had fever and throat pain of 3 days duration. She had mild barking type of cough. There was no cold, rhinorrhea and no watering of eyes.

On examination, bilateral tonsils were enlarged and pharynx was congested, but there were no exudates and no petechiae over the palate. Tongue was normal.

Anterior cervical lymph nodes were mildly tender, but not markedly enlarged.

Q: To treat or not to treat with antibiotics?

In clinical practice, there is a marked overlap of symptoms and signs, and it is sometimes unclear whether we are dealing with GABHS tonsillitis or not. When in doubt, it would be prudent to wait and watch for a day or two, for more features to evolve over time. No harm is done as it has been seen that starting antibiotics late (even as late as 9 days after the onset of symptoms) does not increase the risk of complications of streptococcal infections.

It is also important that attempts to establish the diagnosis of GABHS infection are made in all doubtful cases before starting antibiotics.

Q: How is the diagnosis of GABHS tonsillitis established?

Throat culture is the gold standard for diagnosis of GABHS infection. High sensitivity and specificity make this test the most useful tool. Negative throat cultures, when properly performed and processed, almost rule out the possibility of streptococcal pharyngitis.

However, the test requires about 24–48 hours to obtain a result. Therefore, more rapid testing modalities to take clinical decisions in the form of rapid streptococcal antigen detection tests (RADTs) have been developed. These antigen detection tests are more expensive but results can be obtained immediately in the outpatient setting. The specificity is good but negative results do not rule out GABHS tonsillitis. Therefore, it is recommended that follow-up culture is needed in negative RADT, but if positive, cultures are not needed.

Antistreptolysin-O (ASLO) and other anti-streptococcal antibody tests are not to be performed for the diagnosis of acute tonsillopharyngitis because they do not become positive early in the infection and when positive, indicate past infection.

Q: Who should undergo testing for tonsillopharyngitis?

All patients with clinical features suggestive of bacterial tonsillitis should undergo throat swab culture and/or RADT as needed. However, children with features strongly suggestive of viral tonsillopharyngitis and children under 3 years do not need to be tested or started on treatment. Acute tonsillopharyngitis group A streptococcus tonsillopharyngitis and rheumatic fever are rare in children below 3 years and hence this recommendation. In this group of children, bacterial tonsillitis may be suspected and tested for, when there is a strong family or household contact of GABHS infection and if clinical features are suggestive.

It is not necessary to test or treat asymptomatic contacts in the household of children with proven streptococcal tonsillopharyngitis.

Q: What are the treatment options for GABS tonsillopharyngitis?

Penicillin remains the mainstay of treatment of tonsillopharyngitis. The duration of treatment should be 10 days, except in the case of azithromycin where 5 days is recommended. Large meta-analyses comparing shorter courses with standard 10-day regimen have shown equivalent benefit from 5–6 days of treatment with specific antibiotics. However, current guidelines still insist on full 10 days of therapy.

Dosages of commonly used drugs are listed below in table 2.

TABLE 2: Antibiotic regimens recommended for group A streptococcal pharyngitis

Drug	Route	Dose	Duration
For patients without penicillin allergy			
Penicillin V	oral	Children: 250 mg thrice daily Adolescents: 250 mg four times daily	10 days
Amoxycillin	oral	50 mg once daily (maximum 1,000 mg) or 25 mg (maximum 500 mg) twice daily	10 days
Benzathine penicillin G	Intramuscular	<27 kg: 600,000 U; >27 kg: 1,200,000 U	1 dose

Continued

Continued

Drug	Route	Dose	Duration
For those with penicillin allergy			
Cephalexin	oral	20 mg/kg/dose twice daily (maximum 500 mg/dose)	10 days
Cefadroxil	oral	30 mg/kg once daily (maximum 1 g)	10 days
Azithromycin	oral	12 mg/kg once daily (maximum 500 mg)	5 days
Clarithromycin	oral	7.5 mg/kg/dose twice daily (maximum 250 mg/dose)	10 days
Clindamycin	oral	7 mg/kg/dose three times daily (maximum 300 mg/dose)	10 days

Q: How to treat recurrent episodes and carriers?

Guidelines have been developed for adequate antimicrobial treatment of recurrent bacterial tonsillopharyngitis. Persistent carriers are not at increased risk for suppurative or long-term complications of GABHS like rheumatic fever. Recurrent, documented GABHS infections are rare and may be viral tonsillopharyngitis occurring in chronic carriers of the organism.

Unless documented, bona fide recurrent infections occur, it is not necessary to treat these children aggressively. However, in case of outbreaks in the community, household or class/school, or in case of close family history of rheumatic fever, treatment of the carriers may be considered with any of the regimens below (Table 3).

Q: When should tonsillectomy be considered?

Whenever symptomatic episodes do not reduce in frequency as expected over time and in those individuals in whom no alternative explanation for recurrent group A streptococcus pharyngitis is obvious, tonsillectomy is considered.

These rare patients should be informed the benefits are not always uniform and may be relatively short-lived.

Q: How to manage "ping pong" spread of suspected GABHS infections?

When intrafamily spread is suspected to be the cause of multiple recurrent infections, simultaneous throat swabs from all family

TABLE 3: **Treatment regimens for chronic carriers of group A streptococci**

Route	Drug	Dose	Duration
Oral			
	Clindamycin	• 20–30 mg/kg/day in three doses (maximum 300 mg/dose)	10 days
	Penicillin and rifampin	• Penicillin V: 50 mg/kg/day in four doses (maximum 2,000 mg/day) × 10 days • Rifampin: 20 mg/kg/day in one dose x last 4 days of treatment (maximum 600 mg/day)	10 days
	Amoxicillin clavulanic acid	• Amoxicillin: 40 mg/kg/day in three doses (maximum 2,000 mg of amoxicillin/day)	10 days
Intramuscular and oral			
	Benzathine penicillin G	• 600,000 U for <27 kg and 1,200,000 U for >27 kg	One dose
	Rifampin	• 20 mg/kg/day in two doses (maximum 600 mg/day)	4 days

members are obtained and those with a positive culture or RADTs are treated.

Family pets are not known to contribute to familial spread.

Q: What are the indications for hospitalization?

Most cases of tonsillopharyngitis require outpatient therapy and very rarely if at all need hospitalization. Indications for hospitalization may be:

- Toxic looking child
- Not accepting orally well
- Suspected to have associated complications—peritonsillar abscess or diphtheria.

LEARNING POINTS

- ☞ Accurate diagnosis and rational treatment (drug, dose, and duration) hold the key to prevent sequelae
- ☞ A prudent clinician will utilize rapid streptococcal antigen detection tests (RADT) as and when necessary as these tests are highly sensitive. In an occasional situation wherein the clinical suspicion is high and the RADTs are noncontributory, a throat swab culture is warranted
- ☞ Though Penicillin V is the drug of first choice, amoxicillin being equally effective, palatable, easily available and can be administered in twice daily doses, it is frequently the option in office practice
- ☞ For those with type 1 hypersensitivity reaction to penicillin, cephalosporins are the obvious option
- ☞ Inappropriate use of macrolides is the most common cause of resistant strains of group A β-hemolytic streptococcal in the community
- ☞ Educating parents that the duration of treatment is 10 days always ensures compliance.

SUGGESTED READINGS

1. Shah R, Bansal A, Singhi SC. Approach to a child with sore throat. Indian J Pediatr. 2011;78(10):1268-72.
2. Shulman ST, Bisno AL, Clegg HW, Gerber MA, Kaplan EL, Lee G, et al. Clinical practice guideline for the diagnosis and management of group A streptococcal pharyngitis: 2012 update by the Infectious Diseases Society of America. Clin Infect Dis. 2012;55(10):e86-102.

CHAPTER

5

Retropharyngeal Abscess

Rohit Sasidharan, Jhuma Sankar

CASE 1

- A 2-year-old boy with no significant illness in the past, presented to the emergency with swelling on left side of the neck for 2 days. There was associated fever and redness over the swelling. He had coryza and cough for 3 days prior to the onset of swelling. There was also history of drooling of saliva, noisy breathing, and refusal to feed
- On examination, the child was irritable but vitals were stable. His neck was deviated to the left side and there was a reddish, tender, fluctuant swelling 3 cm × 3 cm palpable in the left anterolateral part of the neck. Multiple enlarged cervical lymph nodes were also palpable. On oral cavity examination, there was drooling of saliva with congested posterior pharynx and anterior displacement of the posterior and left lateral pharyngeal wall. Tonsils were normal. Respiratory system examination revealed only mild suprasternal retractions. Air entry was bilaterally equal and there were no added sounds. Rest of the systemic examination was normal. He was shifted to the pediatric intensive care unit (PICU) for monitoring of airway and post of care for surgical intervention
- During the PICU stay course, the child's respiratory distress worsened with increased suprasternal and subcostal retractions and falling oxygen saturation. He was intubated and mechanically ventilated as there was evidence of bronchopneumonia bilaterally. An urgent contrast enhanced computed tomography (CT) of the head, neck, and chest was ordered to delineate the extent of the abscess
- The CT scan of the head, neck, and chest showed a large retropharyngeal abscess (RPA) measuring 3.7 cm × 3.1 cm × 2.6 cm with inflammatory and phlegmonous changes extending into the left parapharyngeal space and the mediastinum (Fig. 1). Thus, a diagnosis of retropharyngeal wall abscess was confirmed in this case.

Q. What are the likely differentials we could think of in this case?

This child had fever, swelling, and redness of the posterior pharyngeal wall and features suggestive of upper aerodigestive tract infection. The main differentials to be considered are:

- Acute epiglottitis: Epiglottitis is a life-threatening infection characterized by rapidly progressive inflammation of the epiglottis. It usually manifests with high fever, toxic appearance, stridor, muffled voice, dysphagia, and difficulty in handling oral secretions. It can be rapidly progressive and life-threatening. Oral examination should be done in an environment where there is facility for emergent establishment of artificial airway if needed, i.e., in the operation theater. Oral examination may be unremarkable other than pooling of secretions. There will be evidence of edema and inflammation of supraglottic structures

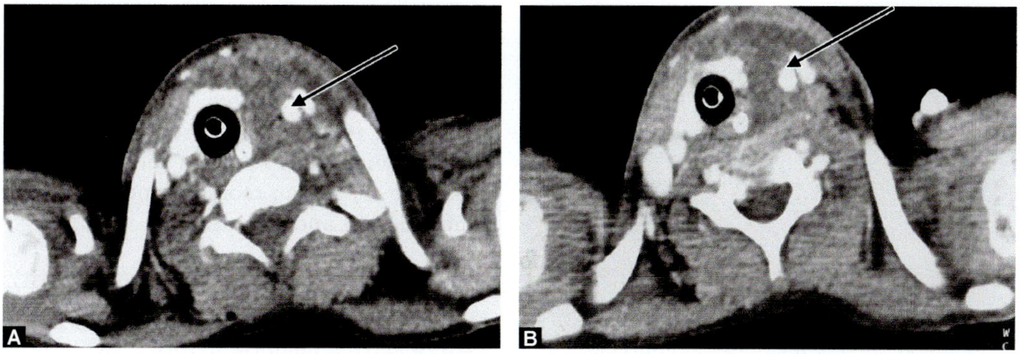

Figure 1: Contrast-enhanced computed tomography shows a large collection in the left parapharyngeal space displacing the trachea to the right (endotracheal tube is seen in the trachea)

- Acute infectious pharyngitis: Pharyngitis due to viral and bacterial infections can present with sore throat, dysphagia, drooling of saliva, and respiratory distress. The presence of edema and cellulitis of the posterior pharyngeal wall mucosa can cause features of upper airway obstruction
- Acute tonsillitis: Acute viral or bacterial tonsillitis can present with the above mentioned complaints. On examination, there will be evidence of enlarged and inflamed tonsils with exudates or membrane covering them
- Peritonsillar cellulitis and abscess (quinsy): Peritonsillar cellulitis is an inflammation of the tissue between the capsule of the palatile tonsils and the pharyngeal muscles, and when there is collection of pus it is called quinsy or peritonsillar abscess. Trismus may limit a complete oral examination. Extremely swollen tonsils with fluctuations and deviation of tonsils to opposite side may be seen along with erythema and exudates over the tonsils
- Retropharyngeal abscess: Usually presents in children less than 4 years with a preceding history of upper respiratory infections. Fever, features of upper airway obstruction, torticollis, and limitation of neck movements may be common presentation. The posterior location of the abscess makes it difficult to visualize on oral examination, but sometimes a bulging posterior pharyngeal wall may be seen
- Lateral pharyngeal abscess: The clinical presentation may be similar to RPA, but the condition is rare. Trismus and swelling below the mandible is more common
- Diphtheria: A life-threatening infectious bacterial pharyngitis should always be kept in mind in children presenting with upper airway obstruction and dysphagia, especially when immunization status is incomplete. Thick pharyngeal membrane and cervical adenopathy (bull neck) are characteristic features.

Q. What are the boundaries of retropharyngeal space?

The retropharyngeal space is also known as retropharyngeal space of Gillette or the posterior space of Grodinsky or the Holoyoke's space. It lies behind the pharynx with the middle layer of deep cervical fascia (buccopharyngeal fascia) forming the anterior boundary abutting the posterior pharyngeal wall. The posterior boundary is the deep layer of deep cervical fascia (prevertebral fascia). These fasciae fuse inferiorly at the level of the first and second thoracic vertebrae. It extends from the base of the skull to the level of tracheal bifurcation. It communicates laterally with the lateral pharyngeal space (Fig. 2).

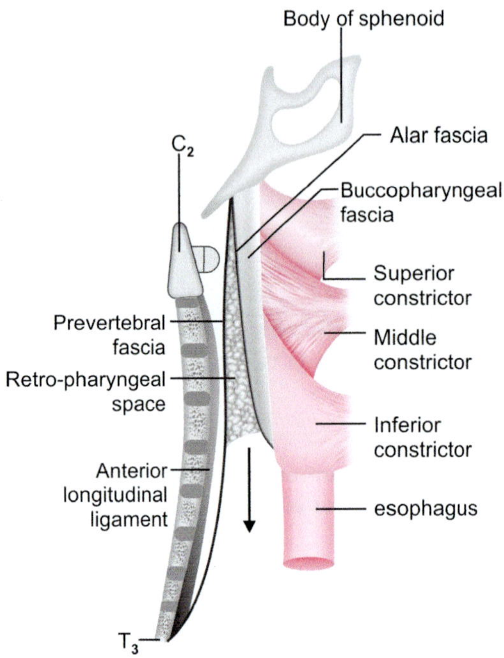

Figure 2: Anatomy of the retropharyngeal space (sagittal section)

Q. What are the contents of the retropharyngeal space?

The retropharyngeal space contains chains of lymph nodes which are arranged in groups of two or four on either side of the midline. These lymph nodes are prominent in young children and involute by the age of 4–5 years, although according to few, involutions occur around puberty. They drain the nasopharynx, adenoids, posterior paranasal sinuses, middle ear, and the Eustachian tube. Infections in these areas may lead to suppurative adenitis and formation of RPA.

Q. How common is retropharyngeal abscess?

Retropharyngeal abscess is a rare entity but requires early diagnosis and treatment as it may be associated with life-threatening complications such as upper airway obstruction, epidural abscess, mediastinitis, carotid aneurysms, or cavernous sinus thrombosis.

Retropharyngeal abscess is most commonly seen in children between ages 2–4 years, although it can occur in children of any age group including infants. With increasing age, there is progressive regression of the retropharyngeal lymph nodes and hence lesser incidence of RPA. It is more common during the winter months and in males.

Q. What are the findings in history and examinations to be elicited in a suspected case of retropharyngeal infection?

The presenting features of RPA are highly variable because of which they present a diagnostic challenge to emergency physicians, pediatricians, and otolaryngologists. The features may be subtle and nonspecific early in the course of illness, while life-threatening symptoms related to inflammation and obstruction of upper respiratory tract may be seen with progression of illness.

The commonly reported symptoms of RPA are:

- Fever
- Neck pain
- Dysphagia/odynophagia
- Sore throat
- Refusal to feed
- Torticollis
- Swelling in the neck
- Drooling
- Respiratory difficulty/stridor.

The initial step in examining a child with suspected deep neck infection is a rapid assessment of the degree of upper airway obstruction. Anxious ill appearing children with drooling, abnormal neck posture, and stridor should be monitored continuously in a setting where emergent artificial airway can be established if necessary such as in an operating room.

The common signs one should look for while examining a patient with RPA are cervical lymphadenopathy, limitation of neck movements, oropharyngeal swelling, torticollis, drooling, and stridor. There should be a high index of suspicion of RPA in a child who cannot fully extend his neck to look up. This is known as "Bolte's sign".

Q. What are the challenges in making a diagnosis of retropharyngeal abscess?

The diagnosis of RPA remains challenging as many patients present with nonspecific symptoms such as fever and neck stiffness. Even though some studies have reported that limitation of neck movements and torticollis are more specific for RPA, diagnosis based solely on history and examination remains a challenge. Hence, a contrast-enhanced CT neck showing evidence of fluid collection with rim enhancement and specific location is used to diagnose RPA in conjunction with the clinical findings.

CASE 2

- A 15-month-old boy, premorbidly normal, presented with an episode of choking with food and was taken to the local emergency department. On clinical examination, there was no evidence of foreign body and the child was sent home. Three days later, the child returned to the emergency department with high grade fever and respiratory distress. Physical examination revealed right cervical swelling and restriction in neck movements. Oral cavity examination revealed a bulging posterior pharyngeal wall and drooling of saliva
- The child underwent blood investigations followed by contrast imaging of the neck. Cervical CT scan revealed a retropharyngeal collection or abscess with "air bubbles" extending from the oropharynx to the cervical-thoracic transition measuring 4 cm × 5 cm. The child was started on intravenous fluid and antibiotics and kept under observation in the PICU.

Q. What is the etiopathogenesis of retropharyngeal infection?

In children and infants, acute retropharyngeal infection is usually nontraumatic caused by suppuration of the retropharyngeal lymph nodes which drain from orpharynx, nasopharynx, nose, paranasal sinuses, adenoids, and tonsils. Rarely, RPA in children can also result from mastoid infection. Retropharyngeal abscess is associated with antecedent upper respiratory infection in one half of the cases. Regional trauma, foreign body ingestion, as a complication of procedure in the oropharyngeal region or immunosuppression, are rare causes in children but common in adults. Retropharyngeal infections progress from cellulitis to organized phlegmon to mature abscess. Early institution of antimicrobial therapy may halt the progression to mature abscess.

Q. What findings do you expect in his blood investigations?

The initial laboratory evaluation in a patient with suspected RPA includes getting a complete blood count with differentials, erythrocyte sedimentation rate (ESR), C-reactive protein (CRP), blood culture for both aerobes and anaerobes, and throat swab for group A streptococcus. Patients with RPA usually have an elevated total count with a predominance of neutrophils and bands and elevated CRP and ESR levels. Blood cultures are rarely positive, but may help in identifying the pathogen. Whenever surgical drainage is done, both aerobic and anaerobic cultures have to be sent immediately to isolate the causative agent.

Q. What are the various imaging modalities available for the diagnosis of retropharyngeal abscess and their findings?

The radiographic evaluation for RPA includes lateral neck radiographs, CT scan of the neck with contrast, and magnetic resonance scan. The imaging strategy depends on the clinical condition of the child and the level of suspicion of RPA. If the patient's condition is stable and the level of suspicion of RPA is low, then a lateral radiograph of the neck may suffice. If suspicion is high, then a CT neck with contrast would be the preferred modality as it gives preoperative insights. Magnetic resonance imaging scan would be helpful during follow-up to identify any residual collection after treatment.

The retropharyngeal space is considered pathologically widened if it is >7 mm at C2 level and >14 mm at C6 level, or if the retropharyngeal space is >50% of the width of the corresponding cervical vertebrae (Fig. 3). Plain lateral neck radiographs showing prevertebral soft tissue thickening, straightening of cervical lordosis due to muscle spasm, presence of gas, or fluid level in the retropharyngeal space are suggestive of the presence of a RPA (Fig. 4).

Contrast-enhanced CT is the radiological modality of choice for evaluating RPA and is highly sensitive but not very specific. It can demonstrate the extension of the abscess to contiguous areas of the neck and chest, identify a nonopaque foreign body if any, may be able to differentiate between cellulitis and abscess in most cases, and identify locculations and position of the carotid artery and internal jugular vein in relation to the abscess for planning a surgical approach.

The CT findings suggestive of an abscess include areas of low attenuation, rim enhancement of the abscess wall, scalloping of the wall margin, tissue edema surrounding the abscess, and a cystic or multiloculated appearance (Fig. 5).

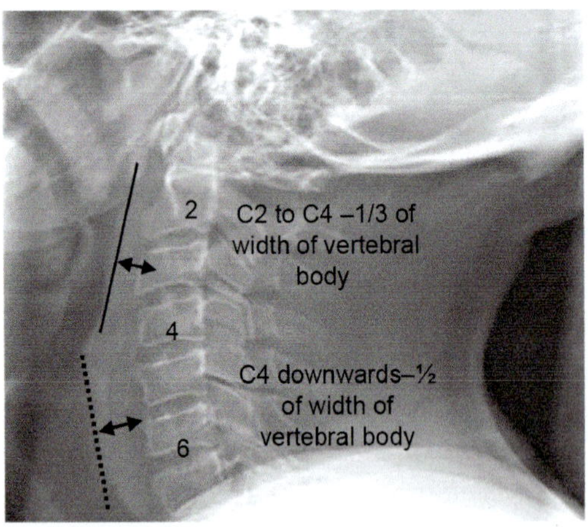

Figure 3: Normal X-ray soft tissue neck (lateral view) shows the expected width of the prevertebral space at different levels. From C2 to C4 (solid black line), the prevertebral space should not be more than one-third the width of the corresponding vertebral body. From C4 downward (dotted black line), it should not be more than the half of the width of corresponding vertebral body

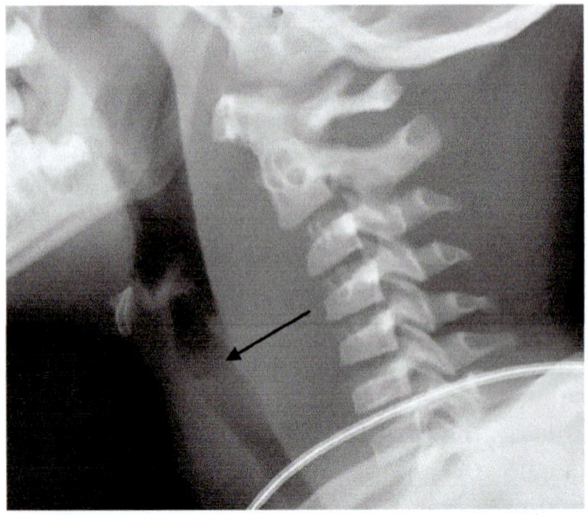

Figure 4: X-ray neck (lateral view) showing widening/thickening of the prevertebral space from C2 downward with the space measuring more than double the size of the corresponding vertebral body suggestive of retropharyngeal collection

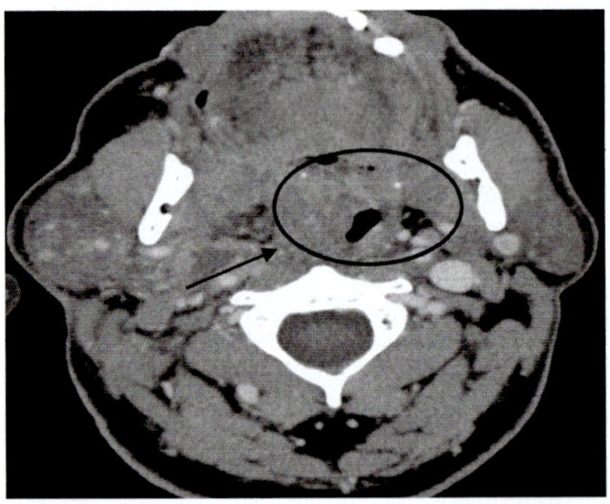

Figure 5: Computed tomography neck showing extensive multiloculated collection located posterior and to the right of oropharynx suggestive of a retropharyngeal abscess

In this child, blood investigations showed only a slight increase in CRP. He was started on ciprofloxacin and amikacin intravenous. On day 2, the child developed worsening of respiratory distress for which he was intubated and had to be put on mechanical ventilation. His antibiotics were changed to amoxicillin-clavulanic acid and clindamycin at this time.

Q. Was the initial antibiotic coverage in this child appropriate? What are the common organisms causing retropharyngeal abscess?

The initial antibiotic coverage in this child was not appropriate as there is no coverage for Gram-positive or anaerobic organism. Retropharyngeal abscess is usually a polymicrobial infection, including aerobes, microaerophilics, and anaerobes. The most common organisms are aerobic *Streptococcus pyogenes* [group A β-hemolytic streptococci (GABS)], viridans streptococcus, *Staphylococcus aureus* [methicillin-resistant *Staphylococcus aureus* (MRSA)], *Klebsiella pneumoniae, Peptostreptococcus,* and anaerobic bacteroides such as *Fusobacterium, Prevotella,* and *Veillonella* species. There has been an increasing incidence of RPA and has coincided with the emergence of GABS and MRSA infections. It has been seen that community acquired MRSA infections may be associated with a more complicated clinical course including mediastinitis, especially in children <2 years with prolongation of hospital stay and duration of antibiotics. Several virulence factors, especially the presence of pore forming Panton-Valentine leukocidin have been attributed to the invasiveness of MRSA.

Q. What would be the appropriate antibiotics to be started in a case of suspected retropharyngeal abscess?

The antibiotic treatment of RPA should be directed against the likely organisms. Early initiation of appropriate antibiotics may prevent the progression from cellulitis to abscess stage. These infections are often mixed and β-lactamase organisms are frequently isolated. The recent emergence of GABS and community acquired MRSA as RPA pathogen makes the antibiotic choice more challenging.

In areas where the incidence of community acquired MRSA is less, the empiric therapy should include high dose of parenteral amoxicillin-clavulanic acid along with an anti-anaerobic such as metronidazole or clindamycin. Alternatively second- or third-generation cephalosporins may be used as second-line therapy in case of penicillin allergy or severe infections. Clindamycin is preferred as it may be effective against community acquired MRSA. In areas where there is clindamycin resistant MRSA, vancomycin or linezolid should be added to clindamycin. Vancomycin may be considered empirically in critically ill children and in those with mediastinal extension while awaiting culture reports. Parenteral therapy is continued until the patient is afebrile and clinically stable after which oral therapy should be continued to complete a 14 days course. The empiric therapy should be amended based on the culture reports if a drainage procedure has been done.

In the intensive care unit, the child was continued on mechanical ventilation for next 48 hours. He continued to have high grade fever, developed features of hemodynamic compromise requiring fluid resuscitation, and vasoactive support. Ear, nose, and throat surgical opinion was taken and the child underwent transoral drainage of pus (7 mL) on day 3 of hospitalization. The pus was sent for aerobic and anaerobic cultures. A transoral drain was kept in situ, intravenous antibiotics and mechanical ventilation were continued.

Q. What is the optimal management of retropharyngeal abscess—medical or surgical?

The optimal management of RPA has been the subject of debate between conservative (medical) versus surgical drainage. The surgical drainage of the abscess has been the treatment of choice for decades. However, recent studies have shown successful conservative treatment of RPA without surgery. The initial modality of treatment should depend on the stage of inflammation, presence of associated respiratory compromise, the presence of drainable fluid, and associated complications. In the early state of the disease, appropriate antimicrobial therapy alone may prevent progression and preclude the need for surgery.

Surgical drainage may be required as a first line therapy if there is associated respiratory compromise or severe septic shock. Surgical drainage may also considered in cases of large mature abscess >2 cm thickness with rim enhancement in CT scan. In all other cases, a trial of conservative antibiotic therapy should be considered first, and surgical drainage is to be considered in the absence of favorable clinical evolution after 48 hours of intravenous antimicrobial therapy.

Q. What are the different surgical approaches for draining retropharyngeal abscess?

Traditionally, external cervical approach has been advocated. But presently, transoral drainage is the preferred modality if the abscess is medial to the great vessels and limited to the retropharyngeal space. With the availability of modern anesthetic technique and better airway management, transoral approach has been found to be relatively safe and effective. Currently, external cervical approach is reserved for abscess extending laterally to the great vessels or to the mediastinum.

Q. What should be the practical approach to the management of a case of suspected retropharyngeal abscess?

A practical approach to the management of a case of RPA is summarized below (Flowchart 1).

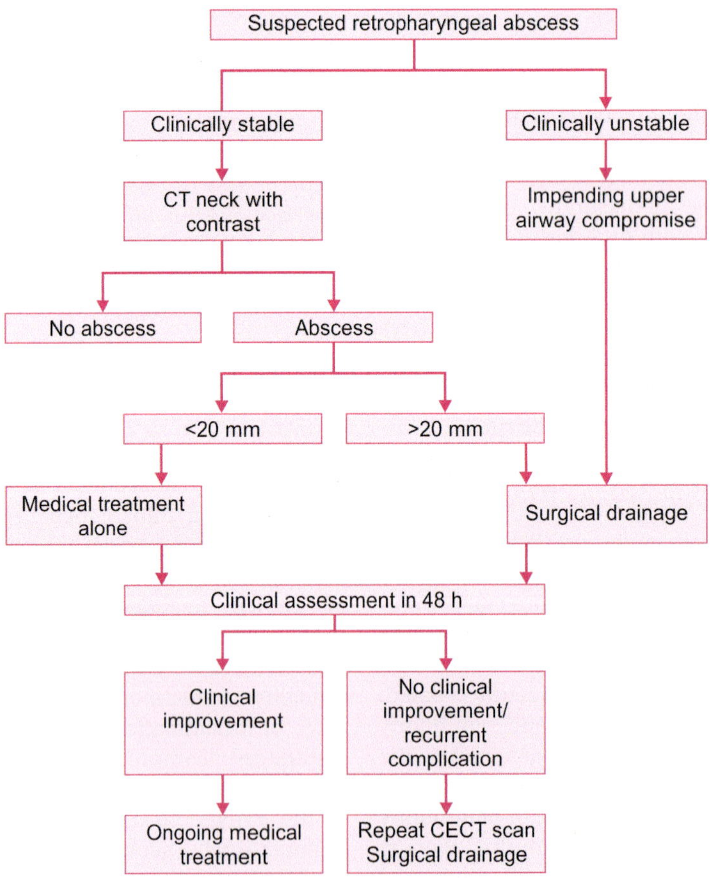

CT, computed tomography; CECT, contrast-enhanced computed tomography.

Flowchart 1: Approach to a child with retropharyngeal abscess

Postoperatively, the child improved, inotropes were stopped and he was weaned off from mechanical ventilation to nasal prongs. The oral drain was removed after 2 days. The pus culture grew K. pneumoniae and S. aureus sensitive to the prescribed antibiotics. Intravenous antibiotics were continued for 7 days and then switched over to oral antibiotics for a total of 14 days. On follow-up, the child was doing well and there were no complications related to the illness or the procedure. An magnetic resonance imaging of the neck showed complete resolution of the abscess.

Q. What are the anticipated complications of retropharyngeal abscess?

Although RPA is a life-threatening condition, complications have become rare because of early detection, timely antibiotic therapy, and early surgical intervention. The most common complications of RPA are:

- Airway obstruction
- Septicemia
- Aspiration pneumonia (rupture of abscess into airway)
- Internal jugular vein thrombosis or thrombophlebitis (Lemierre's syndrome)
- Carotid artery rupture
- Mediastinitis
- Atlantoaxial dislocation.

Q. What is the outcome and prognosis of retropharyngeal abscess?

When detected early and appropriately managed, RPA seldom leads to any long-term consequences. One-fourth of the patients may be managed by antimicrobial therapy alone while others may require surgical intervention. Some children may even require recurrent surgical intervention for persistent fever, recollection of pus, or development of complications. Hence, the duration of illness is highly variable and individualized. These children require follow-up evaluation and imaging to document complete resolution of illness.

LEARNING POINTS

- Retropharyngeal infection in children is a rare aerobic or anaerobic polymicrobial infection
- The incidence of retropharyngeal abscess has been increasing recently in parallel with emerging group A (β-hemolytic) streptococcus infection and methicillin-resistant *Staphylococcus aureus* infections
- Early diagnosis and initiation of appropriate broad-spectrum antibiotics can prevent progression and preclude the need for surgery
- Imaging plays a key role in timely diagnosis of retropharyngeal abscess
- Inappropriate and/or delayed treatment may lead to life-threatening complications and even death.

SUGGESTED READINGS

1. Abdel-haq NM, Harahsheh A, Asmar BL. Retropharyngeal abscess in children: the emerging role of group A beta hemolytic streptococcus. South Med J. 2006;99(9):927-31.
2. Carbone PN, Capra GG, Brigger MT. Antibiotic therapy for pediatric deep neck abscesses: a systematic review. Int J Pediatr Otorhinolaryngol. 2012;76(11):1647-53.
3. Grisaru-Soen G, Komisar O, Aizenstein O, Soudack M, Schwartz D, Paret G. Retropharyngeal and parapharyngeal abscess in children—epidemiology, clinical features and treatment. Int J Pediatr Otorhinolaryngol. 2010;74(9):1016-20.
4. Hoffmann C, Pierrot S, Contencin P, Morisseau-Durand MP, Manach Y, Couloigner V. Retropharyngeal infections in children. Treatment strategies and outcomes. Int J Pediatr Otorhinolaryngol. 2011;75(9):1099-103.
5. Johnston D, Schmidt R, Barth P. Parapharyngeal and retropharyngeal infections in children: argument for a trial of medical therapy and intraoral drainage for medical treatment failures. Int J Pediatr Otorhinolaryngol. 2009;73(5):761-5.
6. Kirse DJ, Roberson DW. Surgical management of retropharyngeal space infections in children. Laryngoscope. 2001;111(8):1413-22.

CHAPTER

6

Adenoid Hypertrophy

Sneha D Varkki, Ajoy M Varghese

CASE 1

A 4-year-old boy was brought by his parents who noted that he snores loudly in sleep almost every day. He had history of mouthbreathing and frequent nasal discharge. He had no history of allergy; he was active and growing well. On examination: alert child, weight and height were >50th centile on growth chart. He had mucoid nasal discharge. Tonsils were enlarged, ears normal, and respiratory system was clear. Clinical diagnosis was considered adenoid hypertrophy causing nasal obstruction.

Q. What are adenoids? Why is it enlarged in children?

Adenoids along with tonsils form part of the Waldeyer's ring of lymphatic tissue at the gateway to the respiratory system. Here an immune response is mounted as antigens enter the body through inhaled or ingested route. Secretory immunoglobulin (Ig)A production is an important function of the adenoid tissue. Being part of the immunological machinery, in children adenoids normally enlarge in size from 3 years to 10 years of age and then regress in size. During this phase of enlargement, it may occupy a disproportionate space in the nasopharynx leading to symptoms and sometimes complications.

Q. What are the effects of adenoid hypertrophy?

Adenoidal hypertrophy causes nasal obstruction, retention of secretions leading to increased local infection, resistance to airflow in the upper airway and ear disease. Symptoms can vary from mild to severe. Extent of obstruction is not only decided by the size of adenoids but also the nasopharyngeal space, tone of the muscles and the adjacent anatomy (Table 1).

Q. Who needs to be screened for adenoid hypertrophy?

During routine visits to the pediatrician, a history of mouth breathing, snoring and sleep disturbances should be taken for all toddlers, preschool and school aged children.

Those children with middle ear disease, recurrent or persistent rhinorrhoea, behavioral concerns like hyperactivity or poor scholastic performance, speech delay, unexplained pulmonary or systemic hypertension should have a screening for adenoid hypertrophy even if typical symptoms of nasal obstruction are not reported.

Sleep disordered breathing is common in children with obesity, craniofacial anomalies, mucopolysaccharidoses and in those who have

TABLE 1: Effects of adenoid hypertrophy

Symptoms/effects	Mechanism
Mouth breathing	Obstruction of nasal airway (Fig. 1)
Snoring	Worsening obstruction due to decreased tone in sleep
Hyponasal speech	Loss of nasal resonance
Swallowing difficulties	Mass effect from enlargement of adenoid and tonsils
Poor appetite	Decreased airflow through nose and poor sense of smell
Growth disturbance	Poor food intake, changes in GH secretion from interrupted sleep
Nocturnal enuresis	Hormonal changes due to sleep disordered breathing
Adenoid facies	Adenoid enlargement causing nasal obstruction and mouth-breathing, affecting dentofacial development
Middle ear disease	Eustachian tube obstruction, bacterial infection and biofilm production on adenoids
Restless sleep, labored breathing at night, short pauses in breathing	Upper airway obstruction and apnea cause hypoxia leading to arousal from sleep
Behavioral/cognitive changes	Due to interrupted sleep
Systemic or pulmonary hypertension	Complication of severe OSA and hypoxia

OSA, obstructive sleep apnea; GH, growth hormone.

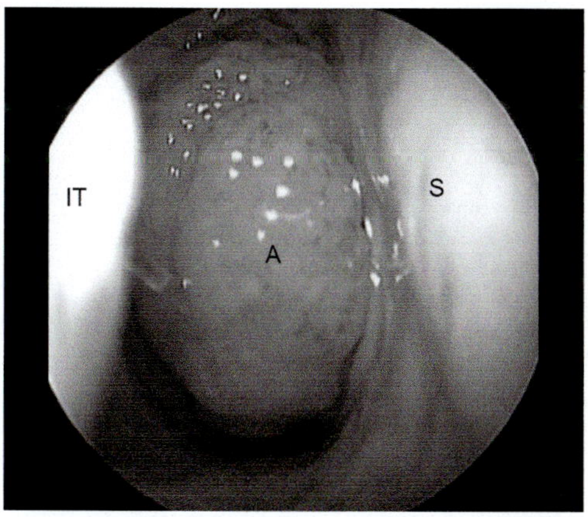

IT, inferior turbinate; S, septum; A, adenoids.

Figure 1: Nasal endoscopic images showing adenoid obstructing choana almost completely ***(For color version, see Plate 1)***

hypotonia from neuromuscular conditions or syndromes. In these patients even relatively small adenoid may obstruct an already compromised upper airway.

Before starting growth hormone therapy in conditions like Prader-Willi syndrome, a detailed evaluation to rule out adenoidal hypertrophy and obstructive sleep apnea (OSA) is indicated. Adenoidal size is noted to increase in these children during treatment.

Q. For the child in case 1, what are the points to be noted on clinical examination?

Child with a diagnosis of adenoidal hypertrophy, following information should be obtained:

- Allergic stigmata
- Growth assessment—weight and height centiles
- Adenoid facies—long thin face with malar hypoplasia, pinched nostrils, open mouth, high-arched palate, shortened upper lip, posterior cross bite and vacant expression
- Craniofacial features which suggest narrow upper airway like retrognathia, flat facial profile
- Presence of palatal submucosal cleft (contra-indication for surgery)
- Tonsillar size and appearance
- Features of rhinosinusitis or middle ear effusion.

Q. What is the usefulness of a lateral nasopharyngeal X-ray in this case?

A lateral soft tissue X-ray of the nasopharynx can demonstrate the presence of adenoid tissue. It is a useful tool for pediatricians to identify significant adenoid hypertrophy. Adenoid nasopharynx ratio (AN ratio) of >0.8 correlates well with clinically significant adenoid hypertrophy. For best results, X-ray is taken at the end of inspiration with the neck slightly extended and mouth open.

Measurements are made as follows

Perpendicular distance from the maximal convexity point on the inferior margin of adenoid to a line drawn along the anterior margin of basiocciput is measured (A). The nasopharyngeal space is measured as the distance between the posterior-superior edge of the hard palate and the anteroinferior edge of the spheno-basi-occipital synchondrosis (N). Adenoids nasopharynx ratio is then calculated as shown in the example below (Figure 2).

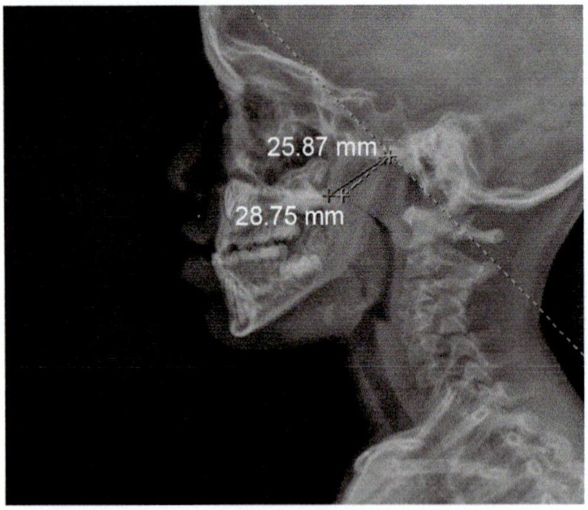

Figure 2: Adenoid nasopharynx ratio (AN ratio): Lateral X-ray of nasopharynx to calculate AN ratio. Green line shows measurement of adenoid size (A). Blue line measures nasopharyngeal space (N)

Q. Child was referred to the ear-nose-throat (ENT) doctor who performed a nasal endoscopy and confirmed the presence of enlarged adenoids. Hearing is normal. Does he need adenoidectomy?

History and examination suggest that the child has adenoid hypertrophy causing symptoms which are not severe. There is no history of OSA, his growth and activities are normal. There are no complications involving the middle ear or the paranasal sinuses. Hence, at this point adenoidectomy is not indicated.

CASE 2

A 5-year-old child had history of mouth breathing, labored breathing, and restlessness in sleep for the past 1 year. He had habitual snoring and, many times a night he was noted to have brief pauseses in breathing. The child was also noted to be disruptive in class and was hyperactive. He had history suggestive of allergic rhinitis and a family history of atopy. On examination: child was active. Height and weight plotted on the 25th centile of growth chart. Blood pressure was normal for age. No dysmorphic features noted. X-ray of the nasopharynx showed large adenoids occluding the nasopharynx. Respiratory and cardiovascular system were normal.

Q. What is the clinical diagnosis?

Obstructive sleep apnea due to adenoidal hypertrophy.

Q. This patient underwent a polysomnogram (PSG) as part of a research protocol. What is a PSG?

Gold standard for objectively documenting OSA is an observed, overnight polysomnography (sleep study). This is a noninvasive test and measures a number of physiologic functions, including electroencephalogram (for staging sleep and detecting arousal from sleep), pulse oximetry, oronasal airflow, and abdominal and chest wall movements. Using pediatric criteria for scoring, respiratory events—obstructive apnea (cessation of oronasal airflow) and hypopnea (reduced airflow) events are identified on reviewing the overnight record. Number of these events per hour of sleep is expressed as apnea-hypopnea index (AHI). In children, it is generally considered that apnea index of <1 is normal, AHI >5 is moderate OSA, and AHI of >10 is severe.

This test is labor intensive, expensive, and not available in most centers. Sleep study is not routinely indicated in the evaluation of a child who has features of obstructed airway in sleep when adenoid hypertrophy has been demonstrated as the cause for obstruction. It is of value in patients with complex medical issues like cardiovascular complications, neurological conditions, syndromic children, and post adenoidectomy patients in whom obstruction persists. It is also valuable in children <2 years with OSA.

Q. In resource-limited setting what are the alternatives to PSG?

Documentation of apnea event with airway obstruction can be done using home video clips or even audio recording. Inpatient overnight observation with pulse oximeter recording and overnight home oximetry can also be utilized to diagnose OSA.

Q. What is the treatment of choice in this case?

Since the child has significant OSA, adeno-idectomy is the treatment of choice.

Q. What additional evaluation is needed in children with severe OSA before surgery?

In addition to routine pre-operative work up like hemogram and bleeding parameters, in high-risk patients, pulmonary hypertension has to be ruled out by echocardiography. Complete evaluation of any underlying medical conditions is necessary.

Q. What are the indications for adenoidectomy?

Indications for adenoidectomy include following:

- Extreme obstruction of the nasopharyngeal airway by adenoids causing OSA
- Moderate nasal obstruction caused by adenoidal hypertrophy with:
    - Recurrent or chronic sinusitis not responding to medical treatment
    - Recurrent acute otitis media (AOM) or chronic otitis media with effusion (OME) in children whom grommet insertion is planned a second time.

Q. What is the role of nonsurgical treatment for adenoid hypertrophy?

Use of intranasal steroids has shown to improve symptoms and reduce adenoidal size. It can be used as initial therapy for mild OSA in otherwise well children. Montelukast, a leukotriene antagonist, a well-tolerated oral drug also has been shown to be beneficial in mild to moderate OSA in children. While 4 mg of montelukast as a single dose is used for children <6 years, 5 mg is used for those >6 years. However, there is no consensus on the dose and duration of treatment.

These agents can also be tried when there are significant risk factors for anesthesia or surgery and when family insists on nonsurgical treatment. In this context, close follow-up of these patients is necessary as evidence for usefulness of these agents in OSA is preliminary and untreated OSA can lead to serious complications. Anti-inflammatory agents have also found a place in the treatment of postsurgical residual OSA.

CASE 3

A 7-year-old boy was brought with complaints of discharge from nose often purulent, recurrent episodes of cough, blocked nose, and snoring at night for 6 months. He got better with antibiotic use, and then it started again. He also had frequent ear pain and parents were concerned about his hearing. On examination: weight and height were <25th centile for age on growth chart. There was mucopurulent discharge from nose and his speech was hyponasal. Ear examination revealed OME. Tonsils were enlarged, but not inflamed. No stigmata of allergy and clubbing. Respiratory and cardiovascular systems were normal.

Q. What is the clinical diagnosis? What other relevant history is to be collected?

Child has clinical features of chronic adenoiditis, possible sinusitis with serous otitis media. Chronic adenoiditis and sinusitis may coexist and often cannot be differentiated from each other in children. Condition is considered chronic when symptoms persist for >90 days. It is important to obtain history of allergic rhinitis and foreign body in the nose. Conditions which predispose to recurrent or chronic sinusitis like immunodeficiency states, ciliary motility defects, gastroesophageal reflux have to be kept in mind while collecting history.

Q. What investigations need to be done?

For a child with suspected chronic adenoiditis following investigations may be done:

- Nasendoscopy to visualize adenoids and to rule out any foreign body or polyps. Purulent secretions in middle meatus are suggestive of sinusitis
- Hearing assessment with pure tone audiometry and impedance audiometry
- Lateral nasopharyngeal X-ray and paranasal sinus X-rays can be helpful
- Computed tomography/magnetic resonance imaging (CT/MRI) imaging is indicated only where complications are suspected or as part of pre-operative work up in selected cases.

Q. What is the next step in management?

Child with chronic adenoiditis or sinusitis needs treatment with β-lactamase stable antibiotics for 3–4 weeks. Topical steroids and saline washes can be used. Adenoidectomy is considered in cases where medical management fails. Rationale for surgery is that bacterial biofilm on the adenoids is thought to be responsible for sinusitis and Eustachian tube dysfunction. In children with allergic rhinitis or asthma, treatment with intranasal steroids may be indicated after surgical treatment.

LEARNING POINTS

- Adenoid normally enlarges in children from 3 years to 10 years before it regresses
- Many factors other than the size of the adenoid decide the severity of symptoms
- Lateral nasopharyngeal X-ray is a useful tool for pediatricians in the evaluation of a child suspected to have adenoid hypertrophy
- Obstructive sleep apnea due to adenoid hypertrophy can cause neurocognitive and cardiovascular complications in children
- Intranasal steroids are mainstay of medical therapy. A few patients may need surgery
- Biofilm production on the adenoids is implicated in the pathogenesis of chronic sinusitis and middle ear disease in children with adenoid hypertrophy. Hence, adenoidectomy has a role in the management of these conditions in children.

SUGGESTED READINGS

1. Friedman Bat-Chen, Goldman RD. Anti-inflammatory therapy for obstructive sleep apnea in children. Canadian Family Physician. Le Médecin de famille canadien. 2011;57:891-93.
2. Fujioka M, Young LW, Girdany BR. Radiographic evaluation of adenoidal size in children: adenoidal-nasopharyngeal ratio. AJR Am J Roentgenol. 1979;133(3):401-3.
3. Mena Viveros N. Biofilms in otolaryngology. Acta Otorrinolaringol Esp. 2014;65:47-52.
4. Muzumdar H, Arena R. Diagnostic issues in pediatric obstructive sleep apnea. Proc Am Thorac Soc. 2008;5: 263-73.

CHAPTER

7

Obstructive Sleep Apnea Syndrome

Rashmi R Das

CASE 1

A 6-year-old boy was brought with complaints of loud snore at night 5 days a week with frequent awakening since the last 6 months. He sleeps in unusual position with the mouth wide opened and head and neck in extended position. There was difficulty in getting up in the morning along with daytime fatigue and occasional morning headache. He is obese and is poor in studies.

Past medical history: Not significant.

Family history: Not suggestive.

Physical examination: His height was between 5th and 25th percentile, body mass index (BMI) was just above 95th percentile. He was noted to have tonsillar enlargement (Fig. 1).

Radiology: The X-ray lateral view of nasopharynx was showing adenoid hypertrophy (Fig. 2).

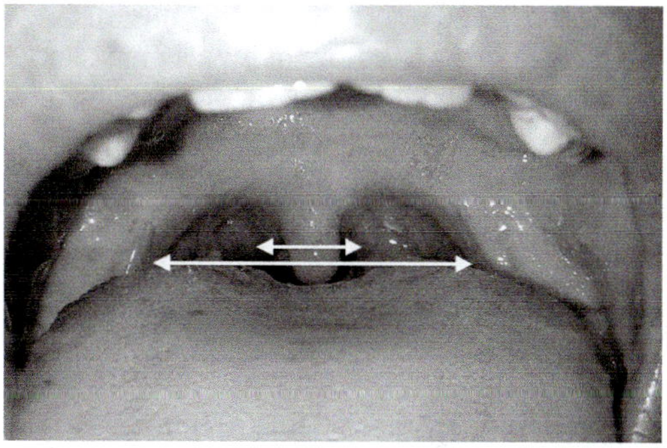

Figure 1: Bilateral tonsillar enlargement *(For color version, see Plate 1)*

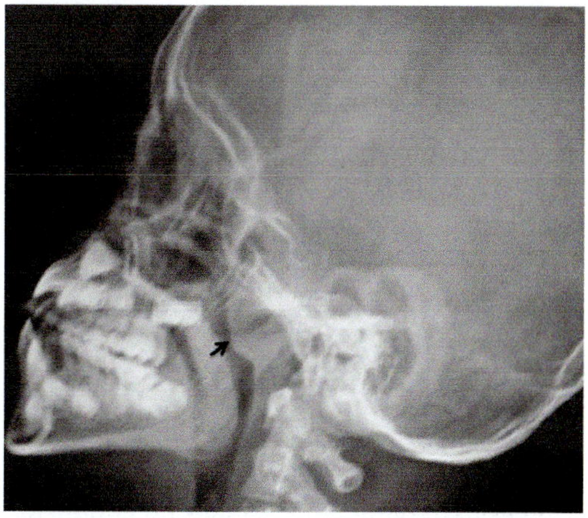

Figure 2: X-ray soft tissue neck showing adenoidal hypertrophy (black arrow)

Q. Does he has obstructive sleep apnea syndrome?

Obstructive sleep apnea syndrome (OSAS) is a type of sleep disordered breathing, characterized either by a prolonged partial upper airway obstruction or an intermittent complete obstruction that adversely affects ventilation or disrupts normal sleep patterns, and accompanied by various other features that include frequent snoring (≥3 nights/week), gasps, snoring noises, witnessed apneas, secondary enuresis, sleeping in unusual position (mouth wide open and/or head and neck in extended position), early morning headache, cyanosis, daytime fatigue or somnolence, behavioral problems (hyperactivity, poor attention span), poor scholastic performance, overweight or obesity, adenotonsillar hypertrophy, adenoid facies, etc. The boy described above is having many of these features and hence meet the criteria for OSAS.

Q. What are the most important points to elicit in his history and physical examination?

- History: A detailed history is the key to eliciting the etiology of OSAS and should include the following elements:
  - Enquire about night time symptoms
    - Snoring (number of nights per week)
    - Sleep pattern at night (good sleep, restlessness, waking up through the night)
    - Breathing pattern during sleep (struggle with breathing or labored breathing, or stop breathing)
    - Sleeping in unusual position (extended head/neck or sitting position)
    - Excessive sweating
    - Bluish discoloration/cyanosis
    - Nocturnal bed-wetting or secondary enuresis
    - Observed episodes of gasps or apneas by parents
  - Enquire about daytime symptoms
    - Behavioral or concentration problem (daytime sleepiness, attention deficit, hyperactivity)
    - Scholastic performance
    - Early morning headache
    - Mouth breathing
    - Growth pattern (normal or abnormal)
  - Ancillary history
    - Nasal block symptoms
    - Recurrent upper respiratory tract infections (nose, throat, and ear)
- Physical examination: A comprehensive physical examination should be conducted with special emphasis on the following:
  - Anthropometry (weight, height, BMI)
  - Adenoid facies (a combination of hypoplastic maxilla, crowded teeth, short upper lip, prominent upper teeth, and high-arched palate)
  - Pierre Robin sequence or isolated micrognathia or retrognathia
  - Nasal examination by headlight or otoscope (septal deviation, choanal atresia, polyps, turbinate hypertrophy)
  - Assessment of nasal airflow by holding a tongue depressor or cold spatula below nose
  - Tonsillar hypertrophy (grading size of the tonsils)
  - Ear (glue ear) and neck examination (lymphadenopathy)
  - Measurement of blood pressure
  - Neurological assessment
  - Syndromic child (Down syndrome, Prader-Willi syndrome, mucopolysaccharidosis, neuromuscular diseases, and craniofacial abnormalities).

Q. How do you interpret his tonsillar enlargement?

Grading of tonsillar size is done in relation to the occupancy of the oropharyngeal airway by the palatine tonsil as shown in the Table 1.

The index case is having grade III tonsillar enlargement.

Q. How do you interpret his adenoid hypertrophy on X-ray?

Adenoid hypertrophy is assessed from the lateral plain X-ray of the nasopharynx (to get an

TABLE 1: Grading of tonsillar enlargement

Grade	Occupancy of the oropharyngeal airway (horizontal measurement between anterior tonsillar pillars)
0	Confined to tonsillar fossa
I	0–25%
II	26–50%
III	51–75%
IV	> 75%

TABLE 2: Assessment of grading of adenoid hypertrophy

Size	Occupancy of the nasopharynx
Small	Nearly 25%
Moderate	Nearly 50%
Large	> 75%

idea about the size and relation to the size of the nasopharynx) as shown in the Table 2.

The index case is having moderate size adenoid hypertrophy as evident from the X-ray.

CASE 2

A 3-year-old girl was brought by her mother with complaints of snoring at night (2–3 episodes/week) along with labored breathing. She sleeps in unusual position with the mouth wide opened and head and neck in extended position. She was developmentally delayed.

Past medical history: Recurrent hospitalizations for medical illnesses.

Family history: Not suggestive.

Social history: She did not play with peers but loved toys.

Physical examination: She had features of Down's phenotype. Her height was between 3rd and 15th percentile, BMI was between 50th and 85th percentile. Nasal examination revealed unilateral choanal atresia.

Radiology: The X-ray lateral view of nasopharynx showed small size adenoid.

Q. How do you interpret her symptoms?

She is having sleep disordered breathing. Sleep disordered breathing refers to the whole spectrum of breathing disturbance during sleep, from primary snoring through to obstructive apnea. Her symptom complex does not fit fully into that of OSAS; however, she is at high risk of developing OSAS. She may have snoring, which is noisy breathing caused by turbulent airflow through the upper airway without the sequelae of obstructive apnea, frequent arousals from sleep or disordered gas exchange.

Q. What are the conditions that carry an increased risk of OSAS?

Following conditions carry an increase risk, and necessitate investigations to rule out OSAS:

- Unclear diagnosis of OSAS
- Syndromic child (Down's, Prader-Willi, mucopolysaccharidosis, Pierre Robin)
- Cerebral palsy
- Craniofacial abnormalities
- Neuromuscular disease
- Achondroplasia
- Obesity
- Grade IV adeno-tonsillar hypertrophy.

CASE 3

A 10-year-old boy was seen for the first time in clinic. His mother reported that he snores loudly at night with frequent awakening, and there were observed episodes of apnea along with bluish discoloration of lips and face. He easily gets fatigued while playing and was obese as well.

Past medical history: History of recurrent sore throat that had been treated multiple times with antibiotics. History of recurrent cough or cold treated with cough syrups and nebulizations.

Family history: Father also had history of snoring during childhood for which he underwent adenotonsillectomy at the age of 9 years.

Social history: Teachers complained that he did not concentrate on his studies.

Physical examination: His height was between 25th and 50th percentile, BMI was >95th percentile. He was noted to have adenoid facies, and there was bilateral grade III tonsillar enlargement. His blood pressure was >99th percentile, and the P2 component of S2 was loud.

Radiology: The X-ray lateral view of nasopharynx was showing adenoid hypertrophy (large size).

Q. What are the factors underlying development of OSAS and does he have any of them?

In the first group of children with no underlying medical diagnosis, they can get obstruction of the nasopharynx by enlarged adenoids and tonsils.

The peak incidence of OSA in this group occurs at 3–6 years of age because of physiological adeno-tonsillar hypertrophy. However, not all the children in this age group develop OSAS. The latter can be explained by the fact that there occurs variation in the pharyngeal muscle tone and anatomical difference in individuals prone to develop OSAS. Besides these, coexistence of persistent allergic (rhinitis) or infective upper respiratory (chronic tonsillitis) conditions in this age group may compound the process leading to OSAS.

In the second group of children, increase in the prevalence of obesity has led to the emergence of OSAS. Though the mechanism is unclear, it may be multifactorial, with an increase in the pharyngeal adipose tissue and decrease in respiratory capacity contributing to factors mentioned above.

In the third group of children, various congenital (craniofacial abnormalities, Down syndrome, neuromuscular diseases) and acquired (cerebral palsy) abnormalities can lead to OSAS. Children with these conditions either have anatomical (narrow pharyngeal airways, abnormal narrow upper airway) and/or functional (reduced pharyngeal muscle tone) abnormalities leading to OSAS.

In the index case, the child is having large adenoids, past history of recurrent sore throat and allergic airway disease. Besides this, he is obese also. All these factors as mentioned above are contributing to the OSAS.

Q. Are history and examination reliable in the diagnosis of OSAS?

A meta-analysis of observational studies has shown that history and examination have poor positive predictive value for OSAS. Because of this, additional investigations are needed to diagnose and treat OSAS.

Q. How are children with OSAS investigated to confirm the diagnosis and severity of the condition?

Besides reliable history and physical examination, children with sleep disordered breathing/OSAS need to be investigated by overnight pulse oximetry (± video recording of the event) and polysomnography. Polysomnography is presently the optimal investigation, and overnight pulse oximetry can be used if the former is not available (however the negative predictive value is low). Polysomnography can measure apneas (cessation in airflow) or hypopneas (reduction in airflow). These two measures are often combined as the apnea-hypopnea index (AHI), which is the total number of apneas and hypopneas per hour of sleep. An AHI of >1 and a minimum oxygen saturation of <92% is considered abnormal and is consistent with the diagnosis of OSAS.

Q. What are the clinical and laboratory features of more severe OSAS?

- Clinical features: Failure to thrive, pulmonary hypertension, cor pulmonale, systemic arterial hypertension, and rarely death are the features of more severe OSAS
- Laboratory features: Includes a combination of the severity of daytime sleepiness and the value of AHI
    - Severity of daytime sleepiness: Assessment can be subjective and objective. Subjective assessment is obtained with "Epworth Sleepiness Scale (range of 0–24, and normal ≤10)".
    - Apnea-hypopnea index:
        - Mild OSAS: 1 to <5
        - Moderate OSAS: 5–10
        - Severe OSAS: >10

The index case has more severe clinic features of OSAS and should undergo the above mentioned investigations on a priority basis.

Q. What are the management options for this child?

The following guideline (Flowchart 1) may be followed while managing children with sleep disordered breathing (snoring, OSAS).

The index case is having OSAS, and there is adeno-tonsillar hypertrophy. So, adeno-

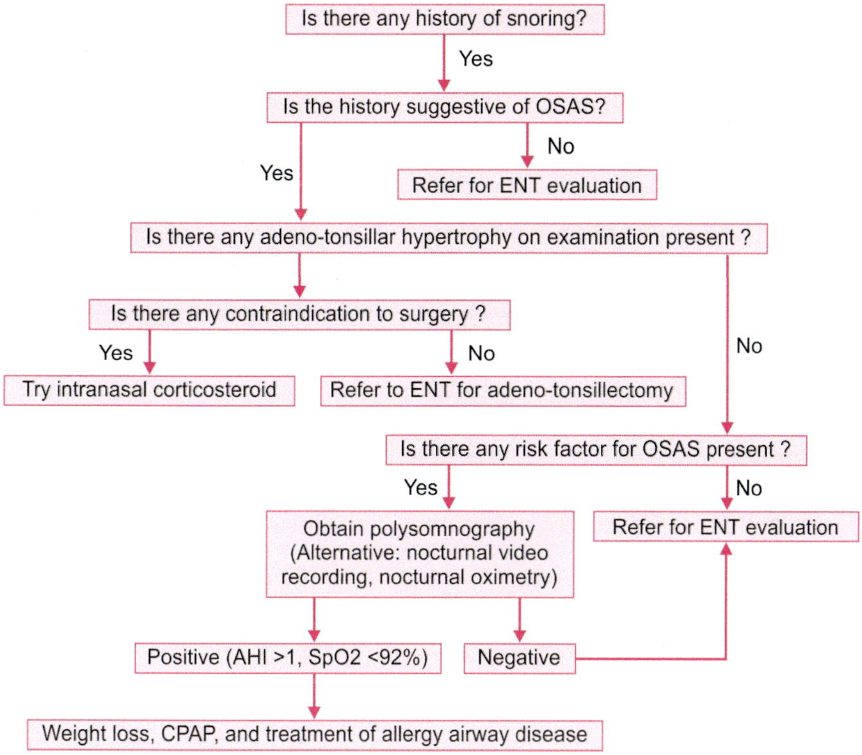

OSAS, obstructive sleep apnea syndrome; SpO2, peripheral capillary oxygen saturation; ENT, ear, nose and throat; AHI, apnea-hypopnea index; CPAP, continuous positive airway pressure.

Flowchart 1: Proposed algorithm for management of obstructive sleep apnea syndrome

tonsillectomy is the first line of treatment for him. He should also be advised to lose weight (as he is obese), if there is a delay in surgery.

Q. Are there any contraindications to adeno-tonsillectomy?

Yes, there are certain absolute and relative contraindications to adeno-tonsillectomy. They are as follows:

- Absolute: No adeno-tonsillar tissue or prior surgery (adeno-tonsillectomy)
- Relative: Small adeno-tonsillar tissue
    - Morbid obesity and very small adeno-tonsillar tissue
    - Bleeding disorder
    - Submucous cleft palate
    - Comorbidities posing risk for surgery.

Q. What are other treatment modalities in case there is contraindication to adeno-tonsillectomy or symptoms recur after adeno-tonsillectomy?

Continuous positive airway pressure (CPAP) is useful if symptoms persist after adeno-tonsillectomy or if adeno-tonsillectomy is not performed. Continuous positive airway pressure is delivered by using an electronic device via a nasal mask, leading to splinting of the airway and improved functional residual capacity. Besides this, weight loss should be advised if the child is obese. Intranasal corticosteroids may be prescribed in mild cases where adeno-tonsillectomy is contraindicated, or if mild OSAS persists after adeno-tonsillectomy.

LEARNING POINTS

- As a part of routine health checkup, pediatricians should ask whether a child snores or not
- In case the child snores regularly and has clinical features suggestive of OSAS, then evaluation should be done including polysomnography
- In case of OSAS due to adeno-tonsillar hypertrophy, adenotonsillectomy is the first line of treatment, and if there is no adeno-tonsillar hypertrophy, other treatment options should be considered
- Intranasal corticosteroids may be considered for children with mild OSAS in whom adenotonsillectomy is contraindicated or with mild postoperative OSAS
- Even mild to moderate OSAS cases can have adverse neurobehavioral outcomes and poor quality of life.

SUGGESTED READINGS

1. Brockmann PE, Schlaud M, Poets CF, Urschitz MS. Predicting poor school performance in children suspected for sleep-disordered breathing. Sleep Med. 2015;16(9):1077-83.
2. Chan J, Edman JC, Koltai PJ. Obstructive sleep apnea in children. Am Fam Physician. 2004;69(5):1147-54.
3. Gozal D, Hakim F, Kheirandish-Gozal L. Obesity and altered sleep: a pathway to metabolic derangements in children? Semin Pediatr Neurol. 2015;22(2):77-85.
4. Grime C, Tan HL. Sleep disordered breathing in children. Indian Pediatr. 2015;82(10):945-55.
5. Marcus CL, Brooks LJ, Draper KA, et al; American Academy of Pediatrics. Diagnosis and management of childhood obstructive sleep apnea syndrome. Pediatrics. 2012;130(3):e714-55.

CHAPTER

8

Croup

Kamal K Singhal, Ravitanya Sodani

> **CASE 1**
>
> An 18-month-old boy was brought to the outpatient department with complaints of barking cough, mild fever, coryza, and hoarse voice for 1 day.
>
> Past medical history: None remarkable.
>
> Physical examination: The child was conscious, playful, and active; color pink; nasal congestion present; stridor audible only on agitation; no chest retractions; auscultation revealed bilateral equal air entry with no added sounds.

Q. When to suspect croup?

Croup is a clinical syndrome that affects children aged 6 months to 6 years. It is characterized by signs or symptoms of upper airway obstruction with presence of inspiratory stridor, barking cough, hoarse voice and in severe cases, respiratory distress. It is frequently associated with a prodrome of coryza, fever, and pharyngitis. Thus, the child in the above case has croup.

Q. What are the etiological agents for croup?

The most common etiological agents for croup are parainfluenza virus and *Rhinovirus.* Other etiological agents include *Enterovirus,* respiratory syncytial virus, influenza virus, human bocavirus, and a co-infection with any of these.

Q. What are the pointers on history and examination to distinguish croup from other causes of acute upper airway obstruction?

The differential diagnosis of croup includes infective and noninfective causes as described in Table 1. Examination of the oropharynx to rule out other differentials, outside the setting where intubation and ventilatory support is not feasible, is not recommended. Nevertheless, examination of the oropharynx in appropriate settings may suggest the diagnosis.

> **CASE 2**
>
> A 3-year-old girl was brought to emergency with complaints of mild coryza for 1 day and sudden onset of difficulty in breathing, barking cough, and hoarseness in voice.
>
> Past medical history: She had been hospitalized once with similar complaints at the age of 2 years and well in-between since then.
>
> Physical examination: The child was agitated agitated, febrile, and pale with stridor at rest. Respiratory system examination revealed marked retraction and absent breath sound on auscultation.

TABLE 1: Summary of differential diagnosis of croup

Differential diagnosis	Indicators on history or examination
Laryngotracheitis or laryngotracheobronchitis	Prolonged expiration, expiratory wheezing
Subglottic stenosis, laryngomalacia, vocal cord paralysis, laryngeal hemangioma	• Young infant (<6 months of age) • Recurrent episodes not responding to treatment • Chronic noisy breathing, persistent hoarse voice or weak cry • History of intensive care unit (ICU) admission and endotracheal intubation
Spasmodic croup	• Recurrent episodes • Absence of prodrome of URI • Symptoms are more transient than viral croup.
Epiglottitis	• Preschool age, rapidly progressing symptoms (fever, difficulty breathing, stridor, sore throat, drooling, dysphagia, pronounced pharyngitis, and throat pain) • Toxic#, sick appearance • Cherry-red, swollen epiglottis • Child in "tripod" or "sniffing position"
Retropharyngeal/ parapharyngeal/ peritonsillar abscess	• Toxic# appearance • Midline or unilateral swelling of the posterior pharyngeal wall • Tonsillar asymmetry or deviation of the uvula • Enlarged cervical lymph nodes, torticollis • Excessive salivation, dysphagia
Bacterial tracheitis	• Toxic# appearance • A rare complication of viral croup—usually by *Staphylococcus aureus, Streptococcus pneumoniae, Haemophilus influenzae,* or *Moraxella catarrhalis*. • Airway assessment may reveal thick pus with ulcerated partly necrotic mucosa in the trachea
Laryngeal diphtheria	• Cervical lymphadenopathy • Presence of membrane • Unimmunized child
Foreign body(FB)	• Sudden onset without viral prodrome, history of choking/gagging while feeding [tracheal foreign body (FB)]; drooling, and dysphagia (large esophageal FB)

#Toxic, not taking feeds, lethargic or very irritable, not interested in surroundings.

Q. How to assess severity of croup?

Various scores have been used to objectively document severity of croup (e.g., Downes and Raphaely, Taussig, Westley, etc.). The Westley scoring system, used most commonly, is illustrated below in table 2. Accordingly, case 1 is mid croup and case 2 is severe croup.

TABLE 2: Westley scoring system for severity of croup

Level of consciousness	Normal (including sleep) = 0; disoriented = 5
Cyanosis	None = 0; with agitation = 4; at rest = 5
Stridor	None = 0; with agitation = 1; at rest = 2
Air entry	Normal = 0; decreased = 1; markedly decreased = 2
Retractions	None = 0; mild = 1; moderate = 2; severe = 3

(Mild croup ≤2; moderate croup 3–7; severe croup >7)

Q. What laboratory investigations are required in a child with suspected croup?

Diagnosis of croup is clinical. In a typical croup, radiological evaluation of upper airway is not indicated. It may be required if history or examination suggests alternative diagnosis such as:

- Retropharyngeal abscess: Increased thickness of posterior pharyngeal wall in lateral X-ray
- Bacterial tracheitis: Ragged tracheal wall in anteroposterior chest X-ray
- Epiglottitis: Thumb sign (thickening of epiglottis and aryepiglottic folds) on lateral X-ray of neck.

The stabilization of the child should take precedence over radiology as these radiological signs (especially in epiglottitis and tracheitis) are not very sensitive or specific. Moreover, there is danger of airway compromise in a sick child being transferred and his neck maneuvered to achieve appropriate radiological view of neck. Blood serologies and microbiological tests are also not useful in croup.

Q. When does a patient of croup merit endoscopic airway assessment?

Endoscopy is indicated in two situations as given below:

1. Indications at presentation in a patient of croup
    - Suspected foreign body aspiration
    - Severe symptoms with difficult intubation: To assist intubation with flexible scope
    - In bacterial tracheitis: Suction with flexible scope may be done to remove viscous purulent secretions, thereby clearing the obstructed lower airway.
2. Indication for airway assessment after stabilization of acute episode
    - Suspected subglottic stenosis, laryngomalacia, vocal cord paralysis, laryngeal hemangioma
    - In patients with documented gastroesophageal reflux: For gastroesophageal reflux (GER)-related laryngopharyngeal changes.

Q. What is the best tool to monitor a child with croup?

Monitoring of the clinical signs and symptoms (mental status, respiratory rate, retractions, and air entry into the chest) is the best tool to monitor a patient of croup. Pulse oximetry alone is not a good method because hypercarbia and not hypoxia is usually associated with laryngeal airway obstruction unless the obstruction is very severe. Nevertheless, pulse oximetry may be helpful if there is associated involvement of tracheo-bronchial tree.

Q. What is the indication for corticosteroids? What is the most appropriate corticosteroid and its dose and route?

All patients with viral croup merit corticosteroids, irrespective of disease severity. Single dose oral dexamethasone is better than single dose oral prednisolone. Inhaled budesonide (2 mg) reduces intensity of symptoms, frequency of hospitalization, and return visits but has not been found to be superior to oral or intramuscular (IM) dexamethasone. Single dose dexamethasone (0.15–0.6 mg/kg, oral/IM, maximum of 8 mg) is indicated. Presently, there is no evidence to recommend repeated doses of corticosteroids. Orally and intramuscularly administered dexamethasone have comparable efficacy. Intramuscular route may be used in patients unable to take medications orally. Combined use of inhaled with oral or parenteral corticosteroids does not yield any additional benefit.

The benefits of systemic corticosteroids at presentation include faster reduction in severity, lesser need for nebulized epinephrine, and reduced need for hospitalization. Furthermore, its use brings down admission days and need for re-admission after discharge.

Q. What is the role of epinephrine, its most appropriate formulation, dose, and route?

Epinephrine acts by causing vasoconstriction, thereby reducing the mucosal edema of the airway. Epinephrine provides short-term (<2 hours) symptomatic relief, thereby allowing time for systemic corticosteroids to act. Thus, patients having at least moderate-grade croup are more likely to benefit with epinephrine. Cheaper and more easily available L-epinephrine is as effective as racemic epinephrine. Dose to be used is 3 mL of L-epinephrine (1:1,000 solution). Clinically significant effect starts at around 30 minutes and lasts about 2 hours. This implies that nebulized epinephrine can be administered every 2 hours (earlier in sever croup) and child should be observed for at least 2–4 hours after last dose of nebulized epinephrine, before discharge from the hospital.

Q. What is the role of heliox?

Presently, there is no evidence to suggest significant beneficial effect of heliox in children with moderate to severe croup.

Q. What is the role of humidified air?

Although used historically, humidified air has no significant beneficial effect in cases of mild-to-moderate croup. Presently, the evidence is insufficient to exclude either a small beneficial or a harmful effect.

Q. What are the indications for hospitalization?

Children with moderate or severe croup who worsen or fail to improve as expected after treatment with epinephrine and corticosteroids should be hospitalized. Admission may also be required for an alternative diagnosis (epiglottitis, bacterial tracheitis, or retropharyngeal abscess) or other comorbidity (dehydration due to decreased intake). Summary of management of croup is described in Table 3.

Q. What are the indications for discharge of a child with croup?

All the following criteria should be fulfilled for considering a discharge:

- Should have received corticosteroid
- Should have been observed for at least 2–4 hours after last dose of nebulized epinephrine
- No stridor at rest, no signs of respiratory distress and sensorium is normal
- No other indication for hospitalization.

TABLE 3: Management summary of croup

Treatment modalities available	Mild croup	Moderate croup	Severe croup
Oxygen therapy to prevent hypoxia <92%	× Not needed	√	√
Tab. Dexa 0.15–0.6 mg/kg orally stat Inj. Dexa 0.15–0.6 mg/kg IM stat Nebulization with budesonide (2 mg) once	√ Tab. Dexa Or Inj. Dexa Or Neb. budesonide	√ Tab. Dexa Or Inj. Dexa Or Neb. budesonide	√ Inj. Dexa
Nebulization with epinephrine 3 mL (1:1,000)	× Not needed	√	√
IV fluids (if dehydrated or low intake)	× Not needed	√	√
Judicious use of antipyretics	√	√	√
Need for admission	× Not needed	√ (not responding to initial management)	√

Tab., tablet; Inj., injection; IV, intravenous; Neb., nebulization; IM, intramuscular.

Q. What would happen to an untreated child with croup?

Although the course of viral croup depends on its severity, mostly it is a self-limiting illness. Wagener et al. studied 527 consecutive patients over a 12 month period. They excluded mild croup (defined as minimal distress and no stridor at rest) as they were routinely managed as outpatients. After excluding this mild croup, they divided patients into three grades. The grade 1 (stridor even at rest without retractions) constituted the majority of the remaining patients (57%). Of the patients with grade 1 severity only one required intensive care. About 19% and 92% of grade 2 and 3 patients required intensive care management, respectively. Percentage of patients requiring intubation in grade 1, 2, and 3 was 0, 6, and 53%, respectively. Thus, most of the patients with croup without significant distress do not need intensive care or artificial airway.

LEARNING POINTS

- Diagnosis of croup is clinical. In a typical croup, radiological evaluation is not indicated
- Clinical signs and symptoms are the best tool to monitor a patient of croup
- Irrespective of severity, all patients with croup should be given corticosteroid
- Patients having at least moderate-grade croup are more likely to benefit with epinephrine.

SUGGESTED READINGS

1. Bjornson CL, Klassen TP, Williamson J, Brant R, Mitton C, Plint A, et al. A randomized trial of a single dose of oral dexamethasone for mild croup. N Engl J Med. 2004;351(13):1306-13.
2. Cherry JD. Croup (Laryngitis, laryngotracheitis, spasmodic croup, laryngotracheobronchitis, bacterial tracheitis, and laryngotracheobronchopneumonitis). In: Feigin RD, Cherry JD, Demmler-Harrison GJ, Kaplan SL (Eds). Textbook of Pediatric Infectious Diseases, 6th edition. Philadelphia: Saunders; 2009. p. 254.
3. Russell KF, Liang Y, O'Gorman K, Johnson DW, Klassen TP. Glucocorticoids for croup. Cochrane Database Syst Rev. 2011;(1):CD001955.

CHAPTER

9

Acute Epiglottitis

Abdus S Bhat, Umar A Qureshi

CASE 1

A 3-year-old unimmunized boy presents to the emergency department in early morning hours, with inspiratory stridor, drooling of saliva and high-grade fever. On enquiring about history, the child had been well till evening when he started having above symptoms which rapidly progressed overnight. On examination, the child was looking toxic and wanted to lean forward rather than lie down. His oxygen saturation was, however, maintained and chest examination revealed stridor.

Q. What is the most likely diagnosis and why?

The most likely diagnosis in the given scenario is acute epiglottitis (AE). The closest differential diagnosis in this case would be acute laryngotracheobronchitis (ALTB). Patients with AE have more fever, are more toxic, have dysphagia, and have more preference for typical sniffing posture than patients with ALTB. Incidence of cough is more in ALTB. Presentation is much more acute in patients with AE. The above patient has high-grade fever, is toxic, does not want to lie down, and duration of illness, >24 hours. Further drooling of saliva is present. All these point toward the diagnosis of AE.

Q. What are the other possible diagnoses?

A number of diseases can have similar presentation as our case above. Table 1 gives a brief idea about the differential diagnosis and differentiating points.

Q. What is AE?

Acute epiglottitis as the name suggests is an acute inflammation of the epiglottis. It is usually associated with inflammation of other structures of the supraglottis including aryepiglottic folds, arytenoid soft tissue, and sometimes the uvula. Classically, the disease does not involve the subglottic or tracheal mucosa. That is why epiglottitis is often referred to as supraglottitis. If not treated in time, death can result from airway obstruction.

Q. What are the causes of AE?

Acute epiglottitis in children is classically caused by *Haemophilus influenzae type b (Hib)*. However, the incidence of AE due to Hib has decreased significantly in countries where vaccination against Hib is being carried out under national immunization programs. In vaccinated children, AE can still occur due to causes other than Hib which are summarized

TABLE 1: Differential diagnosis of acute epiglottitis

Condition	Clinical features	Radiology
Epiglottitis (supraglottitis)	Fever, toxic appearance, "tripod" and/or "sniffing" posture; drooling	Swollen epiglottis "thumb sign" on lateral neck radiograph
Laryngotracheitis (croup)	"Barking" cough, stridor	Tapering of upper airway "steeple sign" on anteroposterior neck radiograph
Bacterial tracheitis	Fever, toxic appearance	Intraluminal membranes and tracheal wall irregularity
Uvulitis	Swelling and erythema of the uvula	Radiographs not diagnostic
Foreign body	History of sudden onset of choking (may be absent); stridor with foreign body lodged in upper airway	Visualization of radio-opaque foreign body
Retropharyngeal abscess	Neck pain, fever, dysphagia, drooling; trismus, midline or unilateral swelling of posterior pharyngeal wall	Widening of the retropharyngeal space and loss of cervical lordosis
Peritonsillar abscess	Typically occurs in older children and adolescents, drooling, trismus, hot-potato voice, swelling of tonsils with deviation of the uvula	Radiographs noncontributory
Angioedema	Rapid onset with swelling of lips and tongue, urticarial rash, dysphagia without hoarseness, possible history of previous attack	Radiographs noncontributory
Congenital anomalies (e.g. laryngeal web, laryngomalacia)	Prolonged course and no systemic symptoms (unless airway narrowing is exacerbated by concomitant infection)	Radiographs noncontributory
Respiratory diphtheria	Gradual onset of symptoms: Sore throat, malaise, and low-grade fever, presence of diphtheritic membrane	Radiographs noncontributory
Thermal or chemical injury	History of exposure, lack of fever or prodromal illness	Radiographs noncontributory

below in Box 1. Risk factors for AE include incomplete or lack of immunization for Hib, immune deficiency, and underlying genetic susceptibility.

Q. What is the pathogenesis of AE?

Inflammation of the epiglottis as a result of infection leads to swelling initially on its lingual side which subsequently progresses to involve the supraglottic structures including arytenoids and aryepiglottic folds. This is because the epithelium and lamina propria is loosely adherent to epiglottic cartilage on lingual surface as compared to laryngeal surface. The swelling does not involve the subglottis as the epithelium is tightly adherent to vocal cords, thereby preventing its spread. The swollen supraglottic structures compromise the caliber of upper airway, thereby leading to stridor. It also leads to dysphagia, which in turn results in drooling of saliva.

Q. What additional things would you look for in history and examination?

Dramatic onset of symptoms is a hallmark of AE. Usually, children are not symptomatic for >24 hours before hospitalization. Classical symptoms in younger children include fever which is of high grade with or without symptoms of upper respiratory tract infection, which is

Box 1: Causes of acute epiglottitis

Infectious causes

- *Bacteria: Haemophilus influenzae type b (Hib)*, H. influenzae types A and F, and nontypeable strain, H. parainfluenzae, Streptococcus pneumoniae, Staphylococcus aureus (methicillin susceptible and methicillin resistant), Pasteurella multocida, Moraxella catarrhalis, Klebsiella pneumoniae, Neisseria* spp., *Enterobacter cloacae,* and *Pseudomonas aeruginosa*¶
- *Viruses*[µ]: Herpes simplex virus type 1, varicella zoster virus, parainfluenza virus type 3, influenza B viruses, Epstein-Barr virus
- *Fungi:* Candida¶

Noninfectious (Traumatic) Causes

- Thermal injury, foreign body ingestion, caustic ingestion

Usually in immunocompromised patients.

*The most common cause in children when an organism is identified.

[µ]Epiglottitis may result from bacterial superinfection.

soon followed by dysphagia, drooling, and respiratory distress (3 D's). The child usually has a toxic look and inspiratory stridor is present. In order to maximize air entry through swollen supraglottic area, the child may assume a tripod posture, wherein the child leans forward supporting his body on extended arms and keeps his or her head in a sniffing position. In cases where airway obstruction is advanced, the child may even present with cyanosis and respiratory arrest. In older children, symptoms are not as severe as in small children.

Q. How would you approach such a case?

One should remember that before attempts at diagnosis are made, airway should be secured on priority in a suspect case of AE where airway obstruction is imminent. Diagnosis of epiglottitis is primarily made on clinical grounds. Direct visualization of supraglottis with or without the help of laryngoscope gives a definitive clue about the diagnosis of AE. Epiglottis will appear as swollen with cherry-red hue, blocking the airway during inspiration. However, direct examination as described above is always fraught with danger of precipitating airway obstruction in young children and should be done cautiously and preferably in an operating room with all facilities of general anesthesia. It should be deferred in patients who do not have imminent airway obstruction as it can itself precipitate obstruction.

Lateral neck radiographs have low sensitivity and specificity as compared to direct visualization. Radiographs are helpful in evaluation of patients in whom AE is a possibility, but other conditions are also likely. Radiographs of the soft tissue of neck in lateral view in AE will reveal a swollen epiglottis protruding from the anterior wall of hypopharynx in the form of a thumb sign. It may also reveal loss of the vallecular air space (a finding that may be underappreciated), thickened aryepiglottic folds, distended hypopharynx, and straightening or reversal of the normal cervical lordosis.

Laboratory studies (blood cultures and blood counts) should not be performed in patients in whom AE is strongly suspected until the airway is secured, because agitation caused by pain may worsen respiratory distress. Most patients with AE have an elevated white blood cell count, but this finding is nonspecific. Cultures of the blood and surface of the epiglottis (in intubated patients) frequently help to identify the microbial pathogen. Epiglottal cultures are positive in 33–75% of patients with epiglottitis. Blood cultures are positive in approximately 70% of children with epiglottitis caused by Hib. In children immunized against Hib, the yield of blood cultures is likely to be lower. Flowchart 1 summarizes the approach to a patient with suspected AE.

Q. How do you manage such a patient?

Airway management

- Patients with AE may present with varying degrees of airway obstruction

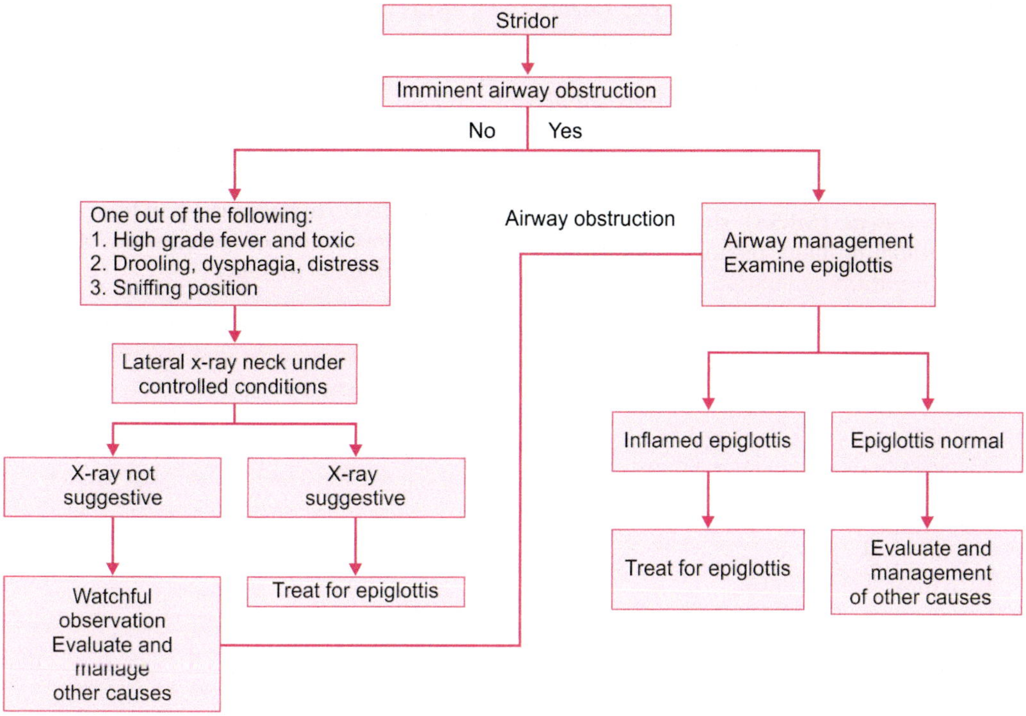

Flowchart 1: Approach to a patient with suspected acute epiglottitis

- Whenever airway obstruction is present or when airway obstruction is imminent, airway should be secured on priority
- In selected cases, where obstruction is not severe patients may be managed without airway in an intensive care unit under close monitoring only when facilities or expertise for placement of artificial airway are available round the clock*
- Intubation in setting of AE should be done cautiously, preferably in an operating room with all facilities of general anesthesia because swollen supraglottic area can pose difficulties for even an expert during intubation
- Airway can be secured either by nasotracheal or orotracheal intubation, tracheostomy or emergency cricothryoidotomy depending upon the clinical condition of the patient, expertise available and the nature of the upper airway
- Surgical cricothyroidotomy may be necessary if neither endotracheal intubation nor tracheostomy can be performed
- When the patient is clinically stable, and the laryngoscopic examination shows reduction in swelling or when leak has started around the endotracheal tube, extubation can be attempted.

**A systematic review in children with AE has shown that mortality can be reduced by putting artificial airway even preemptively given the absence of well-defined criteria that would predict need or no need of artificial airway coupled with high incidence of airway obstruction.*

Antibiotic therapy

- Antibiotic therapy should be instituted as soon as possible to get rid of the underlying etiological organism
- In absence of an epiglottal or blood culture and sensitivity report, an empirical antibiotic policy should be followed depending upon the prevalent organism and sensitivity
- Once culture report is available, the antibiotics can be changed according to the sensitivity pattern

- Empirical antibiotics should cover *Haemophilus influenzae, Streptococcus pneumoniae* and *Streptococcus pyogenes*
- If staphylococcal infection is suspected like in cases of severe sepsis or meningitis, an antistaphylococcal agent having good activity against methicillin resistant *Staphylococcus aureus* (MRSA) should be added. Thus, initial antibiotic regimen would usually contain a third-generation cephalosporin ± vancomycin
- Although there is no well-defined duration of treatment, antibiotics once started should be continued for 7–10 days
- Ceftriaxone should be given at a dose of 50–75 mg/kg body weight intravenously (IV) as a single or two divided doses
- Cefotaxime if used instead of ceftriaxone should be given at a dose of 150 mg/kg/day IV in three divided doses
- Vancomycin should be given at a dose of 40 mg/kg/day in four divided doses by IV infusion over one hour.

Supportive treatment

Includes use of IV fluids, bronchodilators, and antipyretics.

Role of corticosteroids

- Role of corticosteroids in management of acute epiglottitis is controversial and should not be used
- Glucocorticoids may have a role in patients where there is difficulty in extubation after prolonged need for intubation.

Q. What complications can be expected in AE?

Acute epiglottitis can lead to airway obstruction, epiglottic abscess, necrotizing epiglottitis, secondary infection, and death (in less than one percent).

Q. What is the natural course of the disease?

The majority of patients with AE recover without residual airway or other problems if the airway is promptly secured and appropriate antimicrobial therapy instituted. Deaths or injury related to hypoxemia occur from delayed airway intervention or progression of sepsis after institution of therapy.

LEARNING POINTS

- Acute epiglottitis should be suspected in any child with fever, stridor, and rapid onset of symptoms
- Acute epiglottitis can still occur in post vaccination era
- Airway should be secured on priority in all suspected cases of acute epiglottitis (AE) before attempts at diagnosis are made
- Diagnosis is mainly clinical. Direct visualization, lateral neck X-rays, hematology, and microbiology are helpful in selected cases
- Antibiotic therapy and supportive care in addition to airway management are the cornerstone of AE management
- Acute epiglottitis if not suspected and managed in time can lead to death.

SUGGESTED READINGS

1. Damm M, Eckel HE, Jungehülsing M, Roth B. Management of acute inflammatory childhood stridor. Otolaryngol Head Neck Surg. 1999;121(5):633-8.
2. Fenton JE, Glynn F. Diagnosis and management of supraglottitis (epiglottitis). Curr Infect Dis Rep. 2008;10(3):200-4.
3. Friedman NR, Stroud RH. An update on inflammatory disorders of the pediatric airway: epiglottitis, croup, and tracheitis. Am J Otolaryngol. 2001;22(4):268-75.
4. Oropharyngeal examination for suspected epiglottitis. Am J Dis Child. 1988;142(12):1263-7.
5. Ragosta KG, Orr R, Detweiler MJ. Revisiting epiglottitis: a protocol—the value of lateral neck radiographs. J Am Osteopath Assoc. 1997;97(4):227-9.
6. Tibballs J, Watson T. Symptoms and signs differentiating croup and epiglottitis. J Paediatr Child Health. 2011;47(3):77-82.

2
SECTION

Congenital Disorders of Respiratory Tract

CHAPTER

10

Laryngomalacia and Tracheomalacia

Paramesh D H, Salim A Khatib

LARYNGOMALACIA

CASE 1

- First full-term normal delivery (FTND) male, presented with inspiratory stridor soon after birth, associated with chest wall retractions
- Had normal air entry with resting SpO_2 of 96% in room air, required supportive care initially. After 24 hours, the baby started accepting breastfeeds. At times, the stridor was high pitched by agitation and crying, and diminished during sleep. Followed up to 6 weeks baby is thriving well.

Q. What are the causes of purely inspiratory stridor in a well baby?

Common causes for stridor in otherwise normal newborn are as follows:

- Laryngomalacia
- Vocal cord palsy
- Supraglottic cyst, laryngeal cyst
- Subglottic stenosis
- Airway wall hemangioma
- Laryngeal cleft, laryngeal web
- Lingual thyroid
- Hypocalcemia and hypomagnesemia

Q. Possible approach to evaluate baby with inspiratory stridor?

The most common cause is laryngomalacia (60–70%), where it is mild and purely inspiratory stridor. It is with normal cry and feeding well with good thriving starts soon after birth in an otherwise well baby. It is a self-limiting condition and resolves without any intervention by 12–18 months.

If there is any doubt about the cause of the stridor, associated with poor feeding, hoarse cry, extended neck, and poor growth, the following investigations can be considered:

- Chest X-ray: To assess the mediastinum, cardiac size, and position of aorta
- Laryngobronchoscopy: To visualize the airway structures
- Blood tests: Serum electrolytes, metabolic disorders such as hypocalcemia, and hypomagnesemia.

Q. What are clinical manifestations of laryngomalacia?

Laryngomalacia is the term used to describe a condition in which there is partial or complete airway closure caused by an inward folding of the aryepiglottic folds and epiglottis during inspiration.

Laryngomalacia is characterized by following clinical manifestations:

- Purely an inspiratory stridor, if there is any expiratory component, one should seek an alternative diagnosis
- The stridor may be present from birth, but generally becomes apparent by several weeks of age (4–8 months)

- Child has normal cry and thriving well
- The stridor is staccato and crescendo, increasing in loudness and pitch toward the end of inspiration. It is variable and may be absent during sleep
- When laryngomalacia is severe, there may be failure to thrive and poor feeding
- In approximately 5–20% respiratory concerns such as obstructive sleep apnea, tachypnea, dyspnea, respiratory distress, or hypoxia can occur.

Q. What is etiology of laryngomalacia?

Precise etiopathogenesis of laryngomalacia is not known.

- Theory of immature and abnormally collapsible cartilage was further discredited by histological examinations demonstrating normal fibroelastic cartilage tissue in children with symptomatic disease
- Presently, attention has focused on a neuromuscular etiology, consisting of immaturity or abnormal integration of the peripheral nerves, brainstem nuclei, and pathways responsible for swallowing and maintenance of airway patency
- Additional corroboration is provided by histological studies showing significant size difference in the superior laryngeal nerve branches of patients with severe laryngomalacia, compared to age-matched controls
- Subsequent neurological and central nervous system maturation would provide a reasonable explanation for the spontaneous resolution generally seen in the disease.

Q. How to make a diagnosis of laryngomalacia?

- A presumptive clinical diagnosis of laryngomalacia can be made based on the classic symptoms of inspiratory stridor worsened by feeding, agitation, supine positioning, or crying
- A definitive diagnosis can be made accurately by flexible fiber optic laryngoscopy alone in vast majority (88%) (Fig. 1)
- Several anatomical staging systems for laryngomalacia have been proposed which focus on defining the site of collapse:
  - Posterior collapse (from redundant arytenoids mucosa or cuneiform cartilage)
  - Lateral collapse (from shortened aryepiglottic folds)
  - Anterior collapse (from retroflexed epiglottis)
  - Combined collapse (involving multiple areas of anatomic collapse).

CASE 2

- A 5-day-old girl child presented with a history of respiratory noises and at times feeding difficulty
- Examination revealed inspiratory stridor with accessory muscles in action. Clinical diagnosis of laryngomalacia was made and reassured along with positional support for breastfeeding
- Two days later, the baby presented with severe respiratory distress, with all the accessory muscles in action, and increased intensity of stridor with SpO_2 of 88% in room air
- After evaluation, diagnosed to have severe form of laryngomalacia near complete closure during inspiration and underwent surgical intervention—supraglottoplasty and did very well.

Q. Is there any laryngomalacia severity scale?

Based on respiratory symptoms and feeding symptoms, laryngomalacia can be assessed as mild, moderate, or severe (Table 1).

Q. Any additional diagnostic evaluation is necessary?

In mild to moderate severity of laryngomalacia, no additional evaluation is necessary.

- Gastroesophageal reflux disease has been reported in 65–100% of infants with severe laryngomalacia
- Reflux events could then irritate the laryngeal mucosa, causing edema, and thereby worsening the airway collapse. The incidence of synchronous airway lesions is 12–64%.

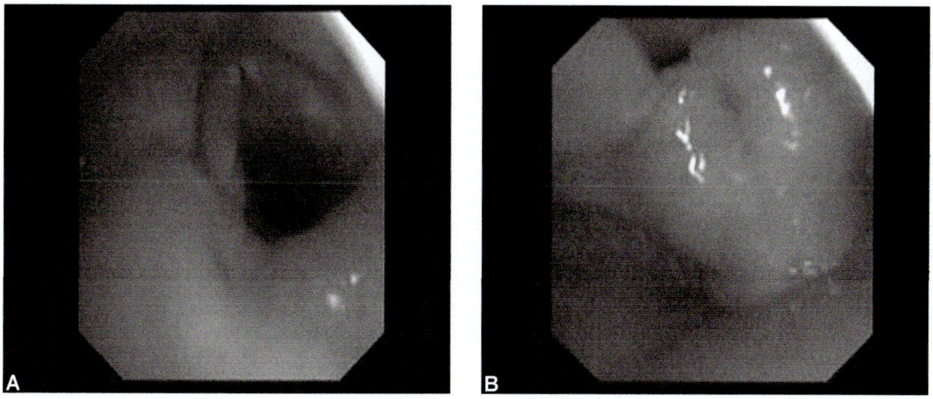

Figure 1: Fiber optic laryngoscopic view of child with laryngomalacia. **A,** during expiration and **B,** during inspiration *(For color version, see Plate 2)*

TABLE 1: **Assessment of severity of laryngomalacia**

Severity level	Respiratory symptoms	Feeding symptoms
Mild	Inspiratory stridor (average resting SpO_2: 98–100%)	Inspiratory stridor with cyanosis or apnea (average resting SpO_2: 86%)
Moderate	Inspiratory stridor (average resting SpO_2: 96%)	Frequent regurgitation or other feeding issues
Severe	Inspiratory stridor with cyanosis or apnea (average resting SpO_2: 86%)	Failure to thrive or aspiration

Q. What are clinical indications for consideration of surgical intervention?

Symptoms of mild to moderate laryngomalacia improve with age. Children with severe disease having respiratory and feeding problems may need surgical intervention (Table 2).

TABLE 2: **Indications for surgery in an infant with severe laryngomalacia**

Respiratory*	Feeding*
• Stridor with respiratory distress • Dyspnea with retractions • Pulmonary hypertension • Severe obstructive sleep apnea	• Episodic cyanosis with feeding • Recurrent aspiration pneumonia • Failure to thrive

*Presence of single manifestation is indication for surgery.

TRACHEOMALACIA

CASE 3

- Baby S, 27-month-old girl presented with history of fever, cold, and cough of 3 days, which rapidly progressed to severe respiratory distress. Her clinical findings, radiological picture, was with acute respiratory distress syndrome. She was treated with oseltamivir and antibiotics. Her ventilation requirement was high and required 4 weeks of ventilation
- She was extubated onto noninvasive ventilation. However, she continued to have inspiratory stridor, and marked recessions which were variable during the course of the day. Bronchoscopy confirmed significant tracheomalacia (portion below cricoid bone)
- Tracheostomy was undertaken and the tracheotomy tube bypassed the malacia part and her distress was reduced.

Q. What is tracheomalacia?

Malacia refers to "softness" of a tissue, typically a bone or cartilage. Collapsibility of the central airways is an important cause of obstruction in childhood respiratory conditions such as tracheomalacia, bronchomalacia, and tracheobronchomalacia (TBM).

Q. What is pathogenesis of tracheomalacia?

To understand pediatric tracheomalacia, it is first necessary to understand the development and structure of the airway as well as airway mechanics.

Airway development

By the third week of gestation the endoderm develops into foregut. The trachea develops from the proximal ventral foregut endoderm while the esophagus arises from the dorsal foregut endoderm. The separation of the two structures is completed by the end of fourth week of gestation. Improper foregut separation of the trachea from the esophagus results in congenital abnormalities such as laryngotracheoesophageal clefts, tracheoesophageal fistulae (TOF), and esophageal atresia (EA) that are associated with tracheomalacia.

The posterior membrane or pars membranacea contains the trachealis muscle, which also changes throughout development. There is an age-related increase in the passive tone, contractility, size and length of the trachealis.

The net effect of the age-related changes to the tracheal rings and posterior membrane is an increase in radius, cross-sectional area (CSA), and circumference of the trachea and a decrease in tracheal compliance. Weakness of either the cartilage or posterior membrane results in increased tracheal compliance and possible compromise of the tracheal lumen during the respiratory cycle.

Q. Can we clinically differentiate between extrathoracic and intrathoracic tracheomalacia?

Extrathoracic dynamic airway collapse causes inspiratory symptoms including stridor, a prolonged inspiratory phase, and low lung volumes.

Intrathoracic airway narrowing whether generalized or localized causes expiratory problems including wheezing, barking cough, a prolonged expiratory phase, and impaired secretion clearance. Children with intrathoracic tracheomalacia can also experience recurrent bacterial bronchitis, cyanotic spells, apnea, and difficulty weaning from respiratory support (Fig. 2).

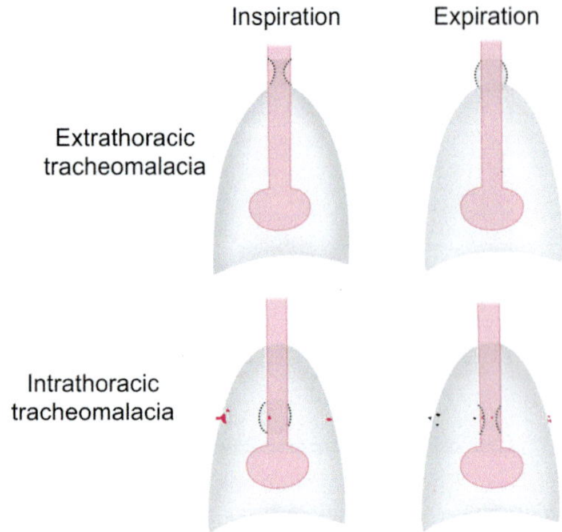

Figure 2: Airway mechanics in intrathoracic and extrathoracic tracheomalacia

Q. How to confirm diagnosis of tracheomalacia?

Tracheomalacia should be suspected in infants at risk when their disease is unusually severe or persistent, where there is wheeze that does not respond to bronchodilators, or where there are episodes of unexplained respiratory distress and cyanosis.

On physical examination, one can appreciate inspiratory stridor with retractions in extrathoracic tracheomalacia and wheezing with retractions in intrathoracic tracheomalacia.

Most authors agree that 50% narrowing of the airways is diagnostic of tracheomalacia by the bronchoscopist during visual inspection (Fig. 3).

More recently, efforts have been made to quantify tracheal collapse accurately using the color histogram method. This technique objectively identifies the airway lumen and determines CSA by accounting for the magnification and distortion of the bronchoscopic image.

Another challenge in the diagnosis of tracheomalacia is that current methods only evaluate the change in CSA without taking the applied transmural pressure into account.

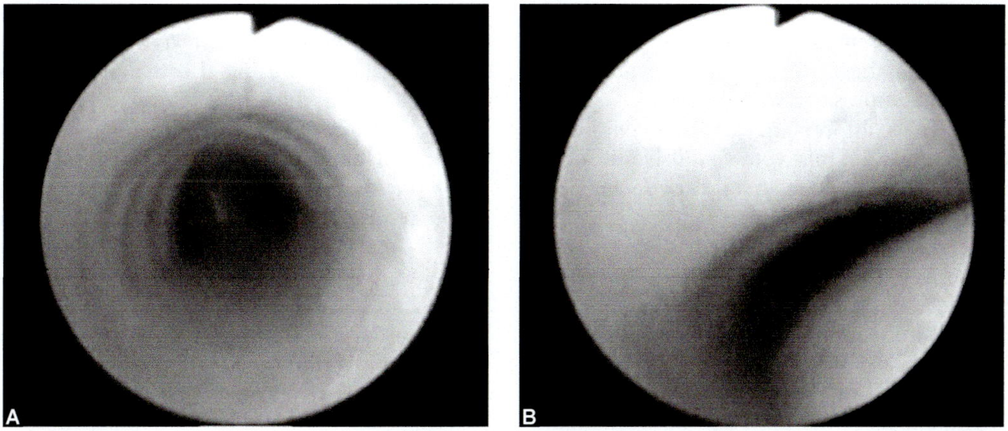

Figure 3: Bronchoscopic findings. **A,** in normal trachea and **B,** in tracheomalacia ***(For color version, see Plate 2)***

CASE 4

- A 1-year-old baby boy, who was diagnosed with large patent ductus arteriosus (PDA) and pulmonary arterial hypertension was referred for evaluation with significant respiratory distress
- His presenting features were shortness of breath, feeding difficulty, and failure to thrive
- On examination, he had hyperinflated chest, recession, and diminished breath sounds in left hemithorax. X-ray confirmed hyperinflation of the left lung
- Bronchoscopy showed narrowing of the left main bronchus in fish-mouth pattern. The computed tomography (CT) scan showed compression of trachea at carina and left main bronchus (Fig. 4). He underwent PDA ligation. He continued to have noisy breathing and check bronchoscopy showed persistent malacia
- A diagnosis of tracheobronchomalacia secondary to compression of airways due vessels was made and symptomatic treatment was given. He slowly showed improvement and his symptoms resolved after 2 years.

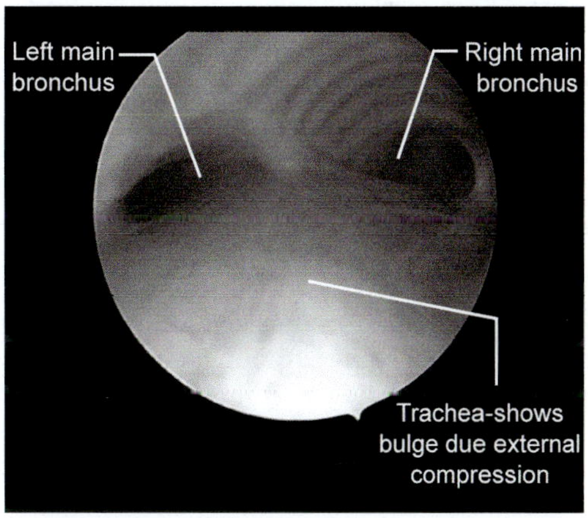

Figure 4: Bronchoscopic findings. Compression of left main bronchus ***(For color version, see Plate 2)***

Courtesy: Anilkumar Sapare, NH Hospital, Bengaluru.

Q. What are the probable causes of tracheobrochomalacia?

Tracheomalacia, or TBM can be primary (congenital) or secondary (acquired). Primary disease is rare.

Primary tracheomalacia was first described by Holinger et al. in 1952, and later defined as weakening of the tracheal wall due to abnormal formation or maturation of the airway.

Secondary or acquired tracheomalacia occurs in the normally developed trachea after some insult such as trauma, external compression, and positive pressure ventilation (PPV), infection or inflammation.

Tracheotomy or prolonged intubation is perhaps the most common cause of acquired extrathoracic tracheomalacia.

The earliest reports of secondary tracheomalacia were described in the 1930s and 1940s and were associated with vascular compression of the central airways, i.e., vascular ring. Later, Gross and Neuhauser noted that this type of deformity of the airways persisted even after the vascular compression was alleviated.

External compression can also occur by axial skeleton as seen in severe scoliosis and pectus excavatum or by space occupying lesions such as goiter, tumors, and cysts.

This baby has congenital heart disease—PDA, pulmonary hypertension with cardiomegaly. The mechanism for the TBM in such children is not well-understood.

Compression of the bronchus (left) by a large heart seems to be the main culprit.

The effects of the TBM can be worsened by increased airway resistance caused by heart failure as well.

The picture below shows narrowing of left main bronchus, which is commonly involved with dilated pulmonary arteries, e.g., pulmonary arterial hypertension, absent pulmonary valve syndrome, and truncus arteriosus.

Treatment

- Tracheomalacia is often self-limited and will resolve or become asymptomatic by the second year of life without intervention
- For patients who are symptomatic of central airways collapse, available treatments include pharmacotherapy, positive pressure application, and surgery
- Pharmacotherapy is directed at increasing the tone of the trachealis muscle, as its contraction has been shown to decrease tracheal compliance. Type 2 and 3 muscarinic receptors play important roles in governing airway smooth muscle tone. Muscarinic agonists—bethanechol, and methacholine directly stimulate airway smooth muscle and improve airway mechanics in children with tracheomalacia
- Patients with tracheomalacia can also be treated with continuous positive airway pressure (CPAP) which provides distending intraluminal pressure which stents open the airway during expiratory maneuvers
- Continuous positive airway pressure can be provided via noninvasive ventilation and via invasive ventilation with either endotracheal intubation or tracheostomy placement. Invasive ventilation can have the added benefit of supporting the malacic tracheal segment with the artificial airway
- Surgical intervention is occasionally necessary to alleviate symptoms and sequelae of tracheomalacia. Aortopexy is a surgical procedure in which the aortic arch is fixated to the sternum. It results in the tracheal lumen being pulled open. It is used to treat severe tracheomalacia or tracheal compression. It is the mainstay of surgical interventions in pediatric intrathoracic tracheomalacia and can provide symptomatic relief
- While patients demonstrate clinical improvement, the collapsible segment of the airway remains. More recently, tracheomalacia associated with TOF has been treated using slide tracheoplasty. This technique removes the affected portion of the airway and can be an attractive method for treatment of short segments of severe tracheomalacia
- In adult patients, silicone stents have been used to stabilize the airway with improvement in respiratory symptoms; however, airway stents are infrequently used in pediatric patients due to the tendency for stents to migrate. While surgical interventions can improve symptomatic tracheomalacia, these methods should be reserved for the most severe cases.

LEARNING POINTS

- ☞ Laryngomalacia is the most common cause of inspiratory stridor in infants
- ☞ Definitive diagnosis can be made by flexible laryngoscopy without sedation
- ☞ Most children can be managed conservatively with close monitoring
- ☞ Additional diagnostic evaluations should be considered in severe form of laryngomalacia
- ☞ Surgical intervention—supraglottoplasty is now considered the mainstay of treatment for severe form of laryngomalacia
- ☞ Tracheomalacia results in excessive dynamic collapse of the central airway that results in clinical symptoms
- ☞ Extrathoracic tracheomalacia causes retractions with inspiratory stridor

- Intrathoracic tracheomalacia causes retractions with expiratory wheeze and impaired airway secretion clearance
- Acquired tracheomalacia occurs in the normally developed trachea due to trauma, external compression, or airway inflammation
- Although tracheomalacia can be suspected by history, physical examination, and supportive radiographic findings, flexible fiberoptic bronchoscopy remains the "gold standard" for diagnosis
- Current treatment strategies involve pharmacotherapy with cholinergic agents, positive pressure ventilation, and surgical repair.

SUGGESTED READINGS

1. Garetz SL, Thorne MC. Laryngomalacia: review and summary of current clinical practice in 2015. Paediatr Respir Rev. 2016;17:3-8.
2. Olney DR, Greinwald JH Jr, Smith RJ, Bauman NM. Laryngomalacia and its treatment. Laryngoscope. 1999; 109(11):1770-5.

CHAPTER

11

Congenital Thoracic Malformations

Prawin Kumar

> **CASE 1**
>
> A 22-year-old primigravid woman underwent level II screening ultrasonography at 21 weeks of gestation and a cystic lesion in fetal lungs was detected.

Q. What could be this cystic lung lesion? What are the differential diagnoses for such type of lung lesions?

Antenatally detected lung lesions can be cystic or solid. In cystic lesion, congenital thoracic malformation (CTM) is the most common lesion.

It is a spectrum of lung disorder resulting from abnormal embryological developmental of lung or its adnexal tissue. It includes:

- Congenital cystic adenomatoid malformation (CCAM)
- Pulmonary sequestration
- Congenital large hyperlucent lung (CLHL)
- Bronchogenic, reduplication, and foregut cyst.

The exact incidence of CTM from developing countries is lacking, from western countries incidence of 4.44/10,000 live birth has been reported.

Q. What are the presentations of CTM?

Congenital thoracic malformation can be detected antenatally in neonatal period or may have late presentation in childhood or even in adults (Table 1). It may be symptomatic or detected incidentally on imaging for another reason.

In this index case also it has been incidentally diagnosed on routine ultrasonography (USG)

TABLE 1: Presentations of congenital thoracic malformation according to age

Antenatal period	Neonatal period	Late presentations (child or adult)
• Intrathoracic mass • Pleural effusion • Fetal hydrops • Oligohydramnios or polyhydramnios • Other associated abnormalities	• Respiratory distress • Stridor (due to airway compression) • Cyanosis in a well-baby • Poor respiratory efforts • Cardiac failure • Incidental findings	• Recurrent infections • Hemoptysis, hemothorax • Bronchiectasis, bronchopleural fistula • Steroid-resistant airway obstruction • Cardiac failure • Cyanosis • Coughing on drinking • Incidental finding of mass or hyperlucent area on X-ray • Malignant transformation

Q. How can we confirm the diagnosis of CTM in antenatal period?

Congenital thoracic malformation can be diagnosed antenatally by:

- Ultrasonography: It is the most common modality and typically used in mid gestation. The lesions may be solid or cystic, later is of two types:
  1. Microcystic (<5 mm): Bright and echogenic without acoustic shadow
  2. Macrocystic (>5 mm): Multiple cysts of variable size.

Limitations

Low specificity, similar appearance of some other lung disease or nonpulmonary lesion so, cannot give definitive diagnosis

- Magnetic resonance imaging: Better description of lesion but not necessary in all cases and also cumbersome
- Definitive diagnosis is only by histopathological examination, but it is usually not needed.

Q. What are the complications which can occur during pregnancy and what are the risk factors for it?

The major complications during antenatal period are pleural effusions, polyhydramnios, hydrops, and pulmonary hypoplasia. Hydrops is a life-threatening condition and mortality is >90% if remains untreated.

Although polyhydramnios and mediastinal shift are considered as ominous signs, but it is the CCAM volume ratio (CVR), which strongly predicts the development of hydrops [CVR = lesion volume (length × width × depth) × 0.52 /head circumference]. CVR value ≥1.6 reliably predicts as high risk for the development of hydrops.

Q. What should be the mode of delivery?

The mode of delivery depends upon underlying condition of fetus, presence of complications, the need for intervention, and treating obstetrician. Vaginal delivery is not a contraindication but need close monitoring as about 10% of the CTM can present just after birth and may require resuscitation or even ventilator support.

> **Case Progression**
>
> In our index case we can inform the parents that serial monitoring with ultrasonography should be done to detect the progress and development of any adverse features that may warrant intervention. Vaginal delivery is as such not contraindicated, but there is need for close monitoring.

Q. If a complication develops, then what are the options available in the perinatal period?

There are two types of interventions—(i) invasive and (ii) noninvasive:

- Medical (noninvasive) therapy:
  - Maternal antenatal steroid: Betamethasone 12 mg intramuscular (IM) two doses 24 hourly
  - Studies have shown reversal of hydrops and survival benefit in up to 50%
- Surgical (invasive) intervention: Thoracocentesis, thoracoamniotic shunt, needle aspiration, surgical resection, radiofrequency ablation, and USG-guided sclerotherapy (ethanolamine, polidocanol)
- Timing of interventions
  - Fetal period (antepartum): Survival rate is 50%
  - Ex utero intrapartum therapy (EXIT): Survival rate is 90%.

Q. What should be the approach in antenatal period?

Natural course of CCAM is well-known. It typically grows from 20 to 25 weeks and then reaches plateaus between 25 and 30 weeks. By third trimester spontaneously regression has been reported and it varies from 30 to 75%. Natural course of others CTM are not well-known.The following algorithm (Flowchart 1) provides an approach to the lesions detected in the antenatal period.

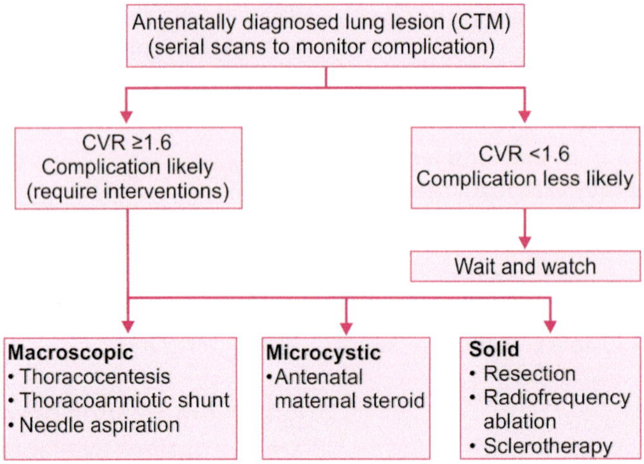

CTM, congenital thoracic malformation; CVR, congenital cystic adenomatoid malformation volume ratio.

Flowchart 1: Algorithm for management of antenatally diagnosed congenital thoracic malformation

Q. What is the natural course and complications of CTM in postnatal period?

Congenital thoracic malformation may remain asymptomatic in 90% of the newborns. Spontaneous regression has been documented in 15–50% of the cases. It can present at any time after birth, even in adult.

The major short-term complications are recurrent infections, hemoptysis, and pneumothorax.

The long-term complications are rare but serious. These include poor lung growth and function, and malignant transformation (pleuropulmonary blastema and bronchioalveolar carcinoma).

Q. How will we approach CTM in postnatal period ? Is there any role of prophylactic surgery ?

The approach is still debatable and will depend on several factors like presence and frequency of symptoms, the expertise of surgeons, and parents' decision.

The justification for prophylactic surgery are:

- Prevention of pulmonary infection
- Prevention of malignancy
- Possibility of better compensatory growth in remaining lung.

The management approach to CTM in postnatal period is described in flowchart 2.

CASE 2

A 7-year-old boy presented with recurrent fever, cough, and fast breathing since 1 month of age, requiring multiple hospitalizations. His serial radiographs since birth were reviewed which showed almost similar findings (Fig.1).

Q. What could be the possible diagnosis in this case?

This child is symptomatic since early infancy and serial radiographs showed repeated consolidation and cystic lesions in same area. So, we should think about congenital lung malformation and CCAM which could one of the possibility in such type of presentation.

Q. What is CCAM and what are the types of it?

Congenital cystic adenomatoid malformation is the most common CTM and mostly (>90%) detected in antenatal period during screening USG. It is usually unilateral and involves the basal lobe on either sides. Stocker initially

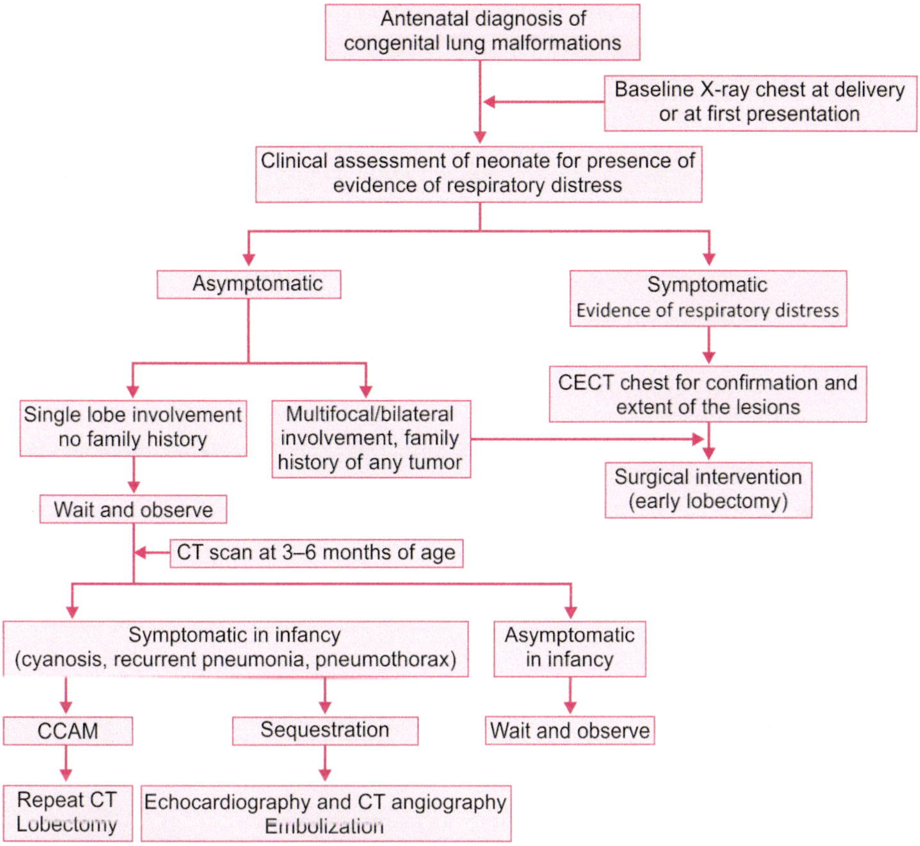

CT, computed tomography; CCAM, congenital cystic adenomatoid malformation; CECT, contrast-enhanced CT

Flowchart 2: Algorithm for management of antenatally diagnosed congenital lung malformations after birth

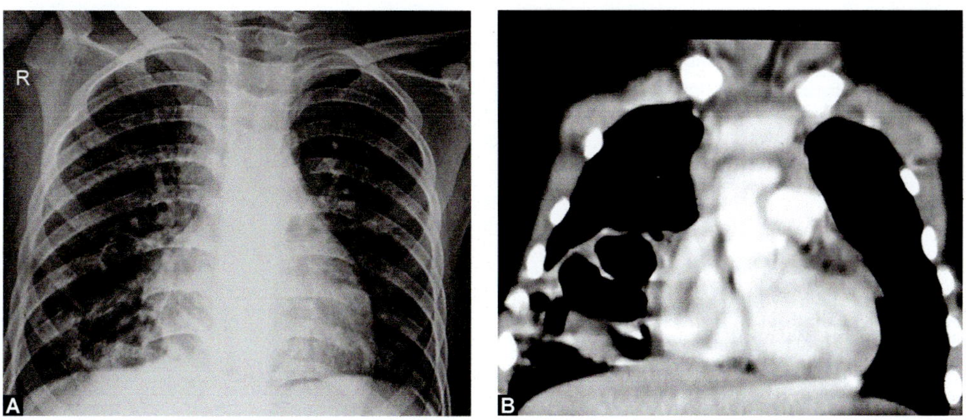

Figure 1: **A,** Chest X-ray: cystic lesion in right middle and lower lobe; **B,** Computed tomography chest: cystic lesions with consolidation in corresponding lobes

TABLE 2: **Classification of congenital cystic adenomatoid malformation**

Type	Incidence	Macroscopic	Microscopic	Remarks
0	Rare (1–3%)	—	• Bronchial-type airway (lined by pseudostratified tall columnar cell and presence of cartilage, muscle, and mucus glands)	• Also known as acinar dysplasia (lethal) • Associated with other anomalies
1	Most common type (>65%)	• Larger (>2 cm) • Usually multiloculated	• Lined by pseudostratified ciliated columnar epithelium • Hyperplasia of mucus cells may be seen	• Usually localized • Best prognosis
2	Second most common (20–25%)	• Consist of multiple small cysts • Give "sponge-like" appearance	• Lined by ciliated cuboidal or columnar epithelium with no cartilage and mucus cells	• Associated with other anomalies (renal, CVS, CNS, diaphragm)
3	Uncommon (8%)	• Appear as solid lesions	• Lined by ciliated cuboidal • Appear like late fetal lung	• Mostly occurs in boys
4	Very rare (2–4%)	• Thin-walled cystic lesions	• Lined by flattened alveolar cells	• Spectrum of lesions from CCAM to type 1 PPB

PPB, pleuropulmonary blastema; CCAM, congenital cystic adenomatoid malformation; CVS, cardiovascular system; CNS, central nervous system.

classified CCAM in three types (macrocystic, microcystic, and mixed lesion) but in 2002, he reclassified it in five types depending on the level of insult during the embryological development (Table 2).

CASE 3

A 5-year-old girl child presented with history of recurrent episodes of fever, cough, and hemoptysis for the last 2 years. Serial chest X-ray showed persistent opacity in right lower lobe (Fig. 2). Computed tomography (CT) scan was suggestive of sequestration. She underwent right lower lobectomy and histopathological examination proved sequestration.

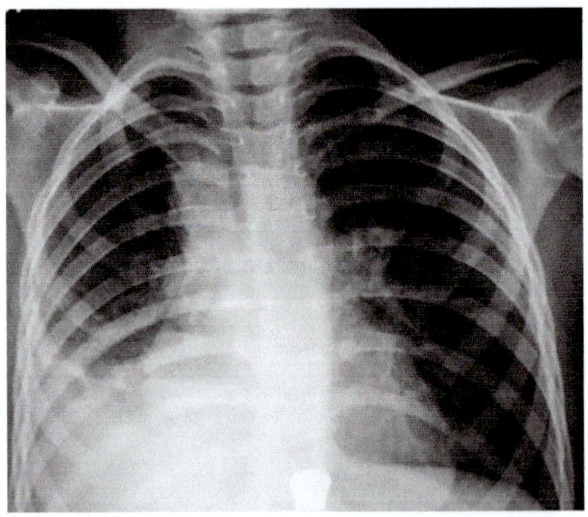

Figure 2: Opacity in right lower lobe with volume loss on same side

Q. What is sequestration and what are the types of it?

Sequestration is a solid CTM which contains solid lung tissue without bronchial communication, and arterial blood supply is from systemic arteries. It is more common in left side and in medial and basal areas. The common presentations are cough, recurrent pneumonia, and hemoptysis. Two types of sequestration are listed in table 3.

CASE 4

A 4-year-old child presented with history of fever, cough, and fast breathing for past 1 week. Chest X-ray showed a hyperlucency on left side (Fig. 3).

TABLE 3: **Types of sequestration**

Characteristics	Intralobar sequestration	Extralobar sequestration
Location	Embedded in normal parenchyma	Separate from normal lung
Pleura	Covered with visceral pleura in continuity with normal lung	It has its own separate pleural covering
Sex	Equal incidence	Common in boys
Age at presentation	At any age (infant to adult)	Usually present in neonatal period
Venous drain	Pulmonary vein	Systemic vein (azygous/portal)
Histology	Lung parenchyma replete with inflammatory tissue and fibrosis	Irregular bronchi and bronchiole with large alveoli
Associated anomalies	Rare	• Common—chest wall, vertebral, heart, renal, and cerebral anomalies • May communicate with gastrointestinal tract)

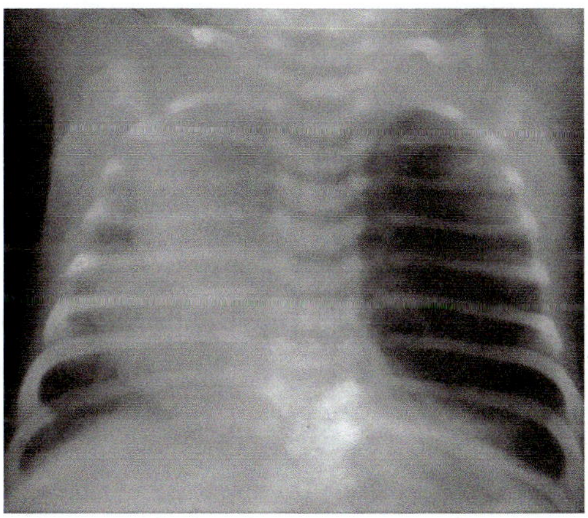

Figure 3: Hyperlucency of left upper lobe with collapse of lingual and lower lobe with mediastinal shift to right

Q. What could be the differential diagnoses for this case?

Unilateral hyperlucency with mediastinal shift may be seen in:

- Pneumothorax
- Pneumatoceles
- Intraluminal obstruction: Foreign body, mucus plug, benign tumor
- Pulmonary hypoplasia or atelectasis
- Swyer-James-MacLeod syndrome
- Congenital lobar emphysema (CLE)

Case Progression

In this case, CECT chest was performed and he was diagnosed as left upper lobe Congenital lobar emphysema.

Q. What is CLE and how it is different from pneumothorax?

Congenital lobar emphysema is now known as CLHL. It is characterized by hyperinflation of one of the lobe of lung but may affect more than one lobe, bilateral or only one broncho-pulmonary segment.

The common locations are:

- Left upper lobe (40–50%)
- Middle lobe (30–40%)
- Right upper lobe (20%).

It is very crucial to differentiate CLHL from pneumothorax (Table 4)

Q. What is the management of CLHL?

When symptomatic, it requires resection of affected lobe; never put a chest tube in CLHL.

TABLE 4: Differences between congenital large hyperlucent lung and pneumothorax

Characters	Pneumothorax	Congenital large hyperlucent lung
Sickness	Patients are usually sick	Relatively stable
In radiograph		
Pulmonary vessels	Not visible in peripheral part	Extend up to the periphery of hyperinflated lung
Pleural line	Separating from lung border is visible	Not visible
Mediastinal shift	Due to pressure from outside the lung	Due to hyperinflation of involved lobe

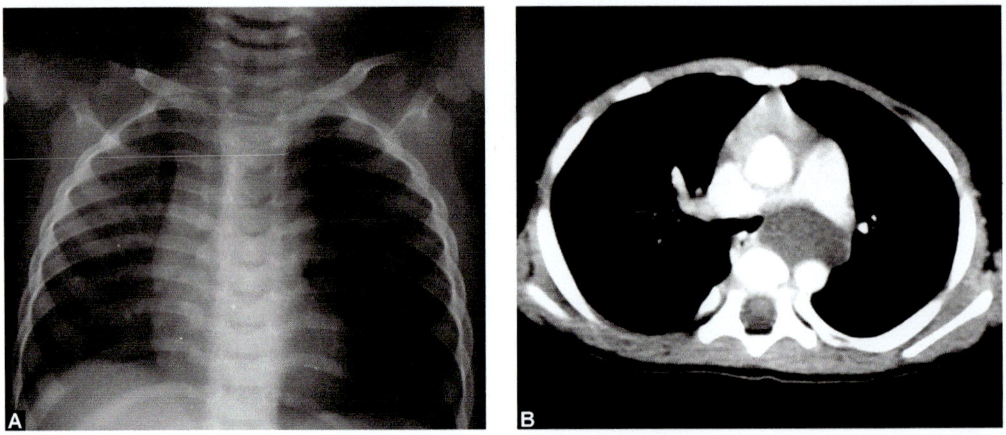

Figure 4: **A,** Chest X-ray showing left pratracheal shadow with tracheal deviation to right side; **B,** contrast enhanced computed tomography revealed bronchogenic cyst causing compression of airway and esophagus

CASE 5

A 3.5-year-old male presented with complaints of recurrent episodes of cough, fast and noisy breathing since 1 year of age, requiring repeated emergency visits. His X-ray and CT chest images are given in figure 4.

Q. What is bronchogenic cyst and what are the presentations?

It is a foregut duplication cyst, located in close relation to carina, esophagus and along the tracheobronchial tree. The presentation is mainly due to compression of surrounding structure (airways/esophagus) or its complication (recurrent infection/hemorrhage).

Q. What is the treatment for bronchogenic cyst?

Treatment options for bronchogenic cysts are:

- Evacuation (percutaneous/transbronchial needle aspiration): This is recommended in the presence of tension cyst which can expand rapidly and even lead to death due to cardiorespiratory compromise
- Complete or partial resection (thoracoscopic or open surgery): It can be lobectomy, segmentectomy, or only removal of the cyst.

LEARNING POINTS

- Antenatal detection of congenital lung lesions need serial evaluation as it often disappears spontaneously but sometime may lead to fatal complication
- After birth early baseline investigation with computed tomography scan even in asymptomatic case is must as X-ray chest may be deceptive

- ☞ If a child presents with persistent or recurrent lung finding in the same lobe, should think about congenital thoracic malformation (CTM)
- ☞ Once diagnosed, the approach should be systemic as it often associated with anomalies of other organs
- ☞ In absence of clear guideline, the approach to management should be based on individual case and expertize and also consider parents views
- ☞ Natural course of the CTM is still not well-known so long-term follow-up should be done.

SUGGESTED READINGS

1. Abel RM, Bush A, Chitty LS, Harcourt J, Nicholson AG. Congenital lung disease. In: Wilmott RW, Chernick V, Boat TF, Wilmott RW, Bush A, Deterding RR, Ratjen F (Eds). Kendig and Chernick's Disorders of the Respiratory Tract in Children, 8th edition. Saunders Elsevier; 2012. pp. 317-57.
2. Chikkannaiah P, Kangle R, Hawal M. Congenital cystic adenomatoid malformation of lung: report of two cases with review of literature. Lung India. 2013:30:215-8.
3. Davenport M, Eber E. Long-term respiratory outcome of congenital thoracic malformations. Semin Fetal Neonatal Med. 2012;17;99-104.
4. Khalke N, Johnson MP. Management of perinataly diagnosed lung lesions. Semin Pediatr Surg. 2013;22:24-9.
5. Ng C, Stanwell J, Burge DM, Stanton MP. Conservative management of antenatally diagnosed cystic lung malformations. Arch Dis Child. 2014;99:432-7.
6. Stanton M, Njere I, Ade-Ajayi N, Patel S, Davenport M. Systematic review and meta-analysis of the postnatal management of congenital cystic lung lesions. J Pediatr Surg. 2009:44;1027-33.
7. Stocker JT. Congenital pulmonary airway malformation: A new name and an expanded classification of congenital cystic adenomatoid malformation of the lung. Histopathol. 2002;41:424-31.

CHAPTER

12

Congenital Diaphragmatic Hernia

Swati Dublish, Vivek Manchanda, Pooja Abbey

CASE 1

A 30-week primigravida was diagnosed to have a space occupying lesion in chest of the fetus during a scan for fetal development. She has presented to you with her report for your opinion.

Q. What are the differential diagnoses for the fetus?

The differential diagnoses for a space occupying lesion in chest are congenital diaphragmatic hernia (CDH), congenital cystic adenomatoid malformation (CCAM), and bronchopulmonary sequestration (BPS).

Q. How to differentiate the three lesions from each other on the basis of imaging?

These can be differentiated by ultrasound or fetal magnetic resonance imaging (MRI). In the developed world, up to 59% of fetus with CDH are identified on antenatal investigations. On ultrasound, CDH can be suspected by the absence of intra-abdominal stomach bubble and presence of polyhydroamnios, presence of intrathoracic stomach bubble, mediastinal shift, small fetal abdominal circumference, or rarely fetal hydrops. Fetal MRI can depict all the herniated organs including the herniated kidney in CDH obviating the need for extensive postnatal imaging (Fig. 1). The contours of the diaphragm can be clearly traced in sagittal and coronal sections.

Congenital cystic adenomatoid malformation is rare and is characteri zed by a multicystic mass of pulmonary tissue with abnormal proliferation of bronchiolar structures that connect to the normal bronchial tree. The vascular supply of CCAM is from the pulmonary artery with drainage into the pulmonary veins.

Bronchopulmonary sequestration results from an abnormal accessory tracheobronchial bud arising from the foregut. Sequestration may be extralobar and intralobar. It has its own vascular supply from the systemic circulation and if a vessel arises from the aorta, the lesion is presumed to be a sequestration.

Q. What are the antenatal prognostic markers for CDH?

There have been many studies describing following as the possible poor prognostic markers:

- Presence of chromosomal anomaly
- Syndromic associations like Beckwith-Wiedemann syndrome
- Presence of associated major cardiac anomalies like double outlet right ventricle
- Absence of a hernia sac
- Presence of liver in chest- intrathoracic liver has a mortality of approximately 55%
- Left ventricle to right ventricle ratio

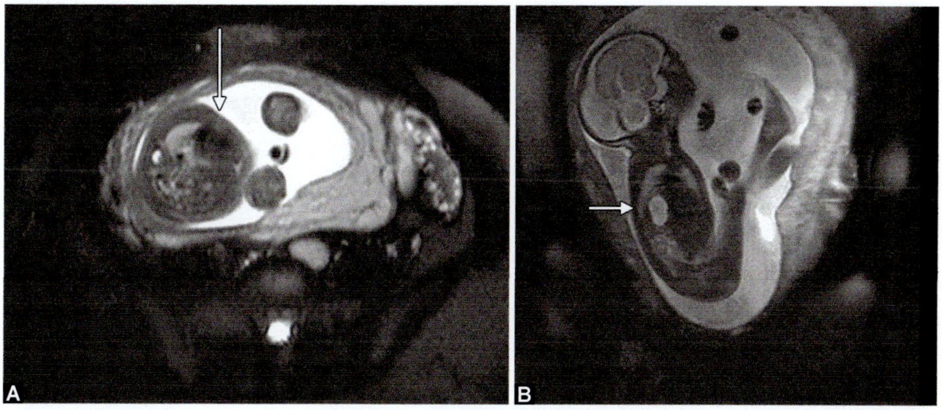

Figure 1: Prenatal magnetic resonance imaging images of a fetus with left congenital diaphragmatic hernia (CDH). Axial T2-weighted images through the fetal chest. **A,** Reveals displacement of the heart (long arrow) toward right by a left-sided CDH, which is better seen on the sagittal oblique image. **B,** the T2-bright stomach bubble (short arrow) is herniating into the fetal chest

- Modified McGoon index (pulmonary artery to aorta ratio) of <1.2
- Lung to head ratio <1
- Total lung volume <18 mL
- Percentage predicted lung volume <15%
- Left-sided hernia has a poorer prognosis compared to right
- A predictive score has been suggested called "CDH-congenital prognostic index (CDH-CPI)". It consists of four groups: (i) genetics, (ii) cardiac, (iii) hernia, and (iv) lung with ten parameters. A score of <8 carries poor prognosis.

Prenatal diagnosis is not possible in those diaphragmatic hernias where the defect is small and the herniation occurs just at delivery (Figs 2 and 3).

Q. What are the fetal interventions possible for CDH?

All fetal interventions are complicated with premature rupture of membranes and preterm delivery with its consequences. Still, with the hope to improve survival in fetus with severe pulmonary hypoplasia, intra-uterine surgery is done. Initially, the open repair of diaphragmatic hernia was used to correct the defect, but the results were not promising. With better understanding of the pathophysiology of the disease, the focus of fetal intervention has shifted from repair of diaphragm to inducing growth of lung and preventing mortality due to pulmonary hypoplasia. The various techniques described are open surgical tracheal occlusion; endoscopic external tracheal occlusion; and endoscopic endoluminal tracheal occlusion. The tracheal occlusion causes fluid accumulation in the lungs and thereby inducing lung growth and development. These procedures are done at 27–32 weeks of gestation. It is mandatory to remove the occlusive device by ex-utero intrapartum treatment (EXIT) procedure, so the mothers need to be in vicinity of the surgical center in case premature delivery occurs. Few small randomized controlled trials have shown benefit of fetal endoscopic tracheal occlusion procedure in fetus with severe pulmonary hypoplasia [with lung to head ratios (LHR) <25%].

CASE 2

An unbooked woman delivered in the emergency labor room and had no antenatal investigations. The newborn child had severe respiratory distress with cyanosis, tachypnea, tachycardia, and prominent hemithorax with minimal air entry, a displaced apex beat indicating mediastinal shift, and scaphoid abdomen—suggestive of diaphragmatic hernia, which is later confirmed on imaging (Fig. 4).

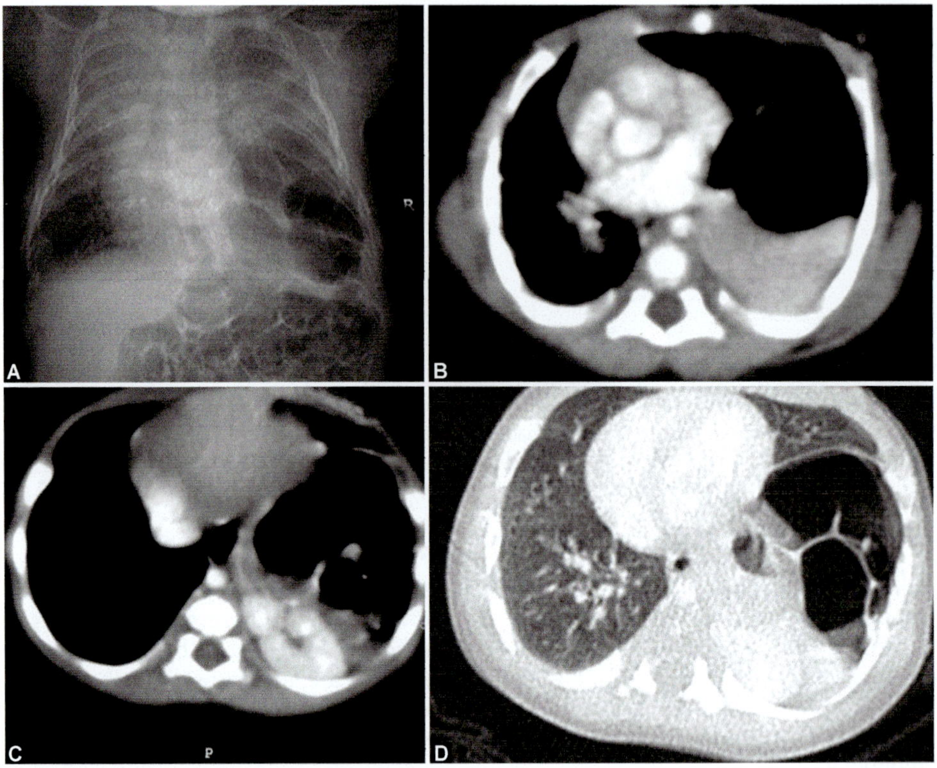

Figure 2: Contrast-enhanced computed tomography chest of a female child with respiratory distress and left-sided diaphragmatic hernia. **A,** Topogram shows loss of definition and apparent elevation of the left hemidiaphragm, with presence of bowel loops in the left lower hemithorax. There is mild mediastinal shift toward right side. **B** to **D**, Axial computed tomography sections reveals presence of the spleen, left kidney, and splenic flexure, respectively, in the left lower hemithorax

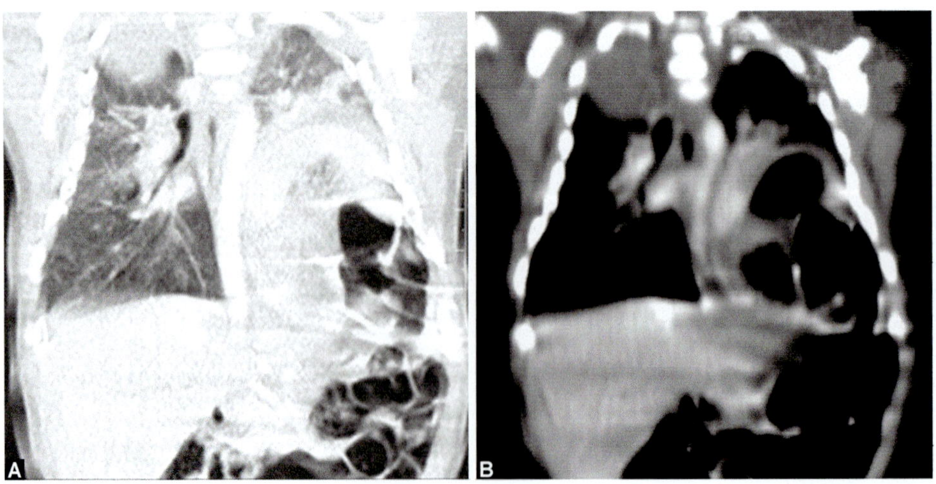

Figure 3: Coronal reformatted computed tomography images of the same patient (as Fig. 2). The intrathoracic herniation of the spleen and splenic flexure of colon are well-depicted. There is passive atelectasis of the underlying left lung

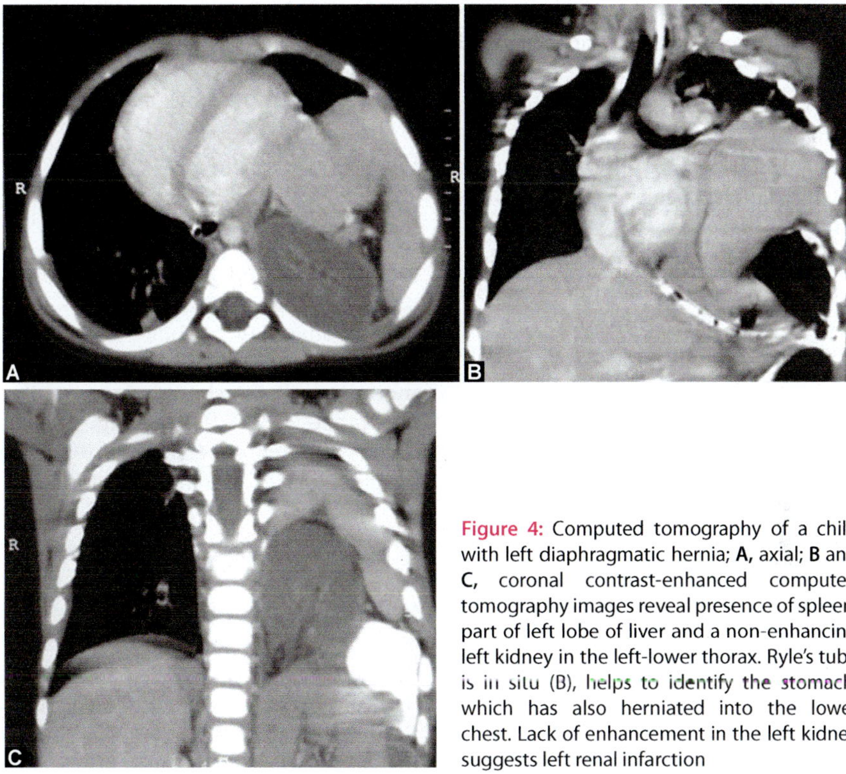

Figure 4: Computed tomography of a child with left diaphragmatic hernia; **A**, axial; **B** and **C**, coronal contrast-enhanced computed tomography images reveal presence of spleen, part of left lobe of liver and a non-enhancing left kidney in the left-lower thorax. Ryle's tube is in situ (B), helps to identify the stomach, which has also herniated into the lower chest. Lack of enhancement in the left kidney suggests left renal infarction

Q. What are the principles of early management?

Congenital diaphragmatic hernia is a medical emergency rather than surgical. The birth of the baby after antenatal diagnosis should prompt delivery of the baby in a center with expert neonatal ventilation and pediatric surgical facilities. The initial therapy after child birth is aimed at respiratory and hemodynamic stabilization of the baby.

After the baby is born, he needs to be assessed for pulmonary hypoplasia. If the baby is tachypneic or cyanotic, immediate intubation needs to be done. Bag and mask ventilation is to be avoided as the leaked air will distend the stomach in the chest and cause further pulmonary compromise.

Q. What are the postnatal surgical options for treatment of CDH?

The baby is taken up for surgery after hemodynamic stabilization and not before first 24–48 hours have been elapsed the time required for adapting from fetal circulation to newborn circulation. If the baby develops persistent pulmonary hypertension (PPHN), the management of PPHN takes precedence over surgical repair. Surgery can be delayed for 7–10 days.

Open and minimally invasive approaches can be utilized. The diaphragm may be approached either through abdomen or through thorax. The abdominal approach gives advantage of easy reduction of hernia contents, inspection of contents (in case of incarceration, obstruction, or strangulation) and performing simultaneous correction of associated malrotation. The abdominal approach is mandatory in case of complications. The thoracic approach has the advantage of better visualization (especially on right side), and ability to identify and preserve phrenic nerve. Minimally invasive techniques (laparoscopy and thoracoscopy) have been utilized through either approach with much improved visualization, pain, and cosmesis. Robotic surgery has been a new advance with promising future.

The surgery is aimed at repair of the defect in the diaphragm. Herniorrhaphy using simple interrupted or continuous sutures is done. If the defect is large, it may not be possible to approximate the edges of the defect. In such cases, the patch closure is done using prosthetic mesh [made from prolene, polytetrafluoroethylene (PTFE) or expanded polytetrafluoroethylene (ePTFE)] or local tissue flaps. The mesh closure allows tension-free repair but has a possibility of complication due to adhesions and infection.

Morgagni hernia should not be repaired through the laparoscopic route in neonates with respiratory distress due to the risk associated with CO_2 pneumoperitoneum.

CASE 3

A newborn diagnosed as left congenital diaphragmatic hernia was intubated right after birth and was on conventional ventilation for 48 hours of life. Her saturations did not improve despite being on high peak inspiratory pressure (PIP) and fraction of inspired oxygen. The arterial blood gas showed metabolic acidosis and preductal to postductal saturation difference of >10% on pulse oximetry.

Q. How will you manage this child?

If the baby does not maintain adequate oxygenation, further increments in the ventilator support may be required with the principle of "gentle ventilation" or "permissive hypercapnia" to prevent trauma to already compromised hypoplastic lungs.

High-frequency ventilation (preserves end expiratory volume and avoids alveolar overdistension) is preferred in order to keep the ventilatory pressures to minimum. Ventilation is done to avoid peak inspiratory pressure >25 mmHg and positive end-expiratory pressure >5 mmHg with aim to keep preductal oxygen saturation >90% and pH within physiological range while allowing $PaCO_2$ to go up to 60 mmHg.

The clinical features of high pulmonary vascular resistance include severity of oxygenation failure characterized by an oxygenation index of >15 despite optimization of lung recruitment, presence of lability of systemic oxygenation and a preductal to postductal saturation difference of >10% on pulse oximetry (SpO_2). Oxygen lability refers to decrements in oxygenation associated with agitation or handling and is suggestive of excessive pulmonary vasoreactivity.

Hemodynamic stability should be maintained with the judicious use of fluids and inotropes. PaO_2 should be maintained in the range of 60–100 mmHg. Inhaled nitric oxide therapy or extracorporeal membrane oxygenation (ECMO) may be utilized.

Q. What are the pulmonary complications in CDH?

Some degree of pulmonary hypoplasia along with changes in the surfactant system and decrease in the cross-sectional area of pulmonary vasculature occur in CDH. Pulmonary artery hypertension can occur due to muscularization of intra-acinar pulmonary arteries. Left ventricular hypoplasia can be seen in very severe cases. Pulmonary blood flow may be reduced due to small cross sectional area of vascular bed and pulmonary vasoconstriction.

Q. What are the causes of mortality in patients with CDH?

Congenital diaphragmatic hernia has an incidence of 1:2,200 to 1:4,000 with a survival of 50–80% and typically occurs in posterolateral hemidiaphragm. Associated anomalies including chromosomal and cardiac anomalies are a major cause of medical termination of pregnancy. Stillbirth may occur in a baby with CDH due to pulmonary insufficiency secondary to lung hypoplasia and inability to maintain adequate oxygenation. In the first few hours of life, a newborn will usually adapt to changes in pulmonary vasculature. But, in baby with CDH, there is pulmonary arterial hypertension and possibility of PPHN which may lead to hypoxemia and death of the baby. A baby on the ventilatory support is at risk for barotrauma and tension pneumothorax, thus worsening the respiratory compromise.

LEARNING POINTS

- Congenital diaphragmatic hernia is a common congenital abnormality which can be diagnosed on antenatal investigations, both maternal ultrasonography and fetal magnetic resonance imaging
- Various prognostic markers are available based on the antenatal investigations to help in determining the prognosis and offering appropriate counseling to the parents
- Focus is shifting from postnatal management to antenatal interventions to prevent complications like pulmonary hypoplasia, but this approach is associated with risks of premature rupture of membranes and preterm labor
- In postnatal management, hemodynamic stabilization of the baby and management of persistent pulmonary hypertension (if present) take precedence over surgical management.

SUGGESTED READINGS

1. Danzer E, Kim SS. Neurodevelopmental outcome in congenital diaphragmatic hernia: evaluation, predictors and outcome. World J Clin Pediatr. 2014;3:30-6.
2. Diemert A, Diehl W, Glosemeyer P, Deprest J, Hecher K. Intrauterine surgery—choices and limitations. Dtsch Arztebl Int. 2012;109:603-8.
3. Jain A, McNamara PJ. Persistent pulmonary hypertension of the newborn: advances in diagnosis and treatment. Semin Fetal Neonatal Med. 2015;20:262-71.
4. Jain V, Agarwala S, Bhatnagar V. Recent advances in the management of congenital diaphragmatic hernia. Indian J Pediatr. 2010;77:673-8.
5. Le LD, Keswani SG, Biesiada J, Lim FY, Kingma PS, Haberman BE, et al. The congenital diaphragmatic hernia composite prognostic index correlates with survival in left-sided congenital diaphragmatic hernia. J Pediatr Surg. 2012;47:57-62.
6. Merrell A, Kardon G. Development of the diaphragm, a skeletal muscle essential for mammalian respiration. FEBS J. 2013;280:4026-35.
7. Ozcan U, Altan E, Abbasoglu L. Space occupying lesions in the fetal chest evaluated by MRI. Iran J Radiol. 2012;9:122-9.
8. Zhang Q, Macartney J, Sampaio L, O'Brien K. High frequency jet ventilation during initial management, stabilization, and transport of newborn infants with congenital diaphragmatic hernia: a case series. Crit Care Res Pract. 2013;2013:937871.

3

SECTION

Wheezing Disorders in Children

CHAPTER

13

Wheezing in Preschool Children

Kana Ram Jat

CASE 1

A 15-month-old girl child presented with an intermittent history of cough and wheezing since 6 months of age. She had four episodes till the time of presentation and each episode was preceded by colds. There were no symptoms in between the episodes. The child had no history of atopy and allergic rhinitis. No member in family had any history of asthma or atopy. On examination, she was thriving well and general and systemic examinations were normal.

Q. How wheezing can be defined and how common it is in preschool children?

Wheeze can be defined as a musical, high-pitched and continuous sound that originates from the chest during expiration resulting from narrowing of intrathoracic airways and limitation of expiratory flow. Reliability of parental reporting is not always good as parents may interpret other respiratory sounds as wheeze. Wheezing in preschool children is not uncommon as almost one-fourth preschool children has at least episode of wheezing by 9 months of age and almost half by 6 years of age. Wheezing in preschool children often misdiagnosed as pneumonia with unnecessary use of antibiotics and wheezing is frequently undertreated.

Q. How to evaluate the case 1 who is having recurrent preschool wheezing?

All preschool children with wheezing should be evaluated by thorough history and examination (Box 1) followed by focused investigation as suggested by history and examination.

Box 1: Features to be evaluated in history and examination in preschool children with wheezing

History

- Is wheezing really present?
- Was child born preterm and required prolonged oxygen therapy?
- Did symptoms started at birth or later on?
- Was onset sudden or gradual?
- How is child growing and developing?
- Is there history of frequent, large volume, or oily stools?
- Is there history of feeding difficulties?
- Do symptoms change with position?
- Is there frequent rhinitis and ear discharge?
- Is there family history of cystic fibrosis, immuno-deficiency, or tuberculosis?
- How frequent are respiratory symptoms (wheezing)? (Does child remain well between episodes?)
- Are there symptoms related to other organ systems?

Continued

Continued

- What is severity of symptoms?
- What are triggers?
- Are symptoms more during night? (which part of night-just after sleep or early morning)
- Is there any response to β-2 agonist therapy?
- Does child have personal history of eczema?
- Is there any family history of asthma, allergic rhinitis, and atopy?

Physical examination

- Signs of respiratory distress, pulse oximetry (if available)
- Anthropometry: For failure to thrive
- Clubbing
- Look for any allergy markers
- Chest examination:
  - Any deformity
  - Wheezing
  - Crepts
- Cardiovascular system examination
- Look for organomegaly.

CASE 2

A 2-year-old boy had recurrent episodes of cough, wheezing, and respiratory difficulty since 3 months of age. Some episodes were preceded by colds and some triggered by cold foods and season change. Elder sibling was a 6-year-old boy and asthmatic. On examination, he was thriving well but have respiratory distress with bilateral expiratory wheeze.

Q. What are differential diagnoses of wheezing in preschool children?

A variety of conditions can cause wheezing in preschool children as shown in box 2. Wheezing due to congenital malformations is present since birth. Foreign body aspiration is most common between 1 year and 5 years of age.

Q. How wheezing in preschool children can be classified?

There is lack of consensus to classify wheezing in preschool children. The famous Tucson study reported three preschool wheezing phenotypes: transient early wheezing, persistent early-onset wheezing, and late-onset wheezing. But this

Box 2: Differential diagnosis for wheezing in preschool children

Wheezing secondary to underlying condition

- Infections:
  - Viral: Respiratory syncytial virus, rhinovirus, etc.
  - Atypical: Chlamydia, mycoplasma
  - Bacterial pneumonia
  - Tracheitis
  - Retropharyngeal abscess
  - Tuberculosis
- Suppurative lung diseases
  - Cystic fibrosis
  - Primary ciliary dyskinesias
  - Bronchiectasis
- Anatomic abnormalities
  - Central airway abnormalities
    - Laryngomalacia, tracheomalacia, and/or bronchomalacia
    - Tracheoesophageal fistula (specifically H-type fistula)
    - Large laryngeal cleft (resulting in aspiration), laryngeal web
  - Airway compression from outside
    - Vascular ring
    - Mediastinal lymphadenopathy
    - Esophageal foreign body, esophageal anomalies (e.g., enteric cyst)
  - Congenital malformations
    - Bronchial cyst or lung cyst
    - Congenital lobar emphysema
    - Aberrant tracheal bronchus
    - Sequestration
  - Intraluminal foreign body
  - Adenoidal hypertrophy
- Aspiration syndromes
  - Gastroesophageal reflux disease
  - Pharyngeal/swallow dysfunction
- Others
  - Immunodeficiency
  - Bronchopulmonary dysplasia
  - Interstitial lung disease, including bronchiolitis obliterans
  - Anaphylaxis
  - Inhalation injury-burns
  - Vocal cord palsy
  - Hypocalcemia
  - Congenital heart disease with left-to-right shunt

Wheezing without underlying condition

classification is of little clinical use as child needs to be followed up prospectively to label one of these phenotypes. The European Task-Force in 2008 suggested classifying wheezing in preschool children as episodic (viral) wheeze (EVW) and multitrigger wheeze (MTW). Episodic (viral) wheeze occurs as discrete episodes of 1–4 weeks duration and child is well between episodes and each episode is usually preceded by a viral respiratory infection. Multitrigger wheeze presents with discrete episodes of wheezing triggered by viral infections but child also has wheezing in between symptoms in response to various triggers like excessive laughing or crying, exercise, smoke, cold air. For clinical purpose, we can classify wheezing having a specific underlying disorder and wheezing without any underlying disorder. The second group may further classified as EVW and MTW.

Q. What investigations are needed in case 1 and case 2 above?

If a specific condition is suspected on detailed history and examination, investigate for that disorder (Table 1). If a specific condition is not suspected on history and examination, even chest X-ray is not required unless symptoms are abnormally severe, recovery is very slow or incomplete (resulting in prolonged or repeated hospital admission) and parents are very anxious. Eosinophil count, skin prick test, and total IgE are not of any use and are not recommended. Tests for gastroesophageal reflux may be considered for children especially to whom wheezing started <1 year of age. In other cases, investigations are needed only for frequent and severe wheezing which respond poorly to treatment and require multiple hospitalizations.

TABLE 1: Suggested investigations for a child with wheezing as per specific history and examination

History/examination	Suspected conditions	Suggested investigations
Child was born preterm and require prolonged oxygen requirement	Bronchopulmonary dysplasia	CXR and/or computed tomography of the chest
Symptoms started at birth or soon thereafter	Congenital anomalies	ENT evaluation, bronchoscopy
Child is failure to thrive	Cystic fibrosis (CF), immunodeficiency	Sweat test, Ig levels, HIV
There is frequent, bulky, or oily stools	Cystic fibrosis	Sweat test
Child has feeding difficulty	H-type fistula, GERD, laryngeal cleft	CXR, barium study, GER scan, ENT, bronchoscopy, pH study
Symptoms are changing with position	Airway malformation, adenoids, obstructive sleep apnea	ENT evaluation, bronchoscopy, X-ray soft tissue neck, sleep study
Continuous rhinitis and frequent ear discharge since early infancy	Primary ciliary dyskinesia	FeNO/nasal NO, electron microscopy
Family history of cystic fibrosis, immunodeficiency, or tuberculosis	Corresponding disease	For corresponding disease
Clubbing	Immunodeficiency, CF, HIV infection	Sweat test, Ig levels, HIV
Murmur, loud p2	Congenital heart disease	CXR, echocardiography

FB, foreign body; CXR, chest X-ray; HIV, human immunodeficiency virus; Ig, immunoglobulin, FeNO, fractional exhaled nitric oxide; ENT, ear, nose, throat; GERD, gastroesophageal reflux disease.

Case Progression

Both of the above cases had no features of underlying specific disease on detailed history and examination. Case 1 may be classified as episodic (viral) whee and case 2 may be classified as multitrigger wheeze.

Q. Mother of case 2 asked, "Does my child have asthma?" How to reply this query?

There is no consensus when to label asthma in preschool children. As per Global Initiative for Asthma 2015 guidelines, asthma in preschool children is considered if there are recurrent episodes of wheezing or coughing with exercise, laughing, or crying in absence of apparent respiratory infection. There is history of atopy or asthma in family and symptoms improves within 2–3 months of controller medications and worsens after cessation. If a preschool child fulfills all above criteria, then we can label it as asthma. But it is only after use of controller medications and not at first instance. In Case 2, we can tell mother that child has features suggestive of asthma but it will be difficult to label asthma at this point of time and we will follow the child with treatment. We can use terms EVW and MTW initially and can label asthma in follow up.

Q. Mother's next question: Will my child develop asthma later in life?

It is difficult to say which preschool children with recurrent wheezing will have asthma at later age; we just can stratify risk to some extent. There are many asthma predictive indices out of which asthma predictive index (API) (Table 2) is most commonly used.

Asthma predictive index is defined as loose index if there is any wheezing episode during first 3 years of life along with one major or two minor criteria and as stringent index if there are frequent wheezing episodes during first 3 years of life along with one major or two minor criteria. With positive loose index there is 2–5 times more likely to have asthma at 6–13 years of age and risk increases to 4–9 times with stringent index. The API had good negative predictive value of 91.6% but poor positive predictive value of 47.5–51.5%.

TABLE 2: Asthma predictive index (API)

Major criteria	Minor criteria
• Parental asthma • Physician diagnosed personal eczema	• Physician diagnosed allergic rhinitis • Wheezing without cold • Eosinophilia ≥4%

Q. Can we prevent children with preschool wheeze from developing asthma later in life?

In Prevention of Early Asthma in Kids (PEAK) trial, the inhaled steroids were beneficial during treatment but had no effect on long-term outcome, once stopped. So, at present there is no drug to prevent development of asthma larer in life among preschool wheezing.

Q. How best preschool children with wheezing can be treated?

An approach to preschool children with recurrent wheezing is shown in flowchart 1. If a specific disorder is suspected based on detailed history and examination, investigate for it and treat if the condition is confirmed. If no specific underlying disorder is suspected in history and examination or no disorder is identified after appropriate investigation, we can classify the wheezing as EVW or MTW. The distinction between EVW and MTW may not be always easy in many preschool children and sometimes EVW may turn into MTW and vice versa. Therefore, frequency and severity of wheezing episodes should be criteria for treatment rather than wheezing phenotype. If wheezing episodes are severe enough to require multiple hospitalizations, episodes are occurring once or twice every month, there is frequent sleep disturbances and child is symptomatic in between episodes, it should be treated.

Best treatment is inhaled corticosteroids (ICS) in low to moderate doses (200–400 μg of budesonide or equivalent per day) via metered-dose inhaler with spacer and mask. A trial of 3 months with good compliance and proper inhalational technique should be given before determining the response. The individual

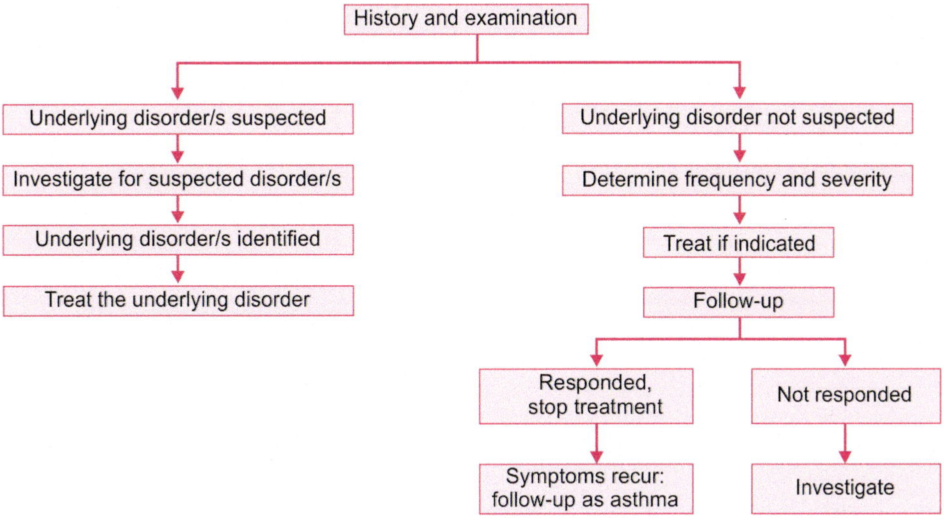

Flowchart 1: Approach to treat wheezing in preschool children

episodes of wheezing should be treated with inhaled or nebulized short-acting β agonists with oral steroids in very severe episodes. If child responds to ICS, we can stop treatment after 3 months. If symptoms recur, he or she may be labelled as asthma and should be treated and followed accordingly. If child does not respond with ICS, stop them and investigate further as appropriate. There is lack of evidence for or against the use of leukotrience receptor antagonists (montelukast) either daily or intermittent in preschool children with recurrent wheezing in both EVW and MTW phenotypes.

LEARNING POINTS

- By 6 years of age, almost one-half of children will have had at least one episode of wheezing
- Misdiagnosing and undertreating preschool wheezing may cause significant mortality/morbidity
- Once specific causes of preschool wheeze have been ruled out, they should be assessed for frequency and severity
- The majority of children (60%) with wheezing before age of 3 years will have resolution of wheezing by age of 6 years
- High risk of persistent asthma: History of parental asthma, personal history of atopy and allergen sensitization, wheezing outside of illness, and elevated blood eosinophils
- Inhaled steroids are mainstay for treatment of wheezing in preschool children, but are not useful in altering natural course.

SUGGESTED READINGS

1. Brand PL, Baraldi E, Bisgaard H, Boner AL, Castro-Rodriguez JA, Custovic A, et al. Definition, assessment and treatment of wheezing disorders in preschool children: an evidence-based approach. Eur Respir J. 2008;32(4):1096-110.
2. Bush A, Grigg J, Saglani S. Managing wheeze in preschool children. BMJ. 2014;348:g15.
3. Castro-Rodriguez JA, Holberg CJ, Wright AL, Martinez FD. A clinical index to define risk of asthma in young children with recurrent wheezing. Am J Respir Crit Care Med. 2000;162(4 Pt 1):1403-6.
4. Castro-Rodriguez JA, Rodrigo GJ. Efficacy of inhaled corticosteroids in infants and preschoolers with recurrent wheezing and asthma: a systematic review with meta-analysis. Pediatrics. 2009;123(3):e519-25.
5. Global Initiative for Asthma. (2015). Gina report, global strategy for asthma management and prevention 2015. [online] Available from http://www.ginasthma.org/local/uploads/files/GINA_Report_2015_May19.pdf. [Accessed Feb, 2016].

CHAPTER

14

Bronchiolitis

Nishant Verma

CASE 1

History: A 6-month-old male child was brought to the emergency room with complaints of low grade fever, cough, and rhinorrhea for the last 3 days, and difficulty in breathing and poor feeding for the last 1 day.

Past medical history: The child was born at 30 weeks of gestation, had a birth weight of 1,100 g, and required a neonatal intensive care unit stay of 3 weeks for prematurity.

Family history: There was no history of asthma or atopy in the family members.

Physical examination: The child was alert, had a respiratory rate of 88/minute with significant retractions and nasal flaring. His SpO_2 on room air was 88%. Chest auscultation revealed wheezing over both the lung fields. Cardiac auscultation is normal.

Q. What are the differential diagnoses of this case?

The differential diagnoses include bronchiolitis, asthma, pneumonia, and chronic lung disease. Table 1 summarizes the points for and points against for these differential diagnoses in this child.

Q. What are the etiological agents responsible for bronchiolitis?

Respiratory syncytial virus (RSV) is the most common causative organism for bronchiolitis, accounting for about 50–60% cases. Other viruses which have been implicated as causative organisms include—rhinovirus, parainfluenza viruses, influenza virus, adenovirus, coronavirus, human metapneumovirus, and human bocavirus.

Q. How should this child with bronchiolitis be investigated?

Chest radiograph is abnormal in a majority of children with bronchiolitis, and it may reveal diffuse hyperinflation of the lungs, flattening of the diaphragm, patchy or peribronchial infiltrates, patchy atelectasis, and rarely consolidation. However, none of the above mentioned findings is diagnostic of bronchiolitis. Radiography should be, therefore, reserved only for children who have a severe disease requiring intensive care unit (ICU) admission or when some diagnosis or airway complication like pneumothorax is suspected. There is limited role of obtaining total and differential white blood cell counts as they do not predict serious bacterial infection in infants with bronchiolitis. Virological testing to identify the causative virus also does not have any role in the treatment as no antiviral agent is approved for treatment of bronchiolitis. Thus, none of the laboratory or radiological investigations is diagnostic of bronchiolitis and over-reliance on these investigations adds to unnecessary cost, radiation exposure, and discomfort to the

TABLE 1: Differential diagnosis of the case

Differential diagnosis	Points in favor of the diagnosis	Points against the diagnosis
Bronchiolitis	• Young age (peak incidence of bronchiolitis is between 2 months and 6 months of age) • Presence of prodromal symptoms • Alert child • Presence of wheezing (chest auscultation in bronchiolitis may reveal prolonged expiratory phase, and wheeze and crackles throughout the lungs)	None
Asthma	• Presence of wheezing	• Very young age of onset • No family history of asthma
Pneumonia	• Presence of respiratory distress	• Alert child • No high-grade fever • No evidence of bronchial breath sounds on auscultation.
Chronic lung disease	• History of preterm delivery • Presence of bilateral lung signs on auscultation	• Very short history (a child with chronic lung disease will be symptomatic even between the episodes of exacerbation) • Absence of clubbing

child without having any effect on the treatment decisions.

It is important to remember that the diagnosis of bronchiolitis is predominantly clinical. A detailed history should be taken to analyze the child's symptoms and the impact of these symptoms on his feeding (as respiratory distress prevents adequate oral fluid intake and causes dehydration). A meticulous clinical examination should be performed to assess the child's responsiveness, hydration status, and degree of respiratory distress. An effort should also be made to identify various risk factors and comorbidities which may put the infant at a higher risk for severe disease [the risk factors include younger age (<6 months), prematurity, underlying chronic lung disease, congenital heart disease, or immunocompromised state].

Q. What is the typical clinical course of bronchiolitis?

In most of the children, the disease is self-limiting and of mild severity, not requiring hospitalization. Recovery starts after 3–5 days, but low-grade symptoms may persist till 4 weeks. However, a small proportion of infants, especially those with risk factors (congenital heart disease, chronic lung disease, immunocompromised, neuromuscular disease, etc.) may develop a severe disease and require hospitalization.

Q. What is the role of pulse oximetry in management of infants with bronchiolitis?

Pulse oximetry is a convenient method to measure the percentage of hemoglobin bound by oxygen (SpO_2) which can be easily performed even in the emergency room or outpatient department. However, continuous pulse oximetry is not recommended in these children as it adds to the discomfort of the child, leads to false alarms, and prolongs the length of stay in the hospital. Supplemental oxygen is indicated in infants with bronchiolitis only if their SpO_2 is <90% at room air. As the infant improves, and is able to maintain SpO_2 >90% on room air, the supplemental oxygen can be stopped.

Q. What is the role of bronchodilators in the management?

In majority of cases, bronchiolitis is a mild self-limited illness which does not require any treatment. Even in children with moderate to severe bronchiolitis, no other intervention apart from supportive care, has shown to improve the clinical outcome. Thus, a conservative, "minimal handling" approach is beneficial. Bronchodilators which have been studied in bronchiolitis include inhaled and oral salbutamol, inhaled epinephrine, and inhaled ipratropium bromide. Studies have shown that use of these drugs may improve clinical symptom scores, but they do not affect disease resolution, need for hospitalization or the length of stay. So, the evidence does not support the routine use of any of these agents either in the emergency department setting, or the inpatient setting. However, in exceptional cases, where an infant with bronchiolitis is deteriorating rapidly, a trial of inhaled bronchodilators (epinephrine or salbutamol) may be undertaken to provide some transient benefit.

Q. Does this infant with bronchiolitis require hospital admission?

A majority of children with bronchiolitis can be managed with supportive care at home; however, some children require inpatient care and monitoring. The indications for hospital admission in a child with bronchiolitis include the following:

- The child has a toxic appearance with refusal to feed, lethargy and features of dehydration
- Children with significant respiratory distress, as evident by presence of any of these features: Nasal flaring, grunting, intercostal, subcostal, and suprasternal retractions, respiratory rate >70 per minute, or apneic episodes
- Evidence of hypoxia: Presence of cyanosis or SpO_2 <90% at room air
- Lack of a trained care-provider at home.

As the infant described in the case above has features of significant respiratory distress as well as evidence of hypoxia, he requires hospital admission for supportive care and monitoring.

Q. What supportive care should be provided to this infant?

Supportive care is the corner stone in management of children with bronchiolitis. It includes the following components:

- Parental education: As majority of cases of bronchiolitis are mild and can be managed at home, educating the parents or caregivers is very important. They should be educated about adequate feeding and early identification of signs of deterioration (such as increasing difficulty with breathing, chest-indrawing, or problems with feeding)
- Fluid administration: Infants with bronchiolitis are at risk of dehydration because of their increased needs (related to fever and tachypnea) and reduced oral acceptance. There hydration status should be carefully assessed and if found inadequate, nasogastric or intravenous fluids should be supplemented
- Nasal suctioning: If the nostrils are blocked, instillation of saline nose drops followed by gentle suction may help the infant
- Supplemental oxygen: Well-humidified oxygen should be supplemented if the infants' SpO_2 falls persistently <90%. The oxygen should be provided by the help of either nasal prongs or face mask or hood
- Mechanical ventilation: A small proportion of infants with severe bronchiolitis continue to deteriorate despite all the supportive care. These infants require admission to an ICU and may require intubation and mechanical ventilation.

Q. Are there any other therapeutic interventions which may be useful in managing infants with bronchiolitis?

A number of novel therapeutic interventions have been studied in bronchiolitis, but most of them have proven ineffective. Use of nebulized hypertonic saline (3% NaCl) in hospitalized children with bronchiolitis has been found to be associated with reduced length of stay. So, nebulized hypertonic saline can be tried in infants with bronchiolitis who require hospitalization. Its use in emergency department is not indicated. The interventions for which there is no supportive evidence and hence, are not indicated in the management of bronchiolitis include steroids (inhaled or oral), antibiotics, montelukast, inhaled furosemide, and chest physiotherapy. Box 1 provides a summary of the interventions used for management of bronchiolitis.

Q. What is the role of palivizumab for prevention of bronchiolitis in infants?

Palivizumab is a monoclonal antibody active against RSV. It is indicated for children who will be younger than 12 months at the start of RSV season (September to March in India) and have any one of the following risk factors: (i) born at <29 weeks of gestation, (ii) suffering from hemodynamically significant heart disease, or (iii) suffering from chronic lung disease of prematurity (defined as preterm infants <32 weeks gestation who require >21% oxygen for at least the first 28 days of life). For the infants who qualify for the prophylaxis, a maximum 5 monthly doses (15 mg/kg/dose) is recommended during the RSV season. Apart from palivizumab, other measures to prevent severe bronchiolitis include exclusive breastfeeding for 6 months, promoting hand hygiene, and protection from environmental tobacco-smoke exposure.

Box 1: Summary of interventions used for management of bronchiolitis

- Interventions which are proven to be effective
  - Supportive care (supplemental oxygen, intravenous fluids)
- Interventions which are possibly effective
  - Nebulized hypertonic saline (for hospitalized patients only)
  - Inhaled adrenaline
- Interventions which are ineffective and not recommended
  - Oral/inhaled salbutamol
  - Montelukast
  - Inhaled/systemic corticosteroids
  - Chest physiotherapy
  - Antibiotics
  - Inhaled furosemide

LEARNING POINTS

- Bronchiolitis is a viral, lower respiratory tract infection which affects children <2 years of age
- The diagnosis of bronchiolitis is based purely on history and physical examination
- Chest radiography is not routinely indicated for management of children with bronchiolitis
- Children with bronchiolitis who have significant respiratory distress, or evidence of hypoxia, or toxic appearance require hospitalization for supportive care and monitoring
- Supportive care is the cornerstone in management of bronchiolitis
- Pulse oximetry should be used to assess the need for supplemental oxygen in these children (oxygen should be administered if SpO_2 is persistently <90%)
- There is no evidence to support the use of antibiotics, steroids, or salbutamol for bronchiolitis
- Nebulized 3% NaCl and epinephrine may have some role in the management of bronchiolitis
- For prevention of Respiratory syncytial virus bronchiolitis, palivizumab should be administered during the first year of life to infants born at <29 weeks of gestation, or infants with hemodynamically significant heart disease, or chronic lung disease of prematurity.

SUGGESTED READINGS

1. Gadomski AM, Scribani MB. Bronchodilators for bronchiolitis. Cochrane Database Syst Rev. 2014;6:CD001266.
2. Ralston SL, Lieberthal AS, Meissner HC, Alverson BK, Baley JE, Gadomski AM, et al. Clinical practice guideline: the diagnosis, management, and prevention of bronchiolitis. Pediatrics. 2014;134:e1474–e1502.
3. Verma N, Lodha R, Kabra SK. Recent advances in management of bronchiolitis. Indian Pediatr. 2013;50(10):939-49.
4. Wohl MEB. Bronchiolitis. In: Chernick V, Boat TF, Wilmott RW, Bush A. (Eds). Kendig's Disorders of the Respiratory Tract in Children, 6th edition. Philadelphia: Saunders Elsevier publishers; 1998. pp. 423-32.
5. Zhang L, Mendoza-Sassi RA, Wainwright C, Klassen TP. Nebulized hypertonic saline solution for acute bronchiolitis in infants. Cochrane Database Syst Rev. 2013;7:CD006458.

CHAPTER

15

Bronchial Asthma

Narendra K Bagri

CASE 1

A 7-year-old boy was brought to the pediatric outpatient department with varying symptoms of cough and chest tightness for the last 1 year. These symptoms were more prominent at night with at least one nighttime awakening per week and often precipitated by exercise and change in weather requiring hospitalization and used to subside after nebulization. There was past history of atopic dermatitis during infancy and family history of allergic rhinitis in father.

Physical examination: The child was stable with respiratory rate of 20/min, saturation of 95% at room air, and chest examination was normal.

Q. Does this child has bronchial asthma?

Bronchial asthma is a chronic airway inflammation characterized by recurrent respiratory symptoms such as cough, wheeze, and breathlessness, along with variable expiratory airflow limitation. Historically, the child in discussion seems to suffer from bronchial asthma.

Q. What are the important clues in history and physica l examination?

History of respiratory symptoms beginning from early childhood along with atopic dermatitis and a family history of allergic rhinitis increases the probability of bronchial asthma. This pattern is consistent with the most common phenotype of asthma known as "allergic asthma", which shows eosinophilic airway inflammation and responds well to inhaled corticosteroids (ICS). The less common asthma phenotype includes "nonallergic asthma", which shows paucigranular pattern on sputum examination and shows a poor response to ICS.

The probability of having bronchial asthma is increased with following features: Multiple symptoms of airway obstruction (wheeze, shortness of breath, cough, and chest tightness) which shows:

- Diurnal variation: Often worse at night or in early morning
- Variability: Vary over time and in intensity
- Triggers: Viral infections, change in weather, exercise, allergen exposure, laughter, irritants (e.g., smoke or strong smells).

Physical examination

Clinical examination in patients with asthma is often normal between the episodes. Expiratory wheezing on auscultation is the most common finding, but this may not be present always or heard only on forced expiration or may be absent in severely reduced airflow as in severe exacerbations due to severely reduced airflow. Evaluation of upper airway may reveal signs of allergic rhinitis or nasal polyposis. The diagnosis of bronchial asthma predominantly rests on characteristic history and variable expiratory airflow limitation.

Q. The symptoms of this child are consistent with asthma, what is the most appropriate next step to confirm your diagnosis?

Asthma is a clinical diagnosis based on characteristic symptomatology as in our index case. However, the pulmonary function tests (PFTs) are used to document the expiratory airflow limitation and variability. Presence of any one the following will suggest asthma—(i) increase in forced expiratory volume in one second (FEV1) of >12%, 20 minutes after 200–400 µg salbutamol, (ii) excessive variability (>13%) in twice-daily peak expiratory flow (PEF) over 2 weeks, or (iii) fall in FEV1 >12% after exercise (5–10 minutes of vigorous running).

> *Note:* *PFTs are not mandatory for diagnosing asthma, and treatment of asthma may be started if the clinical suspicion is strong. Spirometry is difficult to perform <5years of age and it may be affected if child had exacerbation at the time of testing.*

Q. The clinical diagnosis of asthma in index case was also supported by spirometry, the FEV1/forced vital capacity (FVC) of the child in question is 0.78 and there is 13% increase in FEV1 after bronchodilator test. How do you plan the management of this child?

The goals of asthma management are:

- Achieving good symptom control and normal activity levels
- Minimizing future risk of exacerbations, fixed airflow limitation, and side-effects of medications
- Reducing the need for reliever

Three main categories of medications for long-term treatment are:

1. Controller medications: Used regularly to reduce airway inflammation and prevent future exacerbations and decline in PFT, e.g., ICS
2. Reliever (rescue) medications: Used for controlling breakthrough symptoms and for prevention of exercise-induced bronchoconstriction, e.g., short-acting β-agonists (SABA)
3. Add-on therapies: These may be considered for poorly controlled asthma despite optimized treatment with high-dose controller medications and addressing modifiable risk factors, e.g., anti IgE.

Q. On interrogation, it was found that the child is having asthma symptoms on most days of a week including at least one night awakening . What should be the treatment for this child?

The long-term management of asthma depends on the severity of symptoms. Based on the symptoms, it is classified into four levels and treated accordingly (Tables 1-3). Based on symptomatology, this 7-years-old male child should be started with step 3.

Apart from the drugs, the following "non-pharmacological interventions" should be advised for better asthma control:

- Avoid exposure to smoking
- Encourage physical activity
- Avoidance of medications causing broncho-spasm, e.g., β-blockers
- Avoidance of indoor allergens
- Weight reduction and healthy diet
- Breathing exercises
- Vaccinations: Pneumococcal and influenza.

Q. The child was initiated on medium-dose budesonide ICS along with need-based SABA. What are the drug-delivery options, what advice would you give to reduce side effects? When would you call this child in follow-up?

The available drug-delivery devices are depicted in table 3.

The local/systemic side effects of ICS can be minimized by:

- Ensuring correct inhaler technique and device: Always use pressurized metered dose inhaler (pMDI) with spacer

TABLE 1: Stepwise treatment plan for asthma

Step down if well-controlled for atleast 3 months

Assess control #

Step-up after checking technique, adherence, environmental control, and comorbid conditions

Presentation and classification	Preferred initial treatment
Intermittent Asthma symptoms or need for SABA <2/month • No nocturnal symptoms in last month • FEV1% predicted ≥80% • No risk factors for exacerbations*	**Step 1** • SABA as needed • No controller

Mild persistent
• >2/week day-time symptoms and ≥1/month nocturnal symptoms
• FEV1% predicted ≥80%
	Step 2
	• Low-dose ICS
	• Other options:
	  ○ LTRA or
	  ○ Low-dose theophylline
	• Step 2 also considered when:
	  ○ Infrequent symptoms but >1 risk factors for exacerbations*
	  ○ Need of OCS in last year
	  ○ History of admission in PICU for asthma

Moderate persistent • Daily day-time symptoms and ≥1/week nocturnal symptoms • FEV1% predicted ≥80%	**Step 3** • Medium-dose ICS • Low-dose ICS + LABA/LTRA • Other options: ○ Medium/high-dose ICS + LTRA/theophylline
Severe persistent • Daily day-time and nocturnal symptoms • FEV1 <60%	**Step 4** • Medium to high dose ICS + LABA/LTRA • Other options: ○ OCS
Severe persistent uncontrolled on step 4	**Step 5** • Consider anti IgE (omalizumab) • Sputum-guided treatment (adjust treatment based on sputum eosinophilia >3%) • OCS (<7.5 mg/day prednisone equivalent): be cautious of side-effects
Initial presentation with an acute exacerbation	Short course of oral corticosteroids and start controller treatment with: • High-dose ICS or • Moderate-dose ICS/LABA

*Potentially modifiable independent risk factors for exacerbations: Uncontrolled asthma symptoms, high SABA use (increased mortality if >200-dose canister/month), inadequate ICS, poor adherence, incorrect technique, FEV1 <60% predicted, major psychosocial problems, allergen exposures, comorbidities: Obesity, rhinosinusitis, confirmed food allergy, sputum or blood eosinophilia, ever intubated or in intensive care unit for asthma, >1 exacerbation in last year.

#Asthma control = Control of symptoms

In the past 4 weeks, has the patient had following due to asthma:

- Daytime symptoms more than twice/week?
- Any nocturnal symptom?
- Reliever needed for symptoms more than twice/week?
- Any activity limitation?

Based on the response to above questions the level of asthma control is defined as:

- Well-controlled: None of the above
- Partly-controlled: 1–2 of the above
- Uncontrolled: 3–4 of the above

ICS, inhaled corticosteroids; OCS, oral corticosteroids; PICU, pediatric intensive care unit; SABA, short-acting β-agonists; LABA, long-acting β2-agonist; FEV1, forced expiratory volume in one second; LTRA, leukotriene receptor antagonist.

Source: Modified from GINA guidelines 2015.

TABLE 2: **Doses of drugs used**

Drug	Low dose (µg/day)	Medium dose (µg/day)	High dose (µg/day)
ICS			
Fluticasone	100–250	>250–500	>500
Budesonide-DPI	200–400	400–800	>800
Budesonide inhalation solution	250	500	1,000
Beclomethasone	100–200	200–400	>400
Ciclesonide	80–160	>160–320	>320
LTRA: Montelukast (<4 years 4 mg HS, 5–14 years = 5 mg HS, >14 years = 10 mg HS)			
"Omalizumab" subcutaneous injection: 150–375 mg SC every 2–4 weeks based on serum IgE levels			
Theophylline: 10 mg/kg/day			

LTRA, leukotriene receptor antagonist; ICS, inhaled corticosteroids; HS, at bedtime; DPI, dry powder inhaler.

TABLE 3: **Inhalation device and aiding tools**

Inhalation device	Comments
Pressurized metered-dose inhaler (pMDI) with spacer	• Ideal for all age groups • Advantage of spacer: ○ Eliminates need of actuation and inhalation ○ Limits drug deposition in oropharynx and reduces local side-effects ○ Good drug delivery to peripheral airways ○ Can be used for younger children with face mask
Dry powder inhaler (DPI)	• For children >6 years • Needs generation of adequate inspiratory flow • More oropharyngeal drug deposition • Cannot be used in acute settings
Nebulizer	• Used in acute settings • Can be used for children unable to use pMDI with a spacing device

- Rinsing oral cavity after using ICS (in cooperative children)
- Using minimum-effective dose of ICS.

The follow-up should be planned, 1-3 months after starting treatment, every 3-4 months thereafter. Emergency home action plan should be given for managing acute exacerbation and advice regarding when to seek emergency care should be explained.

Q. Using the above tool for assessment of asthma-control, the child was found to have well-controlled asthma at 3 months follow-up. Can stepping down be considered at this stage? When can you consider stopping the ICS?

As the child's asthma is well-controlled after 3 months of ICS, stepping down of the treatment may be considered.

General guidelines for stepping down:

- For whom?
  - Well-controlled asthma and stable PFT >3 months
  - In presence of risk factors for exacerbations or fixed airflow limitation, stepping-down should be done under close supervision
- When?
  - When there is no respiratory infection and patient is not traveling

- How?
  - 25–50% dose reduction at 3-months-interval
  - Controller medications can be stopped after good symptom control for 6–12 months, and patient has no risk factors
- What precaution should be taken?
  - Provide written asthma action plan and schedule a follow-up visit

Q. Six months after initiating step 3 treatment the child developed a viral infection and came to you with increase in symptoms. What will be your approach for stepping-up treatment?

Stepping-up should be considered when asthma symptoms are not controlled despite ensuring the following in follow up visits:

- Good compliance and proper inhaler technique
- Addressing modifiable risk factors, e.g., exposure to smoking.
- Addressing comorbid conditions: Food allergy, rhinosinusitis, gastroesophageal reflux disease, obesity, vocal cord dysfunction, and psychological disorders (depression or anxiety).

How stepping-up can be done?

- Short-term step-up (for 1–2 weeks): This may be initiated by patient as per written asthma action plan or by treating physician during viral infections like in this case or seasonal allergen exposure
- Sustained step-up (for at least 2–3 months): If symptoms are uncontrolled despite ensuring good adherence, proper technique and addressing modifiable risk factors and comorbidities on present, step a therapeutic trial of step-up treatment should be given and the response reviewed after 2–3 months. If there is no response, treatment should be reduced to the previous level, and alternative diagnosis should also be looked for.

> **CASE 2**
>
> The same child was brought to the pediatric emergency at 2 AM with complains of worsening cough and respiratory distress for the last 2 days. He was out of station in a school camp for 10 days and was not taking his controller medications.
>
> Physical examination: The child was in respiratory distress with respiratory rate of 36/min, saturation of 89% at room air, and bilateral wheeze on chest auscultation.

Q. How will you assess the present condition of the child and manage him in emergency department?

The child has developed an acute exacerbation of asthma precipitated by poor adherence to controller medications. The episodes of exacerbations are characterized by an acute increase in symptoms along with decline in lung function. The severity of asthma exacerbation is classified into four stages (Table 4).

Accordingly the child in question has experienced an episode of severe exacerbation

TABLE 4: Severity of acute asthma

Sign/symptom	Mild exacerbation	Moderate exacerbation	Severe exacerbation	Respiratory failure
Alertness	Normal or agitated	Normal or agitated	Agitated	Confused
Respiratory rate*	Slightly increased	Increased	Increased	Undetermined
Accessory muscle use	None—mild	Apparent	Marked	Marked
Dyspnea	Absent or with exertion Speech normal	Moderate: Speaks in phrases, difficult feeding	Severe: Speaks words Refusal to feed	Severe Not able to speak and feed
Color	Normal	Pale	Possibly cyanotic	Cyanotic

Continued

Continued

Sign/symptom	Mild exacerbation	Moderate exacerbation	Severe exacerbation	Respiratory failure
SpO_2 (room air)	>95%	90–95%	<90%	<90%
wheeze	Mild	Apparent	Marked	Silent chest
PEF (% predicted or personal best)	>70%	40–69%	<40%	Unmeasurable
$PaCO_2$	<42 mmHg	<42 mmHg	42–60 mmHg	>60 mmHg

PEF, peak expiratory flow.

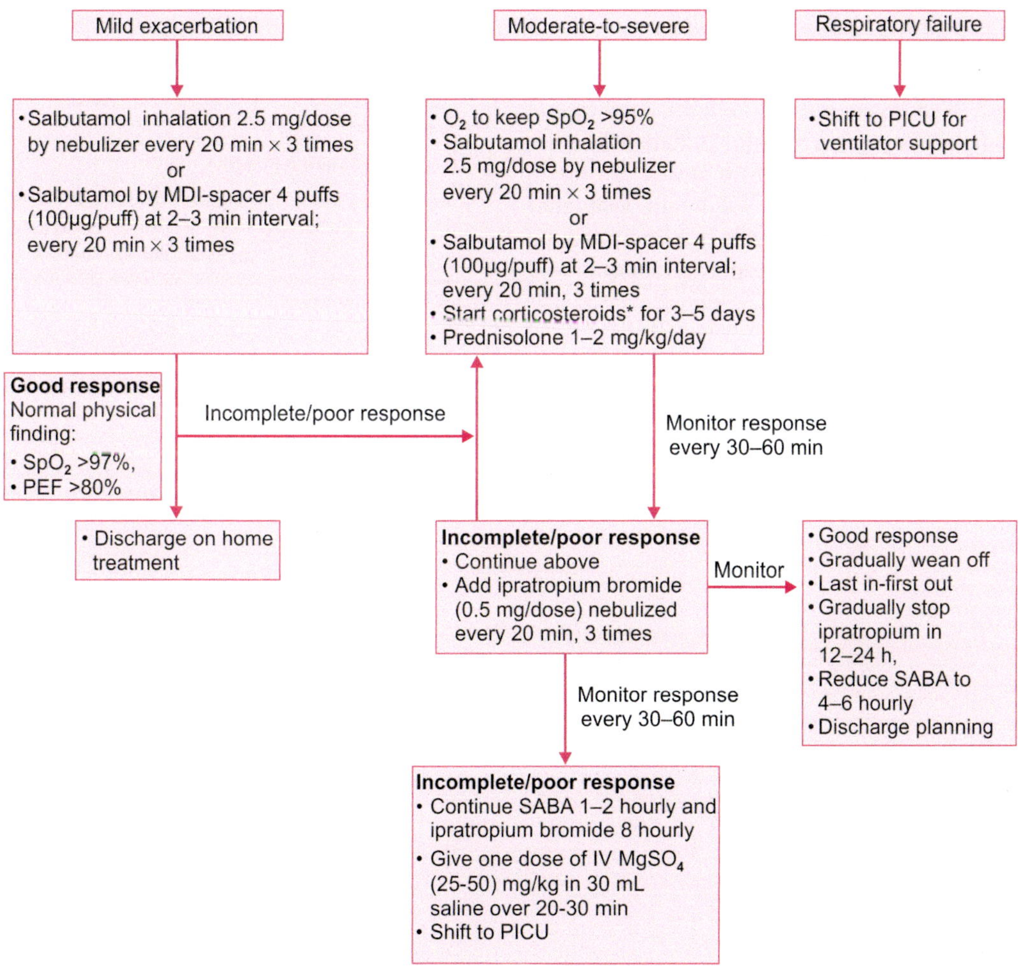

*Corticosteroids: Oral treatment is as effective as intravenous route and requires 4 hours for action. Intravenous (hydrocortisone 5 mg/kg/dose 8 hourly for 3–4 days; initial dose may be 10 mg/kg) should be reserved for patients not able to take orally (e.g., too dyspneic or vomiting) or on mechanical ventilation.

SABA, short-acting β-agonists; MDI, metered-dose inhaler; PEF, peak expiratory flow; PICU, pediatric intensive care unit.

Flowchart 1: Algorithm for management of acute exacerbation of asthma in children of asthma. The following algorithm (modified from global initiative for asthma guidelines) should be followed to treat a child with acute exacerbation in emergency settings (Flowchart 1).

Role of aminophylline and theophylline for acute asthma is not clear. Helium oxygen therapy, antibiotics, and sedatives should not be used for acute exacerbation of asthma.

Q. What should be discharge management after emergency care for exacerbation?

Shift back to as-needed reliever medication. Stop Ipratropium bromide. Initiate ICS prior to discharge in stepped-up doses for up to 2–4 weeks. Schedule a follow-up visit after 1 week and discharge with a written asthma action plan. Ensure proper technique and adherence to treatment.

LEARNING POINTS

- Asthma is one of the most common chronic diseases in childhood
- Diagnosis of asthma is mainly clinical and pulmonary function test may not be required routinely
- Inhaled corticosteroids are mainstay for long-term therapy of asthma
- Proper use of device, technique, and compliance to medications are of utmost importance in management of asthma
- In uncontrolled asthma, look for alternative diagnosis, technique, compliance, and comorbid conditions before stepping-up treatment
- Aggressive management of acute exacerbations is required.

SUGGESTED READINGS

1. Bush A. Diagnosis and management of asthma in children. BMJ. 2015;350:h996.. 2. Global Initiative for Asthma (GINA). (2015). The global strategy for asthma management and prevention. [online] Available from http://www.ginasthma.org [Accessed February, 2016].

CHAPTER

16

Allergic Bronchopulmonary Aspergillosis

Anirban Maitra

CASE 1

A 15-year-old boy was referred to the hospital emergency with ongoing problems. The boy was diagnosed with asthma since he was 4 years of age. He was born after an uneventful pregnancy at term by planned cesarean section. His immediate newborn period was of no concern and he was well until his third birthday when he had his first episode of wheezing triggered by an intercurrent viral infection. He responded to a short course of systemic steroids and inhaled bronchodilators. He had been well until 4 years of age when he had a similar episode severe enough to require admission to the pediatric intensive care unit. He was started on regular inhaled corticosteroids and did well since then. On an average, he had 1 or 2 mild-to-moderate exacerbations a year that was particularly troublesome in the winter and monsoon season. He never required hospital admission and his exacerbations were managed at home by inhaled salbutamol and short courses of systemic prednisolone. In between these episodes, he remained well with no interval symptoms of note.

In the past few days, he had suddenly become unwell with cough, acute onset shortness of breath, and wheezing. Unlike previous episodes, this cough was somewhat productive in nature and coughed a brownish mucus plug. He complained of headache and lost his appetite. He had spiked a low-grade temperature, but had no symptoms of upper respiratory tract infection. His oxygen saturations were 89% in air and 93% in 10 L/min of high-flow oxygen. His respiratory rate was 38/min, heart rate 110 beats/min, and temperature 38.3°C. On examination, he appeared acutely short of breath with widespread wheezing and increased work of breathing (he was using his accessory muscles), but air entry in both lungs was perceived to be equal. There was no significant lymphadenopathy of note, heart sounds were normal, no hepatosplenomegaly on abdominal examination, and no evident skin rash.

Q. What would be your working diagnosis? How would you progress toward managing this child?

The most likely diagnosis is an acute exacerbation of asthma. The child must be provided standard treatment for acute exacerbation of asthma. The child may be discharged home once the child does not need oxygen and is on 4 hourly inhaled salbutamol. Risk factors for this and subsequent exacerbations need to be explored including compliance with his prescribed medications and changes in environment. A follow-up visit needs to be organized to ensure the chest is clear and the recovery is complete.

Case history (continued)

In the follow-up visit after 7 days, the child was still very wheezy and complained of chest tightening. His cough had become more productive with expectoration of mucus plugs. On examination, he had a low-grade temperature, was hypoxic in air, tachypneic, and appeared tired. Chest examination revealed bilateral wheeze and scattered crackles.

Q. How will you approach this child on his second visit?

It is unusual for a child with uncomplicated asthma to have not responded to a decent course of steroids. Box 1 shows quick checklist for nonresponding asthma. He needs to be assessed clinically for oxygen supplementation, hydration therapy, increase in bronchodilators and steroids pending further investigations.

Box 1: Quick checklist for nonresponding asthma

- Check compliance with prescribed regime
- Check device and check technique
- Assess home environment and mitigating factors
- Assess whether this is asthma/asthma exacerbation
- Assess for any comorbidity and complicating factor
- Consider alternative diagnosis

Q. What investigations are indicated at this stage?

Once ensured that his regimen compliance is acceptable, a chest X-ray (CXR) is mandatory at this stage along with further investigations (Box 2).

Box 2: Initial investigations

- Chest X-ray
- Bloods (full blood count, C-reactive protein, eosinophils, urea and electrolytes, total serum immunoglobulin E)
- Sputum for microscopy including Gram stain and culture
- Others as appropriate for alternative diagnosis.

Case history (continued)

The immunoglobulin E (IgE) came back at 800 IU/mL and a number of patchy opacities were noticed in his chest X-ray along with increased prominence of bronchovascular markings. He had hemoglobin of 13.2 g/dL, white cell count of 9,600/mm^3, an absolute eosinophil count of 1,300 cells/μL of blood, normal C-reactive protein, and normal renal and liver functions. His compliance with prescribed medications was considered satisfactory and he admitted having travelled to his ancestral home in a village where he had spent some time engaging in gardening and farming activities. His medications improved the symptoms to some extent, but he continued to be unwell and complained of right-sided chest pain that worsened with respiratory excursions.

Q. How would you interpret these test results and how will it help it to plan further management?

Preliminary investigations suggest eosinophilia, elevated IgE and chest X-ray (CXR) changes. The CXR changes are suggestive of either mucus blockage or infection or both. The history of a recent visit to a farm is indicative of an exposure to helminths or fungus that may explain this eosinophilic state. Given the CXR changes and persistent deterioration of respiratory status, investigating for allergic bronchopulmonary aspergillosis (ABPA) is indicated.

Case history (continued)

Further confirmatory tests were ordered and serology (Aspergillus specific IgE and IgG) supported a diagnosis of ABPA. Sputum for microscopy revealed fungal elements and casts. Skin-prick test for *Aspergillus fumigatus* was not performed due to nonavailability of the kit.

Q. What is ABPA?

Allergic bronchopulmonary aspergillosis is a hypersensitivity reaction to *Aspergillus* species (usually *Aspergillus fumigatus*), an ubiquitous fungi found in the soil that occurs almost exclusively in patients who suffer from asthma or less commonly, cystic fibrosis (CF) and is otherwise immunocompetent.

Q. What is the epidemiology of ABPA?

Allergic bronchopulmonary aspergillosis occurs worldwide and is an important emerging condition in India. The prevalence of ABPA is reported as 1–2% in asthmatic subjects and 2–15% in subjects with CF. It mostly affects teenagers with CF although it has been diagnosed with infants. CF patients with atopy seem to be more vulnerable to ABPA [atopic CF (22%) vs. nonatopic CF (2%)].

Q. What is the etiology and pathophysiology of ABPA?

Most human disease is attributed to *A. fumigatus* although other fungi (*Penicillium, Candida, Curvularia, Helminthosporium,* and *Drechslera*) may also present with a similar illness. Allergic bronchopulmonary aspergillosis is a hypersensitivity reaction to the fungal elements. *Aspergillus* is present intraluminally but is not invasive; hence, ABPA must be distinguished from invasive aspergillosis, which occurs in immunocompromised patients. Allergic bronchopulmonary aspergillosis needs to be differentiated from aspergillomas (collections of *Aspergillus* in patients with established cavitary lesions or cystic airspaces) and from the rare *Aspergillus* pneumonia, which occurs in patients who are on long-term steroids although overlap has been reported.

The first step in ABPA is the colonization of distal airways of subjects with CF or asthma by spores of fungi. Germination of spores releases the antigenic elements that induce IgE-mediated (type 1) and IgG-mediated (type 3) reactions promoting a more intense airway inflammatory than that seen with asthma alone. Exposure to Aspergillus allergen recruits Th2 T lymphocytes that release interleukin (IL)-5 cytokine implicated in the recruitment of eosinophils and B cells. Eosinophilic granules promote intense airway inflammation and B cells target specific antibody production. The humoral immune response elevates *Aspergillus* specific immunoglobulin IgG, IgA, and IgE. Additionally, a neutrophilic inflammatory response is initiated by the release of fungal proteases that induce airway epithelial cells and macrophages to release IL-8 that recruits neutrophils. These neutrophilic granular products perpetuate the inflammatory response. Interleukins (IL-5, IL-8) and other chemokines from eosinophils and neutrophils produce intense inflammatory response that may ultimately lead to bronchiectasis, fibrosis, and airway obstruction.

In the CF airways, the inflammatory response of ABPA is similar to that in asthma with the mutation of the cystic fibrosis transmembrane conductance regulator (CFTR) being an independent risk factor for development of ABPA. cystic fibrosis patients with a genetic susceptibility of increased Th2 CD4+ cell lymphocyte activity (that are Aspergillus specific) demonstrates a greater allergic inflammatory response than in allergic patients sensitized to *Aspergillus* by secretion of cytokines IL-4, IL-5, and IL-13 that promote inflammation. Clinically, ABPA in CF patients herald a most severe progression in all lung function parameters. Especially in a setting of concurrent chronic *Pseudomonas aeruginosa* infection, ABPA causes airway narrowing, gas trapping, and small-airway disease, which affect pulmonary function.

Q. Are there any risk factors for ABPA?

Risk factors for ABPA can be grouped into those who are strongly incriminated in disease causation and those that may be weakly correlated (Table 1).

TABLE 1: Risk factors for ABPA

Strong risk factors	Weak risk factors
• Asthma • CF • Atopy • HLA-DR2- and HLA-DR5-positive	• IL-10 promoter polymorphisms • Surfactant protein polymorphisms • CFTR gene

HLA, human leukocyte antigen; IL-10, interleukin-10; CF, cystic fibrosis; ABPA, allergic bronchopulmonary aspergillosis.

Q. How is ABPA diagnosed?

Allergic bronchopulmonary aspergillosis diagnosis is achieved by a careful history, systematic physical examination and selective investigations in patients with atopy, asthma, and CF who is otherwise immunocompetent.

Q. What are the clinical features of ABPA?

Allergic bronchopulmonary aspergillosis is commonly seen in adolescents and young adults who are known to suffer from atopic conditions (including asthma) and CF, but is otherwise immunocompetent. Clinically, the patient may present with symptoms such as malaise, fever (typically up to 38.5°C), cough, increased wheeze and chest tightening (often confused with asthma exacerbation), purulent sputum containing mucus plugs (brown or black casts), pleuritic chest pains, and hemoptysis. In patients with lung infiltrates or lung fibrosis, physical exam may demonstrate dyspnea, cough, wheeze, and respiratory crackles. In chronic advanced disease, finger clubbing, cyanosis or features of cor pulmonale may be present. In CF patients, ABPA may be associated with CF exacerbation (a marked increase in productive coughing, increased wheezing and chestiness, chest tightness) that often fails to respond to courses of antibiotics and weight loss. However, some patients with CF may have ABPA with no change in their usual symptoms, and the physical exam may be normal.

Q. How do we confirm a case of ABPA?

Once ABPA is suspected clinically in the population at risk, it becomes imperative to confirm the same prior to initiation of specific therapy. This is summarized in box 3.

Box 3: Workup for a suspected case of ABPA

- Initial Investigations
  - SPT for *Aspergillus fumigatus* sensitivity
  - Serum total IgE
  - FBC with peripheral eosinophil count
  - CXR
- Further Confirmatory Investigations
  - Serum *Aspergillus* specific IgE
  - Serum *Aspergillus* specific IgG
  - Sputum microscopy and culture
  - CT chest
  - HLA antigens

ABPA, allergic bronchopulmonary aspergillosis; SPT, skin-prick test; FBC, full blood count; CXR, chest X-ray; HLA, human leukocyte antigen; CT, computed tomography.

Skin-prick test (SPT) for *Aspergillus* is the initial investigation of choice. A positive wheal and flare reaction (>3 mm than control) may be seen in 23-28% of asthmatics and 29% of CF patients and is not in itself confirmatory for ABPA (merely indicates sensitization to *Aspergillus*). Conversely, a negative SPT is helpful in ruling out ABPA. Significantly higher levels of serum total IgE (>417 IU/mL or a fourfold abrupt rise) is an essential response in ABPA. Peripheral blood eosinophilia (>1,000 cells/μL) may be seen in 43–100% cases. Chest X-ray findings do not form part of an essential criterion to confirm ABPA but is often done simultaneously and may provide useful information (Boxes 4 and 5). Infiltrates (atelectasis secondary to bronchoconstriction and mucus plugging) may be visible commonly involving the upper or middle lobe. Advanced stage of ABPA may show fibrobronchiectatic changes in chest X-ray (Fig. 1) These infiltrates may be permanent or transient and is termed as *pulmonary eosinophilia* in the presence of concurrent serum eosinophilia. Others findings involve mucus plugging and bronchiectasis.

Confirmatory tests include elevated levels of serum IgG specific to *Aspergillus* (type 3 immune reaction) and IgE to allergenic Aspergillus protein (Asp f1, f3, 4, or 6 protein). The combination of increased total serum IgE (>417 IU/mL) and increased specific IgE to recombinant Aspergillus allergen f4 and/or f6 allows classic ABPA to be diagnosed with 100% specificity and 64% sensitivity and with a 100% positive predictive value and 94% negative predictive

Box 4: Diagnostic criteria for allergic bronchopulmonary aspergillosis in asthma with central bronchiectasis

- Minimal essential criteria
    - Existing diagnosis of asthma
    - Proximal bronchiectasis dilated bronchi in the inner two-thirds of the chest field on chest computed tomography
    - Immediate cutaneous reactivity to *Aspergillus* species or *A. fumigatus*
    - Elevated total serum IgE (>417 IU/mL or 1,000 ng/mL)
    - Elevated serum-specific IgE and/or IgG to *A. fumigatus*.

Box 5: Diagnostic criteria for allergic bronchopulmonary aspergillosis in asthma without central bronchiectasis

- Minimal essential criteria
    - Existing diagnosis of asthma
    - Immediate cutaneous reactivity to *Aspergillus* species or *A. fumigatus*
    - Total serum IgE concentration >417 IU/mL
    - Elevated serum-specific IgE-*A. fumigatus* and/or IgG-*A. fumigatus*.
    - Chest X-ray infiltrates may be present but are not required for the diagnosis.

value. Sputum examination, although not an essential criterion, is commonly performed and may reveal mucus plugs on gross exam and *Aspergillus* fungal elements and eosinophils. Allergic bronchopulmonary aspergillosis can be categorized as occurring either with or without central bronchiectasis (i.e., occurring within the inner two-thirds of the chest field). This may be confirmed on a high resolution computed tomography (HRCT) chest scan that commonly reveals central bronchiectasis, mucus plugging of the bronchi (finger-in-glove appearance) or bronchiolar mucus impaction (tree-in-bud shadow), pulmonary infiltrates, and peribronchial thickening (Fig. 2). Recently, the International Society for Human and Animal Mycology (ISHAM) has proposed new diagnostic criteria for ABPA as follows (Agarwal et al., 2013).

- Predisposing conditions: Bronchial asthma or cystic fibrosis
- Obligatory criteria (both should be present)
    - Positive SPT or elevated aspergillus specific IgE levels
    - Elevated total IgE levels (>1000 IU/mL)
- Other criteria (at least two of three)
    - Presence of precipitating or IgG antibodies against aspergillus

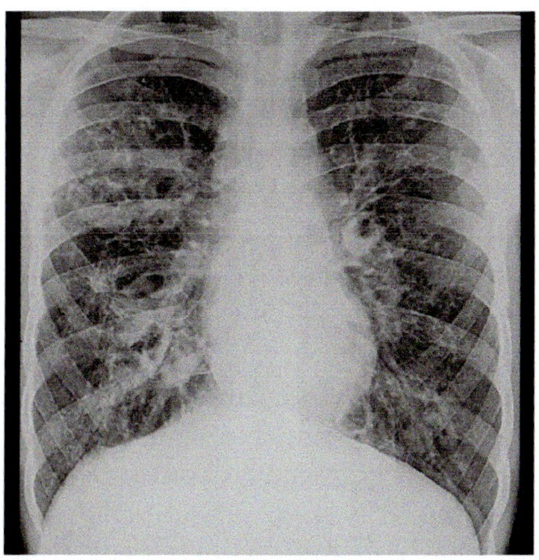

Figure 1: Chest X-ray of a child with advanced stage of allergic bronchopulmonary aspergillosis showing bilateral fibrobronchiectatic changes

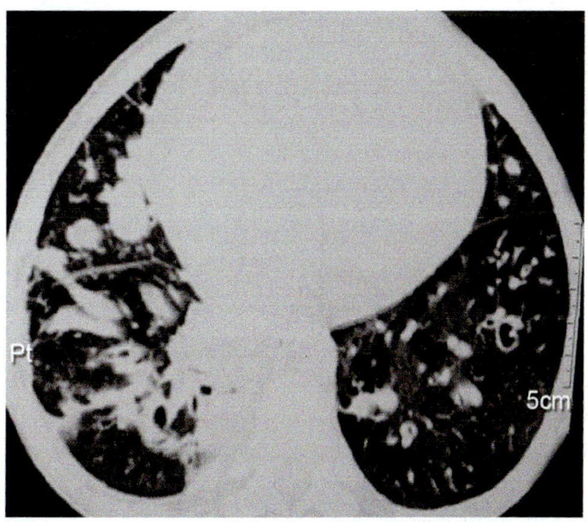

Figure 2: High resolution computed tomography chest of a child with allergic bronchopulmonary aspergillosis showing bronchiectasis (on left side) and hyperattenuated mucus on left side

- Radiographic findings consistent with ABPA (fleeting shadows or findings suggestive of bronchiectasis)
- Total eosinophil count >500 cells/lL

Q. What are the stages of ABPA?

Allergic bronchopulmonary aspergillosis stages are helpful in organizing treatment and for prognostication purposes. They may not progress sequentially (Table 2).

Q. What are the differential diagnoses?

Exacerbation of asthma and infectious exacerbation of CF are the most important differential diagnosis for ABPA and is often hard to separate (Box 6).

Q. Is ABPA preventable?

The doctor has a duty of responsibility to inform high-risk patients to avoid areas of possible exposures to *Aspergillus*. Although ubiquitous, high concentrations of *Aspergillus* may be noted in dead and decaying organic matter such as compost piles. In general, children are advised to avoid mucking out stables, and if they insist on horse riding this must be done out in the open. Furthermore, the patient's home should be assessed for damp and water damage because this can encourage the growth of molds of all types, including *Aspergillus*.

TABLE 2: Stages of allergic bronchopulmonary aspergillosis

Stage	Description	Criteria
I	Acute	All diagnostic criteria present
II	Remission	Symptoms resolved for >6 months
III	Relapse	Recurrence of ≥1 of the diagnostic criteria
IV	Refractory	Corticosteroid-dependent or refractory to treatment
V	Fibrosis	Diffuse fibrosis and bronchiectasis

Box 6: Differential diagnosis for allergic bronchopulmonary aspergillosis

- Asthma exacerbation
- Cystic fibrosis exacerbation
- Chronic eosinophilic pneumonia
- Churg-Strauss syndrome
- Hypereosinophilic syndromes

Q. How do we treat a case of ABPA?

As the process is allergic hypersensitivity reaction, corticosteroids remain the cornerstone of treatment along with optimization of treatment for their underlying asthma or CF. Allergic bronchopulmonary aspergillosis treatment is stage dependent and some variation exists in the dosage of steroids and the addition of antifungals.

Stage I (acute disease) is treated with systemic corticosteroids (prednisolone, given in the morning after food at a dose of 2 mg/kg/day for 2 weeks, then 1 mg/kg/day for 2 weeks, then 1 mg/kg/on alternate day for 2 weeks). Clinical evaluation, CXR, blood eosinophil count, and IgE levels should be checked quarterly for improvement, defined as resolution of infiltrates, ≥50% decline in eosinophils, and 33% decline in IgE. In some cases who do well, the IgE does not fall, so treat the patient not the IgE level. Dose is then gradually lowered over 4–6 months guided by clinical response and IgE. An equivalent dose of dexamethasone may be used instead. Inhaled and nebulized corticosteroids are used by some, but there is no evidence for its use. Pulsed methylprednisolone at 10–15 mg/kg once a day for 3 days every month (maximum dose 1 g) is attractive for the noncompliant patient, and may have fewer side effects, at the cost of more inconvenience. It is an increasingly preferred option, administered usually for 3 months, but may be longer depending on the response.

Patients in stage II disease (remission) require annual monitoring only. Relapse is common within 2–3 years of first episode (stage III) and often high doses of steroids are needed for a long time. Stage I or III patients who do not improve with prednisone (stage IV, occurs when the patient is unable to be weaned off oral corticosteroids and/or there is persistent elevation of serum IgE, along with obstructive and restrictive lung changes) are candidates for antifungal treatment although some centers would use azole antifungals as a routine adjunct to systemic corticosteroids. Patients in stage IV disease are often treated with daily oral corticosteroids, which may need to be given indefinitely.

Itraconazole remains the drug of choice as an antifungal and is a preferred option over ketoconazole that tends to have a higher side effect profile (severe liver injury and adrenal suppression). Itraconazole therapy requires checking drug levels and monitoring liver enzymes and triglyceride and potassium levels. Voriconazole or more recently posaconazole has been used to eradicate *Aspergillus*. In difficult CF cases, nebulized amphotericin (nonliposomal) may be used at a dose of 5–10 mg twice daily after physiotherapy (check for bronchoconstriction and use bronchodilator predose).

Occasionally, prolonged courses of intravenous AmBisome (liposomal amphotericin) may be used in refractory cases. Intravenous caspofungin can also be considered as third line and the anti-IgE monoclonal antibody (omalizumab) may rarely be considered on the basis of case reports.

In stage V, the patient is corticosteroid dependent and has obstructive and restrictive lung changes. They may be dyspneic or cyanotic and have fibrotic, bullous, or cavitary lesions visible on imaging. Serum IgE may be elevated or normal. The bronchial destruction found at this stage makes the prognosis poor with respiratory insufficiency, poor exercise tolerance, and recurrent pulmonary infections commonly associated with this stage

Q. What is the prognosis?

Stage I disease typically responds well to systemic corticosteroids and heals without bronchial destruction. In stage II, typically the patient remains well without any symptoms or infiltrates for >6 months. Stage III disease usually responds to prompt institution of corticosteroids. However, lack of improvement after 2 months of prednisolone treatment suggests a poorer prognosis. More so in the adult population, stage IV is the most common stage at which ABPA is diagnosed. Unfortunately, by this stage the patient has been unable to be weaned off oral corticosteroids without experiencing an exacerbation. In addition, bronchiectasis has already occurred by this point. Stage V is the second most common stage for a diagnosis of ABPA to be made and has the poorest prognosis due to the irreversible restrictive and obstructive lung changes that have occurred by this point.

LEARNING POINTS

- Allergic bronchopulmonary aspergillosis is a hypersensitivity reaction to *Aspergillus fumigatus* mold that has colonized bronchi of patients with asthma or cystic fibrosis
- Exposure of atopic people to fungal spore elements results in the formation of immunoglobulin (Ig) E and IgG antibodies
- It presents as asthma complicated by bronchial obstruction, fever, malaise, expectoration of brownish mucus plugs, peripheral blood eosinophilia, and hemoptysis
- Treatment involves environmental control measures, corticosteroids, and itraconazole
- Early detection and treatment can prevent the development of bronchiectasis or pulmonary fibrosis that otherwise occurs in the later stages of the disease.

SUGGESTED READINGS

1. Agarwal R, Chakrabarti A, Shah A, Gupta D, Meis JF, Guleria R, Moss R, Denning D W and For the ABPA complicating asthma ISHAM working group. Allergic bronchopulmonary aspergillosis: review of literature and proposal of new diagnostic and classification criteria. Clin Exp Allergy. 2013; (43):850-873.

2. American Academy of Allergy, Asthma and Immunology. Allergic Bronchopulmonary Aspergillosis (ABPA)-Pulmonary Disorders (Miles MC, Peters S). Available from http://www.msdmanuals.com/professional/pulmonary-disorders/asthma-and-related-disorders/allergic-bronchopulmonary-aspergillosis-abpa. [Accessed February, 2016].
3. Aspergillus lung disease. In: Balfour-Lynn I (Ed). Clinical Guidelines: Care of Children with Cystic Fibrosis, 6th edition. London: Royal Brompton Hospital; 2014. p. 273
4. Greenberger PA, Miller TP, Roberts M, Smith LL. Allergic bronchopulmonary aspergillosis in patients with and without bronchiectasis. Ann Allergy. 1993;70:333-8.
5. Greenberger PA. Allergic bronchopulmonary aspergillosis. J Allergy Clin Immunol. 2002;110(5):685-92
6. Radojicic C. (2015). Allergic bronchopulmonary aspergillosis. [online] Available from http://bestpractice.bmj.com/best-practice/monograph/836.html [Accessed on February, 2016].

CHAPTER

17

Gastroesophageal Reflux Disease

Gowrishankar NC

> **CASE 1**
>
> A 75-day-old boy was brought for frequent regurgitation. His birth weight was 3.1 kg. On the day of presentation, his weight was 5.2 kg. The baby voided urine 8 times a day and passed soft yellow stools twice a day. Should we counsel the parents or treat the baby?

Q. What is gastroesophageal reflux (GER)?

Gastroesophageal reflux is the passage of contents of the stomach back into the esophagus. It may or may not be associated with regurgitation, vomiting, or both. Physiological GER occurs many times every day in infants, children, adolescents and even adults, but does not cause any symptoms. Physiological GER becomes pathological GER—gastroesophageal reflux disease (GERD) when it causes troublesome symptoms and/or complications. Physiological GER, a self-limiting event, is common post feeds and improves with age.

Q. How physiological GER may be differentiated from pathological GER?

It may appear difficult initially to differentiate physiological from pathological GER but taking time to elicit proper history and following-up, the infant as well will help us to differentiate it. In physiological GER, most of the infants have regurgitation or vomiting but do not have the general warning signs of failure to thrive, esophageal or extra-esophageal symptoms including feeding difficulty, crying spell, and irritability. These infants are otherwise known as "happy spitters".

Children with pathological GER or GERD may have both esophageal and extra-esophageal manifestations. The esophageal manifestations in infants include regurgitation, gagging, choking, and aversion to feed with all these leading to failure to thrive, while pain abdomen may be one of the main features in older children.

In infants with GERD, the extra-esophageal manifestations include failure to thrive, wheezing, stridor, persistent cough, apnea, feeding difficulties, aspiration, regurgitation, recurrent croup while rarer manifestations include apnea or apparent life-threatening events; chronic respiratory diseases; and upper airway problems like sinusitis, otitis media, laryngitis, and dental erosion is seen in toddlers. In older children, it may include cough, hoarseness, stridor, sore throat, asthma, vomiting, wheezing, aspiration, and recurrent pneumonia.

CASE 2

A 5-month-old boy, whose birth weight was 3 kg, was brought for frequent vomiting, cough, incessant cry, not gaining weight (weight on the day of presentation: 4.5 kg), and stridor. Also, he had not attained head control. Should we reassure and follow-up the baby or investigate?

Q. What is possible diagnosis of case 1 and case 2?

Case 1 seems to be physiological GER and needs counseling only. The case 2 is having pathological GER and needs further evaluation.

Q. What are the conditions that may predispose GERD?

The conditions predisposing to GERD are many. Obesity; central nervous system disorders including cerebral palsy, muscle disorders like congenital myopathy, chromosomal aberrations like Down's syndrome, postsurgical status involving the esophagus and diaphragm like esophageal atresia, trachea esophageal fistula and congenital diaphragmatic hernia respectively; conditions causing long-term pulmonary morbidity like bronchopulmonary dysplasia, bronchiectasis, asthma, and cystic fibrosis; and postaccidental caustic injury to the esophagus, form the major chunk of the conditions which predisposes to GERD.

CASE 3

A 4-year-old boy was brought with recurrent episodes of laryngitis, otitis media, and dental caries (not bottlefed at any time in his life). Basic blood investigations, X-ray chest, and immune workup were normal. According to ENT opinion, no intervention was needed then. Can this child have GERD? Do we have to investigate further?

Q. How to investigate this case for GERD?

This child obviously need workup for GERD. The aim of the diagnostic test should be to detect the contents of the stomach refluxing into esophagus. But this reflux is a physiological process. The real crux of the diagnostic tests rests on to differentiate physiological GER from GERD. Hence, the next step is to know the subjects who need to be investigated. Most of the times the clinical picture and the history should be sufficient enough to rule in GERD. Investigations should be done in those who have nonspecific symptoms and those who are predisposed to have GERD. The investigations available include barium study, gastroesophageal scintigraphy, esophageal ultrasound, 24-hour esophageal pH monitoring, esophageal manometry, upper gastrointestinal endoscopy with or without biopsy, and multichannel intraluminal impedance study with pH monitoring.

Q. What is the role of barium study in GERD?

Barium study delineates not only the anatomy of the esophagus, stomach but also the functional status as well (Fig. 1). The contrast study can also demonstrate hiatus hernia and strictures. But the limitation is it neither can differentiate physiological GER from pathological GERD nor can it quantify the reflux episodes. Also, it will not be able to make out if esophagitis is present or not.

Q. What is the role of nuclear scan in GERD?

Nuclear imaging can help to detect aspiration into lungs as evidenced by retention of the radioactivity in the lungs beyond 24 hours (Fig. 2). A silent aspiration also can be made out if radioactivity is detected in lung. At the same time their absence does not imply absence of GERD. It may be useful while evaluating a child with recurrent pneumonia where GERD can be a cause. One of the positive points of nuclear imaging is that it has less radiation, but it is not recommended routinely.

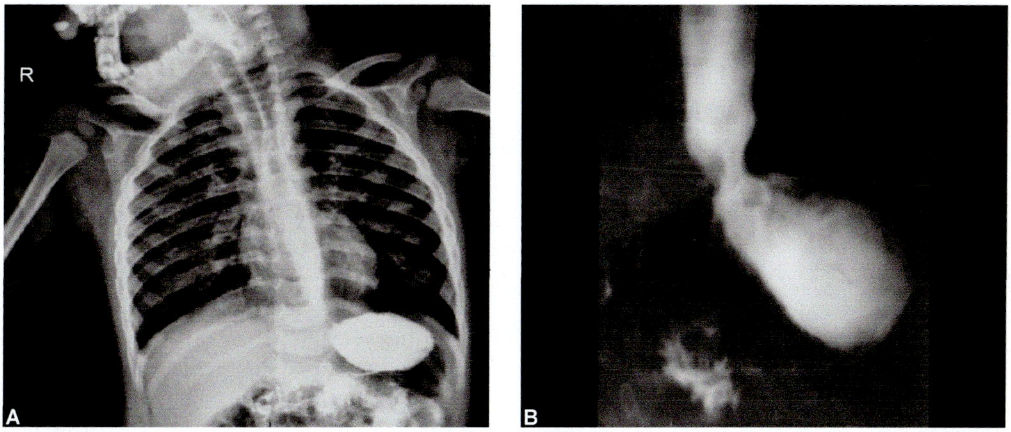

Figure 1: Barium swallow showing gastroesophageal reflux

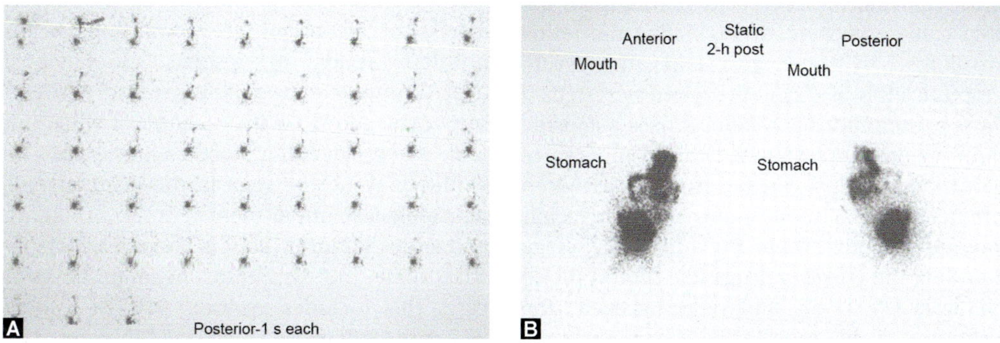

Figure 2: Technetium 99m sulfur colloid esophageal motility scan—positive gastroesophageal reflux

Q. What is the role of upper gastrointestinal endoscopy (UGIE) in GERD?

Upper gastrointestinal endoscopy helps to visualize esophagus directly and makes a diagnosis of GERD when esophagitis is present. The findings include visible mucosal lesions in the esophagus or immediately above the esophagogastric junction, though the findings of erythema of mucosa and irregular Z line are not sufficient to make a diagnosis of reflux esophagitis. Biopsy of the visible mucosal lesions can show basal layer hyperplasia and elongated papillae. But these are nonspecific reactive changes which can be present in other types of esophagitis which include eosinophilic esophagitis, fungal esophagitis, *Helicobacter pylori* gastritis, etc. Hence the positives from UGIE include direct visualization of esophagus for presence and severity of esophagitis and detection of complications which includes ulcer, stricture and Barrett's esophagitis. If GERD is present in the absence of these findings (scopy and histology) it is known as nonerosive reflux disease (NERD).

Q. Is there any role of flexible bronchoscopy in GERD?

Flexible bronchoscopy can help when extra-esophageal manifestations are the main features. The findings of subglottic stenosis, laryngomalacia, laryngeal edema, recurrent respiratory papillomatosis, vocal cord granulomas, or vocal cord nodules can be seen on scopy in those with extra-esophageal manifestations.

Q. Is 24-hour esophageal pH monitoring useful to diagnose GERD?

The 24-hour esophageal pH monitoring helps to investigate a child with suspected GERD under more physiological state by providing more information, especially the "reflux index (RI)" which is the percentage of times the esophageal pH is <4. If the RI is >10 in infant and >5 in children it is suggestive of GERD. The disadvantage of this modality is that it does not detect nonacid or weak acid reflux. Also, the nasal catheter system by restricting the reflux provoking activity can give a negative result. A modification of this is the wireless system—Bravo pH monitoring system. It uses a capsule which needs to be attached to the mucosa of the esophagus and can be of use in children with neurological impairment. Also if the test is done for 48 hours, it has the added advantage of finding the effect of drugs like proton pump inhibitors (PPIs) on acid reflux as well. The usefulness of this monitoring is mainly in the evaluation of those with extra-esophageal symptoms and the response to treatment in difficult to control GERD.

Q. What are newer diagnostic tests for GERD?

Multichannel intraluminal impedance with pH monitoring is a newer method to detect acid and nonacid reflux, duration and direction of the reflux irrespective of the amount of the refluxate. It also distinguishes liquid, solid, and gas reflux. The multiple channels placed in esophagus measures the changes in electrical resistance in the esophagus when there is passage of liquid, solid, or gas across a segment of esophagus. In conjunction with pH monitoring, the temporal association between esophageal pH changes and symptoms is given by this investigation.

CASE 4

A 10-year-old obese boy on inhaled corticosteroids and long-acting β-agonists for moderate persistent asthma presented with recurrent retrosternal chest pain, cough, and hoarse voice. Upper gastrointestinal endoscopy suggested GERD.

Q. What is management for GERD?

Though the symptomatology is not the same between infants, older children, and adolescents, the management principles are relief of symptoms, promote healing of the esophageal inflammation, prevent recurrence and if possible avoid complications. Both nonpharmacological and pharmacological management will be needed. In infancy the results of treatment are rewarding, as the problem tends to resolve spontaneously over time and dietary changes and antireflux measures alone suffice most of the time and rarely needing medications. But this course may not be seen in those infants with neurological impairment. Both in infants and older children certain factors which can accentuate the symptoms need to be taken care. This includes avoiding passive smoking as it causes lower esophageal sphincter (LES) relaxation, and avoiding tight clothing. Food with high-fat content may not only relax the LES, but also delay gastric emptying while small volume frequent feeds may be associated with significant nonacid reflux. Thickened feeds have been found to reduce only the volume of the refluxate. Hence, while managing GERD, due importance needs to be given to feed volume, exposure to smoke, avoidance of reflux-inducing food, and proper positioning of the affected individual so as to control the symptoms. In infants the upright and prone position while awake reduces reflux, but during sleep supine position is recommended because of the risk of sudden infant death syndrome in prone position. In older children, elevation of head-end with left lateral decubitus position during sleep has been found to be of benefit in GERD.

The aim of giving drugs in GERD is to suppress the acid secretion, though both acid and nonacid reflux causes symptoms. The drugs to reduce acid secretion include PPIs and H2-receptor antagonists. Prokinetics which not only increase the LES tone but also improves gastric emptying are given mainly to control vomiting and regurgitation while contact antacids give symptomatic relief in older children and adolescents. At present, none of the drugs are effective in controlling transient relaxation of LES (TRLES) which is the primary mechanism for GERD to occur. Hence, drugs need to be used judiciously in the management of GERD.

Prokinetics should be the first drug when one is dealing with a child with symptoms suggestive of abnormalities in motility and in those who have more regurgitation than pain. Domperidone is a prokinetic which not only improves the motility but also the pressure in LES. Among agents inhibiting acid secretions, ranitidine, a H2-receptor antagonists also available in liquid formulation inhibits acid secretion for about 9–10 hours which heals erosive esophagitis of moderate severity. Proton pump inhibitors inhibit food-induced acid secretion and also, that too for a longer duration. It also heals severe grades of erosive esophagitis. It should be enteric coated to be absorbed in duodenum without any destruction of the drug by acid and needs to be given before the first meal. Most patients require a single daily dose. Though gastric acidity is reduced in all age groups by PPI, its effect in infancy is still debatable as in infants who are fed only on milk predominantly, the refluxate is nonacidic most of the time every day. The currently used PPIs are pantoprazole, lansoprazole, and esomeprazole (Table 1). The duration of treatment is for a period of 12 weeks. The suppression of acid secretion by PPIs is much better than H2-receptor antagonists.

Headache, diarrhea, or constipation can occur as side effects of antacids, whereas increased risk for community-acquired pneumonia and gastroenteritis has been noted in those on prolonged treatment with PPIs and H2-receptor antagonists. If the symptoms do not decrease even at the end of 12 weeks and for those who have persistent vomiting, fail to gain adequate weight, have hiatus hernia and if esophageal stricture as a complication of GERD is present, surgical intervention is suggested only after having a relook at the diagnosis and subjecting them to investigations to rule in or rule out GERD if they have not been done previously. Fundoplication is the commonly done procedure for GERD, but the results are not satisfactory if done early in life (especially <1-year-old children)

TABLE 1: Antacids for management of gastroesophageal reflux disease in children

Drugs	Dosing	Indicated ages
Ranitidine	5–10 mg/kg/day, divided in two to three doses	1 month – 16 years
Famotidine	1 mg/kg/day, divided in two doses	1–16 years
Omeprazole	0.7–3.3 mg/kg/day	2–16 years
Lansoprazole	0.7–3 mg/kg/day	1–17 years
Esomeprazole	0.7–3.3 mg/kg/day	1–17 years

LEARNING POINTS

- Gastroesophageal reflux disease (GERD) in infants, toddlers and older children differs in their presentation
- If the symptomatology is straightforward, management is not difficult
- In those who have extra-esophageal manifestations, investigations may be needed before treatment
- Drugs for management of GERD have to be used appropriately based on the age, symptoms, and complications if present.

SUGGESTED READINGS

1. Benítez CAV. GERD in children: an update. Rev Col Gastroenterol. 2014;29(1):49-55.
2. Boström, Thorsson O, Toth E, Agardh D. BMC Gastroenterology. Clinical value of wireless pH-monitoring of gastro-esophageal reflux in children before and after proton pump inhibitors. 2014;24;14:3.
3. Ferreira CT, Carvalho E, Sdepanian VL, Morais MB, Vieira MC, Silva LR. Gastroesophageal reflux disease: exaggerations, evidence and clinical practice. J Pediatr (Rio J). 2014;90:105-18.
4. Jadcherla SR, Hogan WJ, Shaker R. Physiology and pathophysiology of glottic reflexes and pulmonary aspiration: from neonates to adults. Semin Respir Crit Care Med. 2010;31(5):554-60.
5. Lightdale JR, Gremse DA. Gastroesophageal reflux: management guidance for the pediatrician. Pediatrics. 2013;131(5):e1684-95.
6. Poddar U. Diagnosis and management of gastroesophageal reflux disease (GERD): an Indian perspective. Indian Pediatr. 2013(50):119-126.
7. Vakil N, van Zanten SV, Kahrilas P, Dent J, Jones R,. Global Consensus Group. The Montreal definition and classification of gastroesophageal reflux disease: a global evidence-based consensus. Am J Gastroenterol. 2006;101(8):1900-20.

4

SECTION

Respiratory Tract Infections

CHAPTER

18

Influenza Infections

Indu Khoshla, Vishal Mukhija

CASE 1

A 4-year-old boy presented with moderate grade fever, coryza, and cough since past 2 days. There was a history of similar complaints in a sibling 6 days prior. On examination, the child was active, alert with normal vitals, and no signs of respiratory distress. He had rhinorrhea and mild congestion in throat. On examination, respiratory system was normal.

Q. What infection does this child have?

The child can be clinically diagnosed as viral nasopharyngitis also called "common cold". It is a common self-limiting viral infection causing sneezing, rhinorrhea, and nasal congestion, which progresses to sore throat with systemic manifestations of low grade fever headache and malaise. It is a common syndrome which can be caused by many families of viruses; the common ones are rhinoviruses, respiratory syncytial virus, influenza, parainfluenza, and adenoviruses.

Q. How are the influenza viruses classified?

Influenza viruses are ribonucleic acid viruses of the Orthomyxoviridae family. There are two important antigens on the surface (Fig. 1). Influenza hemagglutinin (H) is a surface glycoprotein that plays a role in attachment to the respiratory epithelial cell surface glycoproteins and initiates the infection. The other antigen is neuraminidase (N), which cleaves these progeny virions bound to the host cell after viral replication and liberates them. There are three genera of influenza viruses:

- Influenza virus A: Responsible for most endemics and pandemics
- Influenza virus B: Infects predominantly humans, does not cause pandemics
- Influenza virus C: Less common. Has only one glycoprotein—hemagglutinin-esterase fusion.

There are 18 different hemagglutinin subtypes and 11 neuraminidase subtypes (H1 to H18 and N1 to N11), which form the basis of further subdividing these genera into serotypes such as H1N1, H2N2, H3N2, and H5N1.

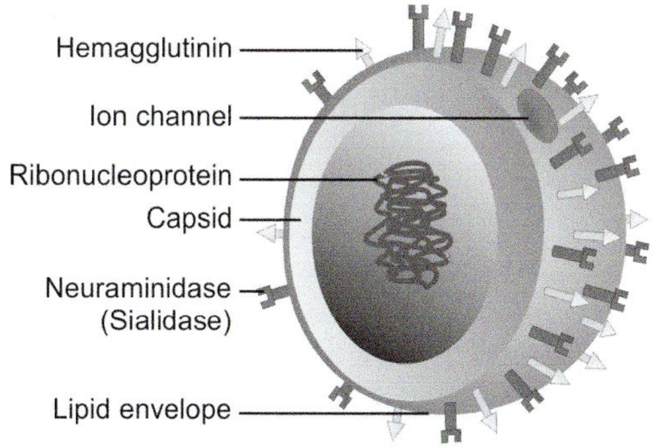

Figure 1: Influenza virus *(For color version, see Plate 1)*

Q. Why do epidemics and pandemics of influenza occur?

Major changes in H and N antigens are known as antigenic shifts, and minor are called antigenic drifts. Antigenic shifts are associated with epidemics and pandemics of influenza A, whereas antigenic drifts are associated with more localized outbreaks. Emergence of any new subtype results in its rapid spread as the human has little (in case of drift) or almost no (in case of shift) immunity to it.

H1N1 was the serotype which caused the pandemic known as the Spanish Flu in 1915. Subsequently, H2N2—Asian flu (1957), H3N2—Hong Kong flu (1968), and H5N1—bird flu (2004) were the major antigenic shifts causing widespread human infections. In 2009, a new influenza A (H1N1) virus called novel H1N1 or just H1N1 emerged and has replaced the H1N1 virus circulating at that time. Currently circulating influenza B viruses are of two lineages—B/Yamagata and B/Victoria.

Q. Are there any clinical pointers in our case to diagnose influenza?

Influenza presents as any viral illness in most immunocompetent persons and is a self-limiting illness. The symptoms also vary with age and previous exposure to the influenza virus. The classic features of uncomplicated influenza virus infection are sudden onset of fever, headache, myalgia, and malaise respiratory symptoms such as cough, sore throat, and rhinitis. In young children, the diagnosis may be missed as symptoms, such as myalgia and headache, may not be apparent. There is no cardinal clinical feature to differentiate influenza from other viral infections conclusively.

CASE 2

A 2-year-old, previously healthy, well-grown child presented with high grade fever, irritability, vomiting, and cough since past 2 days during the winter season. On examination, the child was febrile and sick looking with a respiratory rate of 50/min. There was mild respiratory distress with subcostal and intercostal indrawing and bilateral crackles. Other systems were normal.

Q. Could this child be having influenza?

Influenza outbreaks have a seasonal distribution and occur usually during the winter months in the temperate areas. In tropical countries like India, influenza may occur throughout the year.

One must consider the diagnosis of infection with influenza during influenza season, if the following symptoms or signs are present:

- Febrile infants
- Children with fever and acute onset of respiratory illness (even if these symptoms develop during hospitalization)
- Children with fever and exacerbation of underlying chronic lung disease
- Children with community-acquired febrile pneumonia
- Children with fever [≥100°F (37.8°C)] and severe illness (cough, sore throat, or both in the absence of another known cause of illness).

Q. What is the clinical course of influenza infection in children?

Influenza in otherwise healthy children generally is an acute, self-limited, and uncomplicated disease. In high risk population and occasionally even in healthy children, severe disease requiring hospitalization and even mortality can occur.

Q. Who is at higher risk for severe disease?

The following groups of individuals are at higher risk of severe disease:

- Children <2 years of age
- Adults >65 years of age
- Persons with any chronic pulmonary, cardiovascular, renal, hepatic, hematologic, metabolic, neurologic, neuromuscular, and neurodevelopmental disorders
- Pregnant women
- Morbidly obese [body mass index (BMI) ≥40 for adults or BMI >2.33 standard deviations above the mean for children]

- Residents of nursing homes and other chronic care facilities
- Immunosuppression (including immunosuppression caused by medications or by human immunodeficiency virus).

Q. Is severe disease associated with certain serotypes?

Yes, there is an association between the influenza virus serotypes and the severity of illness. H3N2 influenza A viruses usually cause the most severe disease, followed by influenza B viruses, with H1N1 influenza A viruses causing the least severe disease. However, among young children, H1N1 influenza infections may be more severe than in older children and adults.

Q. What are the complications associated with influenza infection?

The most common complication of influenza in children is otitis media, followed by lower respiratory tract involvement including interstitial pneumonia, laryngotracheitis (croup), bronchitis, and occasionally bronchiolitis. Pneumonia is a major complication of influenza, particularly in high risk patients. If no underlying high risk conditions, influenza pneumonia occurs most frequently in children younger than 2 years. Influenza pneumonia is usually benign and self-limiting. Coinfection with bacteria such as *Staphylococcus aureus* and *Streptococcus pneumoniae* may be particularly severe and rapidly fatal. Other complications, including central nervous system involvement and myositis, are less frequent.

Q. What are the laboratory tests to confirm the diagnosis? Who should be offered this test?

Real time polymerase chain reaction (RT-PCR) done on the nasopharyngeal swab or aspirate is a common test done to diagnose influenza.

Isolation of the virus in nasopharyngeal swab or aspirate by culture or demonstrating a fourfold rise in virus specific neutralizing antibodies in serum are other diagnostic methods used.

Only those who require hospitalization and those at risk of complications should be offered testing.

Q. How should one treat influenza infections and does our case required to be treated?

In most, influenza is a mild illness requiring no specific treatment. Our child has evidence of respiratory distress along with high grade fever in a typical influenza season. He requires hospitalization and further management.

Two classes of antiviral drugs are available for the prevention and treatment of influenza—adamantanes and neuraminidase inhibitors.

Amantadine and rimantadine are adamantanes (also called M2 inhibitors). Adamantanes target the M2 protein of influenza A, which forms a protein channel in the viral membrane that is essential for efficient viral replication. Adamantanes are not active against influenza B viruses or against currently circulating strains of influenza A virus.

Oseltamivir, zanamivir, laninamivir, and peramivir are neuraminidase inhibitors, which prevent the release of virions from the host cell. Neuraminidase inhibitors are active against influenza A viruses (including the pandemic 2009–2010 H1N1 strain) and influenza B viruses. Of these, oseltamivir is readily available and used in children. Categorization of influenza infection and management is shown in table 1.

Q. What is the dosage schedule of oseltamivir?

When indicated, antiviral treatment should be started as soon as possible after illness onset, ideally within 48 hours of symptom onset. However, antiviral treatment might have some benefits in patients with severe, complicated, or progressive illness, and in hospitalized patients when started after 48 hours of illness onset.

TABLE 1: Clinical categories of influenza infection and their management

Category	Presentation	Testing	Hospitalization	Oseltamivir
A	Mild fever, cough, sore throat, body ache, headache, diarrhea, vomiting	No	Home treatment	No
B	Category A plus high-grade fever or category A plus high risk conditions	No	Home confinement	Yes
C	Category A and B plus breathlessness, hypotension, drowsiness, cyanosis, convulsions, bloody sputum, or worsening of underlying chronic condition	Yes	Immediate hospitalization	Yes

Source: Government of India, Ministry of Health and Family Welfare, Department of Health and Family Welfare.

CASE 3

A 10-year-old asymptomatic girl was brought because swine flu had been detected in her mother. Parents were anxious and wished to know about preventive steps that could be taken.

Q. What are the ways to prevent influenza in the child?

Influenza can be prevented by the following approaches:

- Vaccination with inactivated injectable trivalent influenza vaccines or live attenuated nasal influenza vaccine
- Nonpharmacological measures such as isolation and hygiene measures including hand washing.

Q. Do all the available vaccines provide protection against current outbreaks of influenza A (H1N1)?

All the currently available quadrivalent vaccines now have the influenza strain that is antigenically similar to 2009 pandemic swine flu strain, i.e., influenza A(H1N1)pdm09. Hence, all these vaccines do provide protection against currently circulating swine flu strain.

Q. How effective are flu vaccines?

The influenza viruses selected for inclusion in the seasonal flu vaccines are updated each year based on which influenza virus strains are circulating, how they are spreading, and how well current vaccine strains protect against newly identified strains. There are different vaccines for the northern and southern hemispheres and in India the northern hemisphere vaccine is generally followed. The World Health Organization recommends that influenza vaccines for use in the 2016-2017 northern hemisphere influenza season contain the following viruses:

- An A/California/7/2009 (H1N1)pdm09-like virus
- An A/Hong Kong/4801/2014 (H3N2)-like virus
- A B/Brisbane/60/2008-like virus.

Among circulating influenza B viruses, there are two distinct lineages. The B/Brisbane/60/2008-like viruses are from the influenza B/Victoria lineage and represent the predominant circulating influenza B virus. Quadrivalent influenza vaccines contain both a B/Victoria lineage and a B/Yamagata lineage vaccine viruses. It is recommended that quadrivalent vaccines contain the above three viruses and a B/Phuket/3073/2013-like virus, which represents the B/Yamagata lineage viruses The vaccine viruses recommended for the 2016-2017 northern hemisphere influenza season are the same as those recommended last September for the 2016 southern hemisphere influenza season. The recommendation, however, does represent an update to the vaccine viruses used for the 2015-2016 northern hemisphere influenza season which were selected in february 2015. Changes from the prior northern hemisphere vaccine viruses include:

- Replacement of the A(H3N2) component to include A/Hong Kong/4801/2014 (H3N2)-like virus
- For trivalent vaccines, replacement of the influenza B component to include B/Brisbane/60/2008-like virus
- For quadrivalent vaccines, B/Phuket/3073/2013-like virus was recommended as the second influenza B component.

Q. Should vaccine be offered to all individuals?

No, according to Indian Academy of Pediatrics, following group of individuals should be offered the vaccine:

- Children with certain high risk conditions and diseases like chronic cardiac, pulmonary (excluding asthma), hematologic, renal, liver diseases, diabetes mellitus, congenital or acquired immunodeficiency (including human immunodeficiency virus infection), and children on long-term salicylates therapy, etc.
- Healthcare professional including pediatricians
- Laboratory personnel and healthcare workers
- On demand of anxious parents after one-to-one discussion
- Government of India also recommends vaccination for healthcare workers working in close proximity to influenza patients, i.e., in causality, emergency wards, laboratory personnel, etc.

LEARNING POINTS

- Influenza infections can have a varied presentation from a mild infection like a common cold to life-threatening pneumonias
- Most patients require only symptomatic treatment, and specific treatment like antivirals is reserved for children with severe symptoms or high risk factors
- Investigation to confirm viral etiology in the form of real time polymerase chain reaction of a nasopharyngeal swab is required for admitted patients alone
- Annual vaccination is recommended in India for individuals at high risk for exposure or high risk for complications
- Chemoprophylaxis is recommended for contacts as per guidelines.

SUGGESTED READINGS

1. Government of India, Ministry of Health and Family Welfare, Department of Health and Family Welfare. Swine Flu-H1N1 (Seasonal Influenza). [online] Available from: http://mohfw.gov.in/index4.php?lang=1&level=0&linkid=372&lid=3066 [Accessed February, 2016].
2. World Health Organization. (2014). Influenza virus infections in humans (February 2014). [online] Available from: http://www.who.int/influenza/human_animal_interface/virology_laboratories_and_vaccines/influenza_virus_infections_humans_feb14.pdf?ua=1 [Accessed February, 2016].
3. Vashishtha VM, Kalra A, Choudhury P. Influenza vaccination in India: position paper of Indian Academy of Pediatrics, 2013. Indian Pediatr. 2013;50(9):867-74.

CHAPTER

19

Diphtheria

Santosh K Rathia, Jhuma Sankar

CASE 1

A 6-year-old girl, premorbidly normal, partially immunized, was brought to the pediatric outpatient department with complaints of low grade fever, dry cough, sore throat, and odynophagia for the past 4 days associated with neck swelling, voice change, drooling of saliva, and nasal regurgitation of fluids for the past 2 days. She was unimmunized and so were her siblings.

On examination, she was conscious with heart rate of 88/min, respiratory rate 22/min, and oxygen saturation of 96% on room air. Her neck swelling led to a "bull neck" appearance and there was cervical lymphadenopathy. Examination of oral cavity revealed poor oral hygiene, dirty grayish white membrane over both tonsils extending over faucial and posterior pharyngeal wall, which revealed bleeding spots on removal. Examination of the respiratory system revealed only mild suprasternal retractions. Air entry was equal and there were no added sounds. Rest of the systemic examination was normal.

Q. What are the differentials for febrile illness with white membranous tonsillopharyngitis?

Pharyngitis involves a spectrum of inflammatory responses from minimal erythema of the mucosa to diffuse ulceration, exudation, and edema formation. The differential diagnoses include:

- Diphtheria: Unlike acute bacterial tonsillitis, diphtheria is slower in onset with less local discomfort. The membrane extends beyond the tonsils on to the pharynx, soft palate, or even larynx and is dirty gray in color. It is adherent and its removal reveals a bleeding surface. Smear and culture of throat swab confirms the diagnosis
- Membranous tonsillitis: It occurs due to acute pyogenic organisms like group A streptococcus. An exudative membrane forms over the medial surface of the tonsils and look like red swollen tonsils with marked hyperemia of the pillars, uvula, and soft palate
- Infectious mononucleosis: It is caused by Epstein-Barr virus, in this condition both tonsils are enlarged, congested, and covered with membrane causing marked local discomfort. Cervical lymphadenopathy and splenomegaly are additional findings
- Vincent's angina: The disease has an insidious onset with low grade fever. Membrane usually forms over one tonsil can be easily removed, revealing an irregular ulcer on the tonsil. Throat swab will show both the organisms typical of the disease, i.e., fusiform bacilli and spirochetes
- Agranulocytosis: It may present with ulcerative necrotic lesions on the tonsils and

oropharynx. Patient is severely ill in acute fulminant form with granulocytopenia [total leukocyte count (TLC) may be reduced to ≤2,000/mm^3]. In chronic or recurrent form, leukopenia may be present with less marked neutropenia

- Candida infection: Painless curdy white membrane is seen over tonsils and oropharynx. It is seen more often in immunocompromised patient
- Aphthous ulcers: It may involve any part of oral cavity or oropharynx. Sometimes solitary, but may involve the tonsils and pillars
- Leukemia: Children with leukemia (most commonly acute leukemia) usually have anemia, high TLC (sometimes >100,000/mm^3) and show blasts on PS/bone marrow
- Malignancy of tonsils: Persistent sore throat, dysphagia, earache, or lump in the neck are common symptoms. Biopsy confirms the diagnosis
- Traumatic ulcer: An injury to oropharynx may heal by membrane formation within 24 hours of injury.

In the present case, as the child is unimmunized with insidious onset of symptoms and a characteristic pseudomembrane, the initial clinical possibility would be diphtheria, pending laboratory investigations to rule out other causes such as infectious mononucleosis and membranous tonsillopharyngitis due to any other bacteria.

Q. What is the disease burden of diphtheria?

Diphtheria is a major vaccine preventable disease with high morbidity and mortality. About 4,489 cases have been reported in 2012 and estimated deaths in 2011 were 2,500 [World Health Organization (WHO) 2012]. The coverage for diphtheria-tetanus-pertussis 3 (DTP3) was estimated to be 83%. In India, about 2,500 cases had been reported in the year 2012 (WHO 2012).

Q. What is the etiopathogenesis?

Diphtheria is caused by the Gram-positive bacillus *Corynebacterium diphtheriae*. The mode of spread is via respiratory secretions (direct or airborne droplet) or from skin lesions. Humans are believed to be the only known reservoir. Asymptomatic carriers are important for transmission of diphtheria. Immunity (either via natural infection or vaccine-induced) does not prevent carriage.

The major virulent factor in diphtheria is the potent exotoxin. The exotoxin is secreted by toxigenic strains. The exotoxin is a polypeptide containing two chains A and B held together by a disulfide bond. The toxigenicity is obtained by "lysogenic conversion"—a process of bacteriophage-mediated transfer of *tox* gene. Inside the cell, the toxin causes cell death by inhibiting elongation factor 2 required for protein synthesis (Fig. 1). The toxin produces local tissue necrosis and can produce systemic complications affecting the cardiac, neurological, hepatic, and renal systems. The myocardium and peripheral nerves are the most affected.

CASE 2

A 3.5-year-old unimmunized girl presented to the casualty with history of low grade fever and noisy breathing for the past 3 days and was admitted to the pediatric intensive care unit with respiratory failure requiring mechanical ventilation. While intubating, a grayish white membrane extending over posterior pharynx till larynx was noted. With a strong clinical suspicion of diphtheria, the child was given antidiphtheric serum and started on intravenous penicillin. Within 24 hours, her need for ventilation increased and was found to have pulmonary edema and heart failure. Soon after, she developed refractory hypotension despite escalating doses of multiple inotropes. Echocardiographic findings were consistent with acute cardiomyopathy with poor contractility (left ventricular ejection fraction <25%). After 30 hours of admission, she developed multiple cardiac arrests and succumbed despite all resuscitative efforts.

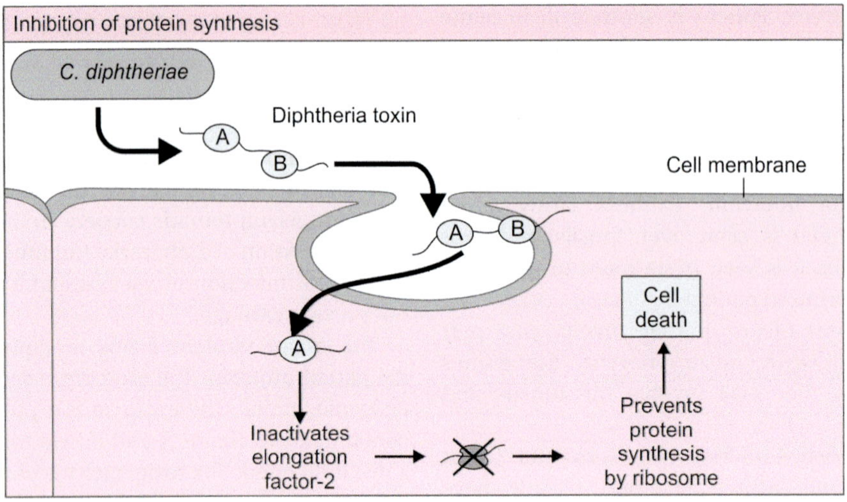

Figure 1: Effect of toxin on protein synthesis

Q. What are the typical clinical features of diphtheria based on anatomical sites involved?

After an average incubation period of 2–4 days, local signs and symptoms of inflammation develop. The onset of symptoms is typically gradual. The most common presenting symptoms are sore throat, malaise, cervical lymphadenopathy, and low grade fever. In >90% cases, the primary foci are the tonsils or pharynx (Fig. 2). The nose and larynx are the next most common sites.

Q. How do we confirm the diagnosis?

Definitive diagnosis is based on culture of respiratory secretions and discharge from cutaneous lesions. Other helpful tests include tests for toxin detection and biochemical tests.

Culture

Cultures should be obtained from the throat and nose including a portion of the membrane (if possible) or swab from beneath the membrane. Transport to the laboratory must be accomplished quickly since the media must

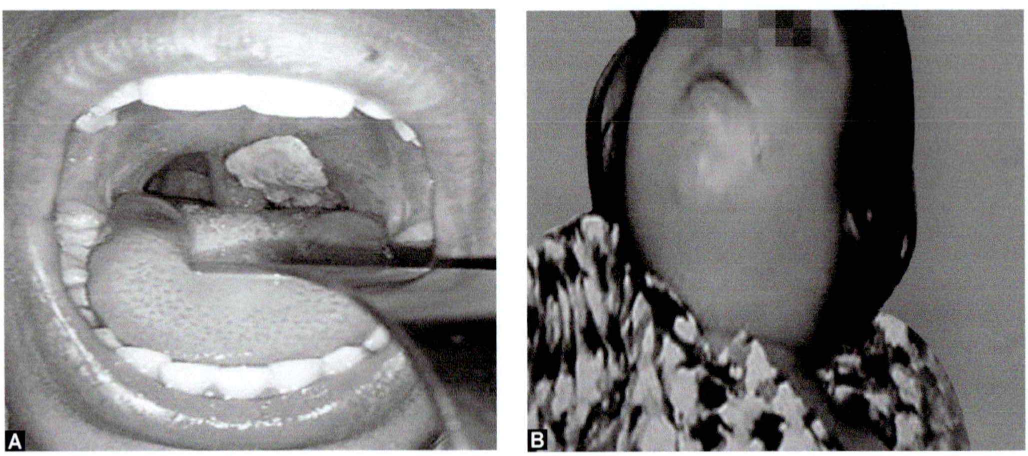

Figure 2: Tonsillar and pharyngeal diphtheria in two patients *(For color version, see Plate 3)*

be inoculated promptly. The characteristic microbiological feature includes presence of Gram-positive rods in typical "Chinese letter pattern" distribution on Gram's stain, black colonies with halos on Tinsdale mediagram stain, and presence of metachromatic granules on Loeffler's media.

Toxin detection

These tests help determine the toxigenic potential of the infecting organism. However, the decision to give antitoxin should not be based on these tests, but purely on basis of clinical profile. The two available tests are:

- Elek test: An *in vitro* assay that detects development of an immunoprecipitin band on antitoxin-impregnated filter paper laid over an agar culture of the organism
- Polymerase chain reaction: Detects subunit A of the diphtheria toxin gene.

Biochemical tests

Corynebacterium diphtheriae is catalase and cystinase positive and urease and pyrazinamidase negative.

Investigations to rule out other causes

At times when cultures are negative along with other corroborative tests, it may be useful to rule out other differentials for exudative tonsillopharyngitis. These may include but are not limited to the following:

- Total, differential counts and blood smear (for agranulocytosis, blasts in leukemia and atypical cells in infectious mononucleosis)
- Throat swab culture (for diphtheria, pyogenic bacteria, Vincent's angina and fungal infection)
- Other specific tests, if warranted such as:
  - Paul-Bunnell test (for infectious mononucleosis)
  - Bone marrow aspiration or needle biopsy
  - Biopsy of the lesion (for local malignancy).

Q. What are the complications of diphtheria?

The important complications of diphtheria include:

- Myocarditis: Typically occurs 7–14 days after onset of symptoms (varying between 1 week and 6 weeks). It is characterized by clinically evident cardiac dysfunction (dyspnea, gallop rhythm and cadiomegaly) in 10–25% patients, electrocardiogram changes (ST-T changes with QTc prolongation) in two-thirds of patients and elevated cardiac enzymes. Severe myocarditis is characterized by complete heart block, arrhythmia, and circulatory collapse
- Renal failure from direct toxin induced acute kidney injury or hypotension related pre-renal azotemia may occur in severe cases and may warrant renal replacement therapy
- Other systemic complications: Nontoxigenic *C. diphtheria* strains have been implicated in cases of endocarditis, mycotic aneurysms, osteomyelitis, and septic arthritis. If toxin production is unopposed by antitoxin, it causes early localized signs to give way to circulatory collapse, respiratory failure, stupor, coma, and death.

CASE 3

An 8-year-old boy, partially immunized, premorbidly normal, presented with low grade fever, nasal crusting, and dry cough since last 1 week. He also had change in voice, and weakness of both lower limbs for the past 24 hours. On examination, the patient had hypotonia with absent deep tendon reflexes and symmetrical weakness of all four limbs. There was palatal palsy with hypernasality of voice and grade II tonsillar hypertrophy with whitish exudates. Swab culture was suggestive of diphtheria.

Q. What are the neurological complications of diphtheria and how do these children present?

Neurological complications occur in approximately 5% of patients and in up to three-fourths of patients with severe diphtheria.

- Neurologic complications parallel the extent of primary infection and are multiphasic in onset, i.e., the severity of disease correlates with the severity of toxin production, as well as the time between the onset of symptoms and administration of antitoxin
- Local neuropathies (paralysis of the soft palate and pharyngeal muscles) are followed by cranial neuropathies (usually oculomotor and ciliary nerves, followed by facial or laryngeal paralyses) usually seen in the fifth week
- Peripheral neuritis develops weeks to months later and can range from mild weakness to total paralysis. The onset of symmetrical polyneuropathy may be from 10 days to 3 months characterized by predominantly motor neuropathy with diminished deep tendon reflexes. Weakness progresses from proximal to distal musculature (unlike other demyelinating illness progressing from distal to proximal) and there may be respiratory paralysis due to diaphragmatic involvement
- Acute flaccid paralysis reporting system can be effectively used for detection of postdiphtheric neuropathies as well.

Q. What are the treatment modalities for diphtheria and its complications? What are the practical points to remember while managing these cases?

The treatment of diphtheria consists of antibiotic therapy, antidiphtheric serum, and supportive care.

Antibiotics

The antibiotics of choice are:

- Erythromycin: 40 mg/kg/day (maximum 500 mg) four times a day for 14 days
- Penicillin G: 25,000–50,000 units/kg (maximum of 1.2 MU) intravenous every 12 hours until the patient can take orally, followed by oral penicillin V (250 mg four times a day) for 14 days.

Corynebacterium diphtheriae is usually susceptible to multiple other agents like macrolides, quinolones, tetracycline, co-trimoxazole, vancomycin, daptomycin, linezolid, and quinupristin-dalfopristin. In the setting of antibiotic resistance, vancomycin, or linezolid are reasonable alternative drugs. Otherwise, antibiogram results should be used to individualize therapy.

Antitoxin

Diphtheria antitoxin is an equine hyperimmune antiserum that binds to and inactivates the diphtheria toxin. Antitoxin is effective before toxin enters the cell and, therefore, must be administered early. The risk of hypersensitivity and/or serum sickness is approximately 10%. The history of prior allergy should be elicited and a scratch test dose of 1:100 dilution should be administered. The test dose may be followed by 0.02 mL of 1:1,000 dilution of antitoxin and then the therapeutic dose. The dose of antitoxin depends upon the site and severity of infection and is to be administered intravenously over 60 minutes so as to inactivate toxin rapidly. The dose recommended by the American Academy of Pediatrics are:

- Pharyngeal/laryngeal disease of <48 hours duration: 20,000–40,000 IU
- Nasopharyngeal disease: 40,000–60,000 IU
- Bull neck or >3 days of illness: 80,000–120,000 IU.

Other supportive measures

Airway management

Airway management is of prime importance due to risk of airway obstruction. Airway obstruction is the commonest complication of diphtheria and is an important cause of mortality. Respiratory failure is anticipated and managed aggressively in cases with extensive pseudomembrane, stridor at presentation, or "toxic bull neck". Intubation may be difficult due to extensive airway edema, mucosal friability, and inadvertent dislodgment of the pseudomembrane. Ideally, intubation should be performed by experienced personnel with an operative backup for tracheostomy for definitive airway management.

Myocarditis

Heart failure should be managed with inotropic support and decongestive therapy. Temporary pacing may be required in few cases and may be life saving. Antiarrhythmic agents may be required in few others. Carnitine has been reported to be beneficial in a study in children comparing carnitine with placebo in reducing the incidence and mortality of diphtheritic myocarditis. However, no definitive recommendations can be made on the basis of this study alone as of now. The decision to administer carnitine should be based on the severity of primary illness and left to the physician's discretion.

Flaccid paralysis

Care of the patient should be similar to management of patients with acute flaccid paralysis with appropriate positioning, splints, physiotherapy, and care of bed sores among others.

Cutaneous diphtheria

The treatment of cutaneous diphtheria consists of antibiotic therapy. Antitoxin is not usually needed as pseudomembranes and cardiac involvement is rare.

> Practical points to remember while managing diphtheria
>
> - *Airway management is of prime importance due to risk of airway obstruction*
> - *The mainstay of therapy is antibiotics and anti-diphtheretic serum in severe cases*
> - *Antitoxin should be administered as early as possible for best effect*
> - *Test dose is required before administering antitoxin in all cases, as risk of hypersensitivity is high*
> - *Antitoxin is not needed in localized cutaneous diphtheria, as pseudomembrane and cardiac involvement are rare.*

Q. What isolation procedures should be followed and what antibiotic prophylaxis should be given to contacts? If a contact is identified to be a carrier without any clinical symptoms, what should be the approach to such a case?

Isolation

Patients with respiratory diphtheria should be isolated with contact precautions for cutaneous disease. Isolation should be continued until two consecutive cultures taken at least 24 hours apart are negative.

Contact prophylaxis

Close contacts (e.g., relatives, friends, and caretakers who regularly visit the home and medical personnel exposed to secretions) should be given antimicrobial prophylaxis. If immunization is not current (last dose within a year), diphtheria-tetanus (DT) should be administered. After cultures have been obtained, contacts should be treated with a single dose of benzathine penicillin G (for children <6 years of age—600,000 units intramuscularly, and for ≥6 years of age—1.2 million units intramuscularly) or oral erythromycin at a dose of 40mg/kg/day for 7–10 days.

Asymptomatic carrier

When an asymptomatic carrier is identified, the following steps are to be taken:

- Antimicrobial prophylaxis is administered for 7–10 days
- An age-appropriate preparation of DT is to be immediately administered if the patient has not received a booster injection within 1 year
- The carrier is placed in strict isolation (for respiratory tract colonization) or contact isolation (for cutaneous colonization only) until at least two subsequent cultures taken 24 hours apart after cessation of therapy are negative

- Repeat cultures are performed at a minimum of 2 weeks after completion of therapy in patients and carriers. If results are positive, an additional 10-day course of oral erythromycin should be administered and follow-up cultures performed
- Even antimicrobial agents fail to eradicate carrier status in 100% of individuals.

Q. In case 2, we saw that despite best efforts and administration of antitoxin at admission, the child succumbed. What are the causes of death in diphtheria in the best settings and what is the optimal timing of administration of therapy?

- Death due to mechanical airway obstruction or cardiac involvement with circulatory collapse occurs in at least 10% of patients with respiratory tract diphtheria
- For patients in whom disease is recognized on day 1 and antitoxin therapy is promptly initiated, the mortality rate is approximately 1%. If appropriate treatment is withheld until day 4, the mortality rate can raise up to 20%.

Q. Is vaccination still the single preventive measure than multiple modalities once fatal disease occurs?

- Diphtheria vaccine is available in the form of DPT/DT and contains 10–25 Lf doses of toxoid. It is used for both primary and booster immunization in children
- In India, the WHO schedule for primary immunization in the form of three doses of diphtheria, pertussis, tetanus at 6, 10, and 14 weeks of age and then two booster doses at 15–18 months and 4–6 years age is followed
- Most infants (94–100%) develop protective antibody titers after primary immunization
- Disease in previously immunized individuals is milder and less likely to be fatal. The duration of immunity after primary immunization has been variously reported in different studies to be ranging from 16 months to 10 years. Therefore, diphtheria vaccine is advised once every 10 years for later age for definitive protection.

LEARNING POINTS

- Diphtheria is a major vaccine preventable disease with high morbidity and mortality
- It should be suspected in any unimmunized child presenting with viral prodrome and the classical pseudomembrane
- Important complications associated with unfavorable outcomes include acute airway obstruction, myocarditis, and polyneuritis
- The mainstay of therapy is antibiotics and antidiphtheritic serum in severe cases
- Antitoxin should be administered as early as possible for best effect
- Close contacts should be given antimicrobial prophylaxis and diphtheria-tetanus if unimmunized
- Diphtheria vaccine available in the form of diphtheria-tetanus-pertussis/diphtheria-tetanus is used for both primary and booster immunization in children.

Acknowledgment

The authors would like to thank Dr Vinay M for helping in editing the manuscript.

SUGGESTED READINGS

1. American Academy of Pediatrics. Diphtheria. In: Pickering LK, Baker, Kimberlin DW, Long SS, editors. Red Book 2012: 2012 Report of the Committee on Infectious Diseases. 29th ed. Elk Grove Village, IL: American Academy of Pediatrics; 2012.
2. Clarridge JE, Popovic T, Inzana TJ. Diphtheria and other corynebacterial and coryneform infections. In: Hausler WJ, Sussman M, editors. Topley and Wilson's Microbiology and Microbial Infections. New York City: Oxford University Press; 1998. p. 347.
3. Efstratiou A, Engler KH, Mazurova IK, Glushkevich T, Vuopio-Varkila J, Popovic T. Current approaches to the laboratory diagnosis of diphtheria. J Infect Dis. 2000;181 Suppl 1:S138.
4. Farizo KM, Strebel PM, Chen RT, Kimbler A, Cleary TJ, Cochi SL. Fatal respiratory disease due to Corynebacterium diphtheriae: case report and review of guidelines for management, investigation, and control. Clin Infect Dis. 1993;16:59-68.
5. Jayashree M, Shruthi N, Singhi S. Predictors of outcome in patients with diphtheria receiving intensive care. Indian Pediatr. 2006;43:155.
6. Kneen R, Nguyen MD, Solomon T, Pham NG, Parry CM, Nguyen TT, et al. Clinical features and predictors of diphtheritic cardiomyopathy in Vietnamese children. Clin Infect Dis. 2004;39:1591.

CHAPTER

20

Pertussis

Bhagwan S Sharma, Mukesh K Gupta

CASE 1

A 3-year-old girl presented with history of paroxysms of cough for 2 weeks preceded by viral prodrome of 2–3 days duration. She was prescribed cough syrup, to which there was no response. She continued to have paroxysms of cough initiated at times by crying or exposure to smoke, at times followed by vomiting and more during daytime. She was also breathless at times and occasionally had an inspiratory loud sound. She was incompletely immunized. On examination, vitals were stable, weight (12.5 kg), and height (91 cm) were between 10th and 25th centiles. Throat and systemic examination, including respiratory system, were normal.

Q. What are the possible differentials in this child?

Fever at the beginning of illness indicates infective origin. Paroxysmal cough since 2 weeks with post-tussive vomiting, inspiratory sound (whoop) in a 3-year-old child who is partially immunized and absolutely normal in between the episodes suggest a pertussis-like illness. Absence of findings in throat examination and absence of lymphadenopathy rules out diphtheria and long history with absence of stridor rules out croup as diagnostic possibility. There was no history of previous episodes of wheezing, allergy, or asthma in the family, thereby making hyper reactive airway disease less likely.

Q. What is pertussis and what are the etiological agents implicated?

Pertussis is an acute infectious disease which usually affects young children and is caused by *Bordetella pertussis* a fastidious Gram-negative coccobacillus. Three other species (*B. parapertussis, B. holmesii,* and *B. bronchiseptica*) can also cause a pertussis-like illness in humans but milder, as they do not produce pertussis toxin. Coinfection of *B. pertussis* and *B. parapertussis* may also occur. Pertussis-like symptoms may also be caused by adenoviruses, respiratory syncytial virus, human parainfluenza viruses, influenza viruses, *Mycoplasma pneumoniae,* and other agents.

It is clinically characterized by insidious onset with mild fever and an irritating cough which gradually becomes paroxysmal with the characteristic whoop, many a times with cyanosis and vomiting. The disease spectrum varies from mild illness without whoop like a usual viral upper respiratory infection to a classical severe illness.

Q. How common is this disease?

Before widespread use of the pertussis-containing vaccines, it was a common childhood disease and a major cause of child and infant mortality. Today as well, it is one of the potentially lethal diseases of the infants and young children who have not been immunized, malnourished, or have other respiratory infections. Routine childhood immunization under Universal Immunization Programme led to a reduction in disease incidence. However, it still remains a public health problem of concern in our country. Globally, there are 20–40 million annual cases with 200,000–400,000 deaths. Reliable epidemiologic data from India is lacking.

Q. How does it spread and how contagious is pertussis?

Following are the salient features of epidemiology of pertussis:
- Transmission: Through respiratory droplets by coughing and sneezing
- Communicability: Maximum in catarrhal stage, secondary attack rate up to 80%
- Infective period: Extends from a week after exposure to about 3 weeks after the onset of paroxysmal stage
- Incubation period: Varies from 3 to 14 days (not >3 weeks)
- Reservoir: Usually human adolescents and adults. Very limited survival outside human body.

Pathogenesis

Bordetella pertussis is not invasive; it produces a local infection and primarily a toxin-mediated disease. It produces a variety of biologically active substances (pertussis toxin, filamentous hemagglutinin, agglutinogens, adenylate cyclase, pertactin, and tracheal cytotoxin), which are responsible for attachment to ciliated respiratory epithelial cells, inhibited clearance of organisms, and local epithelial damage resulting in inflammation and necrosis of the mucosa.

Q. What are the clinical features?

There are three stages in the clinical course (Flowchart 1):
1. Catarrhal stage: It usually lasts for about 10 days and is characterized by insidious onset of congestion, rhinorrhea, low-grade fever, sneezing, lacrimation, anorexia, malaise, and hacking night cough that becomes diurnal later
2. Paroxysmal stage: It lasts for 2–4 weeks and is characterized by one or more of the following:
   i. Intermittent, irritative hacking paroxysmal cough
   ii. Choking, gasping, eyes watering, and bulging of eyes
   iii. Occasional coughing up of mucous plugs
   iv. Post-tussive exhaustion
   v. Coughing in long spasms with the face turning red, or sometimes blue
3. Convalescent stage: Coughing wanes and improves during the convalescent stage.

Each stage lasts about 2 weeks. However, immunized children do better, with shortening of all stages. Conjunctival hemorrhages and petechiae on the upper body are common due to severe spasmodic coughing.

Q. When should one suspect pertussis?

It should be suspected in all patients who have incessant cough for 2 weeks especially if physical examination is unremarkable. Among infants, cough lasting ≥2 weeks with one of

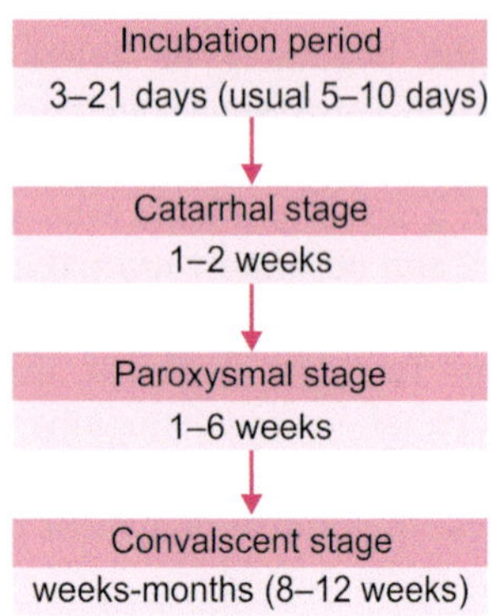

Flowchart 1: Clinical course of pertussis

the following symptoms, such as paroxysms of coughing, inspiratory "whoop", post-tussive vomiting, or apnea (with or without cyanosis) in the absence of a more likely diagnosis, are highly suggestive of pertussis. However, disease presentation varies with age and history of previous exposure or vaccination. In strong epedimeologial linkage, any child with flu-like illness should be suspected for whooping cough irrespective of duration of cough.

CASE 2

A 4-month-old infant was brought with history of cough for 5–7 days and a day before he had one coughing episode when it seemed like he stopped breathing. He was alright 7 days back when his mother noticed him to have congested and running nose. His mother assumed that he got common cold from his siblings. He was younger of the two siblings, developmentally normal, had received two doses of DPT [diphtheria, pertussis (whooping cough), and tetanus] vaccines, and was healthy till the day of presentation. His general and systemic examination was normal.

The fact that he had a possible apneic episode suggested that his illness was not a simple common cold. Since the systemic examination was normal, the central nervous system causes of apnea in infants (meningitis, intracranial bleed, and hypoglycemia) were unlikely. Absence of tachypnea, cyanosis, and intercostal retractions except during the paroxysm of cough, ruled out respiratory failure as a cause of apnea.

Q. What are the possible complications and who are at risk?

Infants under 6 months of age have a higher risk of morbidity and mortality particularly, those who have not received the primary vaccination series against pertussis. Box 1 summarizes the complications.

Q. What are the suggested laboratory investigations?

Table 1 summarizes the available investigations. Figure 1 summarizes timing of various laboratory tests.

Box 1: Complications of pertussis

Complications in young children
- Secondary bacterial pneumonia—most common
- Neurologic complications—seizures, encephalopathy more common among infants
- Otitis media
- Anorexia
- Dehydration
- Pneumothorax
- Epistaxis
- Subdural hematomas
- Hernias
- Rectal prolapse

Complications in adolescents and adults
- Difficulty sleeping
- Urinary incontinence
- Pneumonia
- Rib fracture

TABLE 1: Pertussis laboratory diagnosis

Investigation	Comments
Culture*	• Gold standard
Polymerase chain reaction	• Can confirm pertussis in an outbreak • Highly sensitive • High false-positive rate
Serology (detecting specific anti-pertussis toxin antibodies)#	• Can confirm illness late (2–3 weeks) in the course of infection • Many tests have unproven or unknown clinical accuracy
Direct fluorescent antibody test§	• Low sensitivity and variable specificity • Should not be used for laboratory confirmation • Dependent on the experience of the lab technician

*Not very sensitive (<60%) and is positive during the catarrhal stage and escalating paroxysmal stage. The highest rates are obtained with infants, false negative in those received amoxicillin or erythromycin. A flexible swab kept in the posterior nasopharynx until the patient coughs is one way to obtain the specimen.

#In infants liable to interference with maternal antibodies. The presence of a high level of anti-pertussis toxin antibodies in the serum of a nonvaccinated individual indicates infection.

§Direct fluorescent antibody testing of nasopharyngeal secretions is rapid, but has low sensitivity and variable specificity.

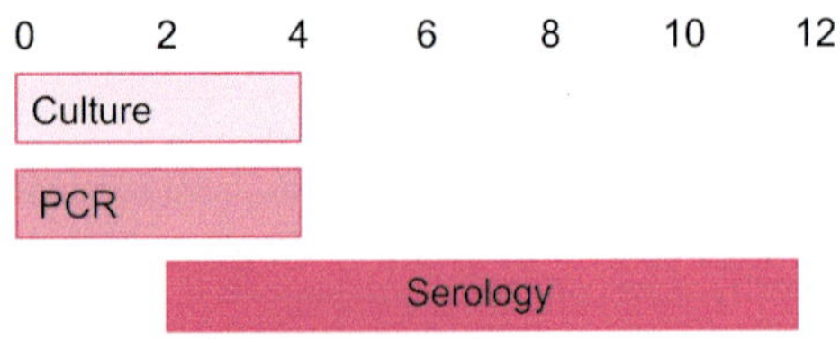

PCR, polymerase chain reaction.

Figure 1: Optimal timing of laboratory testing for diagnosis (weeks)

Q. How do we diagnose this disease?

Box 2 provides the diagnostic criteria for pertussis.

Box 2: Diagnosis of pertussis

Clinical case definition

In the absence of a more likely diagnosis a cough illness lasting ≥2 weeks with one of the following symptoms:

- Paroxysms of coughing
- Inspiratory whoop
- Post-tussive vomiting, or
- Apnea (with or without cyanosis) (for infants aged <1 year only)

Laboratory criteria for diagnosis

- Isolation of *Bordetella pertussis* from clinical specimen
- Positive polymerase chain reaction (PCR) for *B. pertussis*

Epidemiologic linkage

- Contact with a laboratory-confirmed case of pertussis*

Case classification

- Probable: meets the clinical case definition, is not laboratory confirmed
- Confirmed:
  - A case of acute cough illness of any duration with a positive culture for *B. pertussis*
  - A case that meets the clinical case definition and is confirmed by PCR, or
  - A case that meets the clinical definition and is epidemiologically linked directly to a case confirmed by either culture or PCR.

*An illness meeting the clinical case definition should be classified as "probable" rather than "confirmed" if it occurs in a patient who has contact with an infant aged <1 year who is polymerase chain reaction positive for pertussis and has ≥1 sign or symptom and cough duration <14 days (classified as "probable" case).

Source: Centers for Disease Control and Prevention, Vaccine Preventable Diseases, Surveillance Manual. 5th Edition. Pertussis. 2011.

Q. How do you manage a child with pertussis?

Supportive therapy is the mainstay of treatment. The goals of therapy include limiting the number of paroxysms, observing the severity of cough, providing assistance when necessary, and maximizing nutrition, rest, and recovery. Oxygenation, respiratory support, or mechanical ventilation should be provided as necessary. Infants should be carefully observed for apnea, cyanosis, or hypoxia. Table 2 provides the details of antibiotics therapy in pertussis. Antibiotics have a role if started early in the course.

TABLE 2: Antibiotic therapy in pertussis

Drug	Dose, frequency, and duration
Azithromycin (preferred agent for all ages)	• <1 month—10 mg/kg/day once daily for 5 days • ≥1 months infants and children—10 mg/kg on day 1 and 5 mg/kg/day on days 2–5 once daily • Adults—500 mg on day 1 then 250 mg/day on days 2–5 once daily
Erythromycin: associated with infantile hypertrophic pyloric stenosis—not preferred in <1 month	• 40–50 mg/kg/day, maximum 2 g/day, QID for 14 days
Clarithromycin: not recommended <1 month	• 15 mg/kg/day BD for 7 days (maximum 1 g/day)
Cotrimoxazole (TMP-SMZ): alternative agent in those with hypersensitivity to macrolides, contraindicated in <2 months	• Infants >2 months: TMP 8 mg/kg/day, SMZ 40 mg/kg/day • Max adults: TMP 320 mg/day, SMZ 1,600 mg/ • BD for 14 days

*Although antimicrobial agents initiated during the paroxysmal stage do not affect the duration and severity of illness, they can hasten the eradication of B pertussis in the respiratory tract and help to prevent spread. Antibiotics may also prevent or alleviate secondary bacterial infection.

BD, twice a day; QID, four times a day; TMP, trimethoprim; SMZ, sulfamethoxazole.

Q. What are the indications for hospitalization?

Hospitalization should be strongly considered for patients at risk for severe disease and complications. These include all infants <3 months; infants between 3 and 6 months with severe cough spasm; prematurely born young infants; and infants or children with underlying pulmonary, cardiac, or neuromuscular disease. Inpatient care is also required for patients with intractable nausea and vomiting, failure to thrive, seizures, or encephalopathy, or for patients with sustained hypoxemia during paroxysms of cough requiring supplemental oxygen.

Q. Is there any role of chemoprophylaxis?

Since the postexposure prophylaxis of contacts has not been shown to reduce the incidence of culture-confirmed cases or clinical symptoms with additional problems of cost, side effects of drugs, and issue of adherence, in most of the clinical situations, the diagnosis of pertussis in the index case is only presumptive. Therefore, it is restricted only for household and close contacts of the patients. All other contacts should be placed on surveillance and antibiotics started at the first respiratory symptom. Course of antibiotic is to be administered to close contacts within 3 weeks of exposure, especially in high-risk settings (neonates, unimmunized or partially immunized young infants, and individuals with other comorbidities). Drugs and doses are same as in treatment schedule (the effectiveness of clarithromycin has not been proven but is inferred).

Q. How to immunize children against pertussis?

Recommended immunization schedule include:

- Three doses of the trivalent vaccine (DTP or DTaP) or pentavalent vaccine including DTP or DTaP components should be administered at 6, 10, and 14 weeks
- Two boosters are administered at 18–24 months and 4–6 years
- A single dose of Tdap (tetanus, diphtheria, and pertussis) is recommended at the age of 10 years.

Considering the faster waning of immunity with acellular pertussis (aP) vaccines and superior priming with whole-cell pertussis (wP) vaccines, aP vaccines should be avoided for the primary series of infant vaccination. However, aP vaccines may be preferred when there are severe adverse effects with previous dose(s) of wP vaccines or children with neurologic disorders, if resources permit. For the first and second booster doses as well, wP vaccine is preferred. However, considering a higher reactogenicity, aP vaccine/combination can be considered for the boosters in individual cases after one to one discussion. Indian Academy of Pediatrics recommends that if any aP-containing vaccine is used, it must at least have three or more components in the product, the more the better.

Tdap during pregnancy

Indian Academy of Pediatrics/Advisory Committee on Vaccines and Immunization Practices suggests immunization of pregnant women with a single dose of Tdap during the third trimester (during 27 through 36 weeks gestation) regardless of prior vaccination and it has to be repeated in every pregnancy.

Children aged 7–10 years, who are not fully immunized with the childhood DTwP/DTaP vaccine series, should receive Tdap vaccine as the first dose in the catch-up series; for remaining doses use Td vaccine.

Q. Does herd immunity protect most people?

Since pertussis spreads so easily (high communicability), protective immunity decreases over time (waning immunity), and aP vaccines may prevent colonization, we cannot rely on herd immunity to protect everyone.

Q. Do pertussis vaccines protect from severe disease?

A child, who has been vaccinated and gets pertussis, is less likely to have severe infection. Typically, cough would not last as many days and coughing paroxysms, whooping, and vomiting are likely to occur less frequently. When vaccinated children get pertussis, fewer have apnea (life-threatening pauses in breathing), cyanosis (blue/purplish skin coloration due to lack of oxygen), and vomiting.

Q. Do pertussis vaccines protect for a lifetime? If a child has whooping cough, does he still need to be administered a pertussis vaccine?

Considering the disease-related morbidity and mortality, it is essential to vaccinate the children as pertussis vaccines are effective (80–90%). They typically offer high levels of protection for the first 2 years of getting vaccinated, however, protection decreases over time. This is known as waning immunity. Hence, there is a need to administer booster doses time to time as per recommendations. Similarly, natural infection can also protect for few years. Hence, a child who suffered from pertussis should also receive the age appropriate vaccination.

LEARNING POINTS

- Pertussis causes significant morbidity in children
- It can affect from neonatal period to adolescent life
- Diagnosis is mainly clinical and laboratory diagnosis is not always required
- Treatment is mainly supportive and antibiotics have a role if started early in course of the disease
- Vaccinations have good protective value against pertussis.

SUGGESTED READINGS

1. American Academy of Pediatrics. Pertussis. In: Pickering L, Baker CJ, Kimberlin D, Long SS, editors. Red Book: 2009 Report of the Committee on Infectious Diseases, 28th edition. Elk Grove Village, Illinois: American Academy of Pediatrics; 2009. pp. 504-19.
2. Centers for Disease Control and Prevention (CDC). Updated recommendations for use of tetanus toxoid, reduced diphtheria toxoid, and acellular pertussis vaccine (Tdap) in pregnant women--Advisory Committee on Immunization Practices (ACIP), 2012. MMWR Morb Mortal Wkly Rep. 2013;62(7):131-5.
3. Vashishtha VM, Choudhury P, Bansal CP, Yewale VN, Agarwal R, editors. IAP guidebook on immunization 2013-14. National Publication House, Indian Academy of Pediatrics: Gwalior; 2014.
4. Pertussis. In: Andrew Kroger, Jennifer Hamborsky, Charles (Skip) Wolfe (Eds). Epidemiology and Prevention of Vaccine-Preventable Diseases: The Pink Book. 13th ed. Public Health Foundation; 2015.
5. Tiwari T, Murphy TV, Moran J. Recommended Antimicrobial Agents for Treatment and Postexposure Prophylaxis of Pertussis, 2005 CDC Guidelines.

CHAPTER

21

Community Acquired Pneumonia

Dinesh Raj

> **CASE 1**
>
> A 5-month-old child was brought to the pediatric outpatient department with complaints of fever, cough and tachypnea for 3 days. The child was exclusively breastfed and was accepting breastfeeds well. On examination, the child was alert and interested in surroundings, had a respiratory rate of 64/min with no accessory muscle use. Oxygen saturation was 98% on room air. On auscultation, diffuse crackles in most areas were appreciated. The child was started on oral amoxicillin for 5 days and asked to review after 2 days, and early in case of any danger signs.

Q. What does the child have?

The child has community acquired pneumonia (CAP), which is the leading cause of under-five mortality around the world, attributing to at least one-fifth of the deaths. The World Health Organization (WHO) definition of CAP includes presence of cough with tachypnea/respiratory difficulty.

Q. What are the etiologic agents causing community acquired pneumonia?

The etiology of CAP depends on age of the child, season, and geographic location. Viruses are responsible for almost half of the cases of CAP in young children under 5 years of age. Among bacterial causes, *Streptococcus pneumoniae* accounts for almost one-third cases in all age groups. Sometimes, polymicrobial or mixed infection (viral-viral, viral-bacterial, bacterial-bacterial) may be present. Table 1 enumerates the various etiologic agents grouped by age of the child.

TABLE 1: Etiological agents of community acquired pneumonia in various age groups

Age group	Organisms
Under 2 months	• Common: Gram-negative bacteria *(Klebsiella pneumoniae, Escherichia coli), Staphylococcus aureus* • Uncommon: *Streptococcus pneumoniae, Haemophilus influenzae, Ureaplasma*, CMV, HSV
2 months to 5 years	• Common: *S. pneumoniae, H. influenzae, S. aureus, K. pneumoniae, Chlamydiae, Mycoplasma*, viruses (RSV, influenza, parainfluenza, adenovirus, human metapneumovirus) • Uncommon: Measles, varicella, pertussis, *Mycobacterium tuberculosis*
Above 5 years	• Common: *S. pneumoniae, Mycoplasma, Chlamydia* • Uncommon: *H. influenzae, S. aureus, M. tuberculosis*, viruses (adenovirus, EBV, influenza, parainfluenza, RSV, rhinovirus)

CMV, cytomegalovirus; HSV, herpes simplex virus; RSV, respiratory syncytial virus; EBV, Epstein-Barr virus.

Q. What are the usual clinical features of a child with community acquired pneumonia?

Clinical feature of CAP are nonspecific and vary with age and etiological agents. Usually in infants and young children, CAP is preceded by features suggestive of an upper respiratory tract infection, i.e., rhinorrhea and cough. Fever and cough may be variably present. No clinical sign or symptom can be used to diagnose pneumonia definitively. However, tachypnea is the most sensitive and specific sign of CAP with abnormal chest radiographs. Age-related definition of fast breathing as suggested by WHO for the diagnosis of pneumonia is widely acceptable (Table 2). Respiratory rate should be counted for one whole minute, as there may be irregular breathing, particularly in infants. Associated fever may increase breathing rate by 10 breaths per minute with each degree celsius rise in temperature.

Older children may present with abrupt onset fever with chills, cough, and chest pain usually suggestive of bacterial pneumonia. Atypical pneumonia may present with gradual onset of low grade fever, nonproductive cough, malaise, and headache. Auscultatory findings include crackles, bronchial breathing, decreased breath sounds, and wheezing. Presence of wheezing more frequently suggests viral or atypical pneumonia. Chest pain, abdominal pain (due to involvement of lower lobes), and neck pain/rigidity (due to involvement of upper lobes) can be observed by older children.

TABLE 2: Definition of fast breathing as defined by the World Health Organization

Age group	Respiratory rate per minute
<2 months	≥60
2 months to 1 year	≥50
1 year to 5 years	≥40
≥5 years	≥30

CASE 2

A 6-month-old bottle fed infant was brought to the emergency department with complaints of fever and cough for 2 days. Mother also noticed that the child was unable to feed properly and breathing unusually fast. The child was immunized for his age. On examination, the child was febrile to touch, heart rate of 132/min, respiratory rate of 60/min, and lower chest indrawing. Oxygen saturation was 91% at room air. Lung auscultation revealed diffuse crepts and bronchial breathing in right infrascapular region. The child was hospitalized and started on humidified oxygen. Intravenous access was obtained, blood sent for investigations, and intravenous antibiotics were started. Chest radiograph of the child is shown in figure 1.

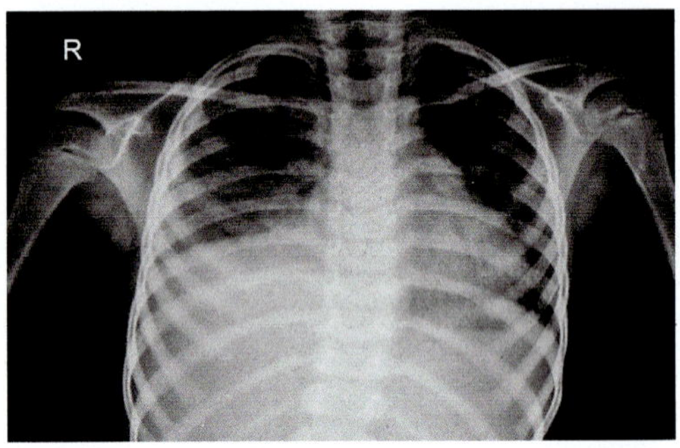

Figure 1: Chest radiograph showing inhomogeneous opacity in right lower zone

Q. How is severity of community acquired pneumonia assessed?

Severity of CAP is related to type and virulence of the microorganism, host susceptibility, and resistance pattern of the organism. Clinical features reflecting increased severity of CAP include accessory muscle use, chest retractions, nasal flaring, head nodding, grunting, cyanosis, altered sensorium, and impending respiratory failure. Apart from that, the child's overall clinical appearance may predict increased severity. Therefore, a "toxic" looking child with tachycardia, respiratory distress, and increased capillary refill should be considered for immediate hospitalization.

There are no validated scoring systems to predict severe CAP with complicated with reasonable sensitivity and specificity. The revised WHO classification now includes only two categories: (i) pneumonia, defined as children having fast breathing and/or chest indrawing which can be managed with oral amoxicillin administered on an ambulatory basis and (ii) severe pneumonia, i.e., children with pneumonia having danger signs needing injectable antibiotics.

Q. What are the indications of hospitalization?

Indications of hospitalization in CAP include:

- Hypoxemia—oxygen saturation below 90% on room air
- Feeding difficulty
- Overall toxic appearance of the child
- Suspected/documented infection with methicillin resistant *S. aureus*
- Failure to respond to oral antibiotics
- Inadequate observation/supervision by family

Q. What laboratory investigations are needed while managing community acquired pneumonia?

Routine imaging is not warranted, especially in those who can be managed as outpatients. However, chest radiograph is useful in confirming the presence of CAP, assessing the extent, identifying presence of any complications, and ruling out other possibilities like foreign body aspiration. It should, therefore, be obtained in all children with severe pneumonia, those needing hospitalization, and when complications are suspected.

Radiographic findings include focal or multifocal alveolar opacities, interstitial changes, and/or pleural effusion. Repeat or follow-up imaging is not required in children having uneventful recovery. However, those with progressively increasing symptoms or clinical deterioration over 48–72 hours should have a repeat imaging.

Moreover, lung ultrasound and/or computed tomography scan may be needed on a case to case basis when complications (parapneumonic effusions, empyema, necrotizing pneumonia, and empyema) are expected.

Blood counts and serum inflammatory markers (C-reactive protein, procalcitonin) may only partly be useful in differentiating between bacterial and viral etiology. Yield of blood culture is very low in CAP; however, it should be obtained in children with severe pneumonia and worsening symptoms. Microbiological isolation is usually difficult in CAP, but may be attempted in children with unusual course and poor response to standard antimicrobials. When indicated, nasopharyngeal aspirate/nasal swabs for viral pathogens or bronchoalveolar lavage can be obtained. For sick children needing mechanical ventilation, tracheal aspirate can be obtained. Viral antigen detection or PCR can be done to identify viruses. Gram staining/culture and antigen detection can be done for bacteria. Isolation of any virus/bacteria from the upper airway does not necessarily prove causation. Urine antigen for *S. pneumoniae* is not recommended due to high false positivity due to nasopharyngeal colonization.

Q. What is the management of community acquired pneumonia?

Case management is the cornerstone of pneumonia control and can be managed as per revised WHO guidelines. It involves classification of the severity of pneumonia using simple clinical signs including fast breathing, chest indrawing and danger signs, and then advocating the appropriate treatment. Treatment essentially includes home care advice, antibiotics for home treatment, or admission/referral to a higher-level health facility. The revised WHO classification recommends oral amoxicillin at 20–40 mg/kg dose twice a day for 5 days for home management of pneumonia. Severe pneumonia should be managed with a combination of ampicillin (or benzyl penicillin) and gentamicin. Children with severe pneumonia who failed on first-line medications should be put on ceftriaxone. For children above 5 years, macrolide antibiotics should be considered, as *M. pneumoniae* and *C. Pneumoniae* more often cause CAP in this age group.

Recently, there are concerns regarding WHO case management, as the diagnostic criteria often leads to overdiagnosis and overtreatment which may complicate the emerging antibiotic resistance. It is, therefore, important to individualize the treatment especially where inpatient facilities are available. Regarding choice of antibiotics, British Thoracic Society guidelines also suggest amoxicillin as the first choice with co-amoxiclav, cefaclor, and azithromycin as alternatives. They suggest intravenous antibiotics if child is unable to take orally (or has vomiting), has signs of septicaemia, or has evidence of complicated pneumonia. The options include amoxicillin, co-amoxiclav, and third-generation cephalosporins. The Infectious Diseases Society of America guidelines recommend amoxicillin as first-line oral therapy for CAP. For inpatient treatment, ampicillin or penicillin G is recommended for fully immunized children and in areas with absence of high level penicillin resistance for invasive *S. pneumoniae*. Otherwise, third-generation cephalosporin is indicated, especially in children with life-threatening infections.

Dehydrated children and those with difficulty feeding should receive intravenous fluids. One-third of the children with CAP may have hyponatremia, so dextrose (normal saline or N/2 in 5% dextrose) may be used with monitoring of serum electrolytes.

There is no consensus on the appropriate treatment duration for CAP. However, for uncomplicated CAP managed as outpatient, 5-day treatment seems appropriate. Children with severe pneumonia managed as inpatients may need slightly longer (at least 5-7 days), and should be decided on a case to case basis. Table 3 is shows commonly used drugs for CAP.

TABLE 3: Commonly used antibiotics and their doses

Antibiotic	Dosage	Dose interval
Amoxicillin	Oral: 30–40 mg/kg/day	12 hourly
Azithromycin	Oral: 10 mg/kg on day 1; 5 mg/kg from day 2 to 5	24 hourly
Ampicillin	IV: 150–200 mg/kg/day	6 hourly
Gentamicin	IV/IM: 7.5 mg/kg/day	24 hourly
Penicillin	IV/IM: 200,000 U/kg/day	6 hourly
Cefuroxime	IV: 100–150 mg/kg/day Oral: 20–30 mg/kg/day	8 hourly 8–12 hourly
Ceftriaxone	IV: 50–100 mg/kg/day	12 hourly
Cefotaxime	IV:100–200 mg/kg/day	8 hourly
Cloxacillin	IV: 50–100 mg/kg/day	6 hourly
Vancomycin	IV: 40–60 mg/kg/day	6–8 hourly
Clindamycin	IV: 40 mg/kg/day	6–8 hourly

IV, intravenous; IM, intramuscular.

CASE 3

An 18-month-old girl child, premorbidly normal, was brought to the emergency department with complaints of fever and cough for 5 days, and difficulty breathing for 1 day. On examination, the child was toxic, febrile, and irritable. Respiratory rate was 54/min, oxygen saturation was 85% on room air, and improved to 92% with supplementation of oxygen. A chest radiograph was obtained which was suggestive of bilateral patchy opacities, multiple thin walled cystic spaces, and pneumothorax with shift of mediastinum. She child was shifted immediately to pediatric intensive care unit and started on ceftriaxone and cloxacillin. A chest drainage tube was inserted which led to partial relief in symptoms. Even after 2 days, she continued to remain tachypneic and developed a pneumothorax on the other side for which immediate needle decompression was done and a chest tube was inserted subsequently. Mechanical ventilation was initiated as she continued to be in distress with borderline oxygen saturation. Subsequent chest radiograph showed hydropneumothorax which did not improve despite manipulating the chest tube already in place. Another chest tube was inserted and she was shifted to high frequency ventilation. Pleural fluid culture grew *S. aureus*. She was started on nasogastric feeds. After 3 weeks of ventilation, she was gradually weaned and extubated.

Q. What are the complications of community acquired pneumonia?

The pulmonary complications include parapneumonic effusion, empyema, pneumothorax, necrotizing pneumonia, lung abscess, bronchopleural fistula, and respiratory failure. Parapneumonic effusion and empyema occur in roughly 0.7% of children with pneumonia. Apart from lungs, metastatic infection can result in meningitis, endocarditis, osteomyelitis, septic arthritis, and abscesses. Sepsis and septic shock may lead to multiorgan dysfunction.

Necrotizing pneumonia is necrosis and liquefaction of pulmonary parenchyma and is a potentially serious complication of pneumonia. The main causes are *S. pneumoniae* (especially serotype 3 and serogroup 19), *S. aureus,* and *Klebsiella pneumoniae.* The patients usually have a toxic appearance and unusually long course.

Q. How is *Staphylococcal pneumonia* different?

Staphylococcus aureus is an uncommon but important cause of CAP, particularly in infants. It may also occur as a complication of seasonal influenza. Children are usually more toxic and sicker at admission. There may be associated pyoderma and/or minor or major injury. It is more common during rainy season. These children may develop complications as discussed above, more often. Therefore, it should be suspected in children who are severely ill and are not improving with standard therapy for CAP. The *S. aureus* isolates are increasingly found to be methicillin resistant *S. aureus* (MRSA). For treatment of suspected staphylococcal pneumonia, cloxacillin should be added to therapy. If MRSA is suspected, vancomycin may be added in place of cloxacillin. A close watch for complications should be done and managed accordingly. Presence of empyema and air leaks often complicates the management of staphylococcal pneumonia.

Q. How can community acquired pneumonia be prevented?

Definite risk factors of CAP include lack of exclusive breastfeeding during first 6 months, malnutrition, low birth weight, lack of measles immunization, indoor air pollution, and overcrowding. *Haemophilus influenzae* vaccination has recently been introduced in many states in universal immunization schedule. Pneumococcal vaccination can also be effective intervention to reduce pneumonia in developing countries, but issues regarding lack of data regarding prevalent strains and high cost need to be sorted out.

LEARNING POINTS

- Community acquired pneumonia (CAP) is the leading cause of under-five mortality around the world attributing to at least one-fifth of the deaths
- Tachypnea is the most sensitive and specific sign of CAP with abnormal chest radiographs
- Case management is the cornerstone of pneumonia control and should be managed as per revised the World Health Organization (WHO) guidelines
- Revised WHO classification includes only two categories: pneumonia, defined as children having fast breathing and/or chest indrawing and severe pneumonia, defined as children with pneumonia having danger signs
- Indications of hospitalization in CAP include hypoxemia (oxygen saturation below 90–92%), respiratory distress, feeding difficulty, toxic appearance, and suspicion of methicillin resistant *S. aureus*
- The complications of CAP include parapneumonic effusion, empyema, pneumothorax, necrotizing pneumonia, lung abscess, bronchopleural fistula, and respiratory failure
- In case of suspicion of staphylococcal pneumonia, cloxacillin/vancomycin should be added.

SUGGESTED READINGS

1. Bradley JS, Byington CL, Shah SS, Alverson B, Carter ER, Harrison C, et al. Pediatric Infectious Diseases Society and the Infectious Diseases Society of America. The management of community-acquired pneumonia in infants and children older than 3 months of age: clinical practice guidelines by the Pediatric Infectious Diseases Society and the Infectious Disease Society of America. Clin Infect Dis. 2011;53(7): e25-76.
2. Geneva: World Health Organization; 2014. Revised WHO Classification and Treatment of Pneumonia in Children at Health Facilities: Evidence Summaries.
3. Harris M, Clark J, Coote N, Fletcher P, Harnden A, McKean M, et al.; British Thoracic Society Standards of Care Committee. British Thoracic Society guidelines for the management of community acquired pneumonia in children: update 2011. Thorax. 2011;66 Suppl 2:ii1-23.
4. Sarthi M, Kabra SK. Pneumonia. In: Kabra SK, Lodha R, editors. Essential Pediatric Pulmonology. 2nd ed. New Delhi; Noble Vision: 2010.

CHAPTER

22

Atypical Pneumonia

Daisy Khera, Mudit Mittal

CASE 1

- A 10-year-old boy was brought to pediatric outpatient department (OPD) for a second opinion as there was no relief in his symptoms of pneumonia, despite taking oral amoxicillin-clavulanic acid for the last 5 days. His mother reported that the child had mild fever, sore throat, and dry cough along with headache and malaise for the last 10 days
- The doctor's prescription noted that 5 days back the patient had normal vitals. He had a macular rash over face, trunk, and extremities associated with urticaria. There was no respiratory distress. Chest examination revealed bilateral crepitations. He had WBC counts of 8250/µL with 45% neutrophils and 51% lymphocytes. At that time his chest X-ray showed bilateral patchy infiltrates
- Over the last 5 days, the symptoms progressively worsened with development of respiratory difficulty on the fifth day. The past and family history was uneventful. Examination revealed heart rate 92/min; respiratory rate 36/min, and axillary temperature 99.8°F. Nasal flaring was present but there were no chest retractions. A dull note was appreciated on percussion of the right side chest. Air entry was decreased on the right side of the chest and bilateral crepitations were heard. There was increased vocal resonance on the right side.

Q. Could this child have atypical pneumonia?

Yes, the clinical presentation is consistent with atypical pneumonia. The term "atypical pneumonia" was first used in 1938 by Reiman to describe several cases of pneumonia which were clinically different from the other commonly described pneumonias (Box 1).

Q. What are the causes of atypical pneumonia?

The viral pneumonias may have the atypical features described above. However, the term atypical pneumonia is classically used for pneumonias caused by atypical organisms.

Box 1: Features suggestive of atypical pneumonia

- Insidious onset
- Less virulent course than typical pneumonia
- Interstitial inflammation of lungs and hence patchy infiltration on chest radiographs
- Absence of peripheral leukocytosis
- Absence of growth of microbes on routine cultures
- Failure to respond to penicillins and other antibiotics routinely used for community acquired pneumonias

Common:

- *Mycoplasma pneumoniae*
- *Chlamydophila pneumoniae, Chlamydophila psittaci, Chlamydophila trachomatis*
- *Legionella pneumophila.*

Uncommon:

- *Coxiella burnetii*
- *Francisella tularensis*
- *Bacillus anthracis*
- *Yersinia pestis.*

Q. How common are atypical pneumonias?

Atypical organisms such as *Mycoplasma pneumoniae* are implicated in 15–30% cases of community acquired pneumonia—*Chlamydophila pneumoniae* in 6% cases and *Legionella pneumophila* in a minority of cases of infants and children.

A Finnish study found that in children younger than 5 years of age, the incidence of *S. pneumoniae* infection was 8.6/1,000 per year and mycoplasma infection was 1.7/1,000 per year. In children aged from 5 to 15 years, the incidence of *S. pneumoniae* fell to 5.4/1,000 while that of mycoplasma rose to 6.6/1,000. Though the organisms *M. pneumoniae* and *C. pneumoniae* commonly cause community acquired pneumonia in school age children and teenagers, they may infect preschool age children more commonly than generally recognized. In one study, the age of patients with atypical infection ranged from 9 months to 13 years, with 47% occurring in those aged younger than 5 years.

Q. How can one reach an etiological diagnosis in cases of atypical pneumonia?

In a suspected atypical pneumonia one should look for clinical and epidemiological clues pointing toward an etiological agent. The laboratory investigations should be ordered on the basis of these clues or pointers.

Q. What are the clues in this patient suggesting a diagnosis of atypical pneumonia?

There are many epidemiological and clinical pointers in this patient which suggest a possible *M. pneumoniae* infection.

Epidemiology

Mycoplasma pneumoniae is the causative agent of *Mycoplasma pneumonia*. It is transmitted by respiratory droplets during close contact with high secondary attack rates of 70–75%. It has an incubation period of 2–3 weeks. The incidence of infection is about 4 per 1,000 children per year. *Mycoplasma pneumonia* is more common in the age group of 6–18 years but it is being increasingly recognized in younger children.

Clinical features

Approximately 20% of *M. pneumoniae* infections are asymptomatic. In symptomatic patients, the disease usually starts as an influenza-like syndrome with the predominant symptoms being low grade fever, malaise, headache, sore throat, and cough; vomiting and diarrhea may be present in up to 20% patients. On physical examination, the children may have crepitations (40–73%), wheezing (35%), or small areas of dullness on percussion suggestive of atelectasis or pleural effusion.

Mycoplasma infection is associated with various nonrespiratory features like skin rashes, arthralgia, myalgia, otitis media, sinusitis, hemolytic anemia, and nervous system involvement (aseptic meningitis, encephalitis, cerebellar ataxia, transverse myelitis, peripheral neuropathy, psychosis, and Guillain Barre syndrome).

Usually most of the patients remain ambulatory, but some patients may require admission because of respiratory distress. The radiographic features are nonspecific. The most common radiographic findings are perihilar opacities (60%) (Fig. 1), reticulonodular infiltrates (40%), segmental or lobar consolidation (28%) (Fig. 2), and pleural effusion (8%).

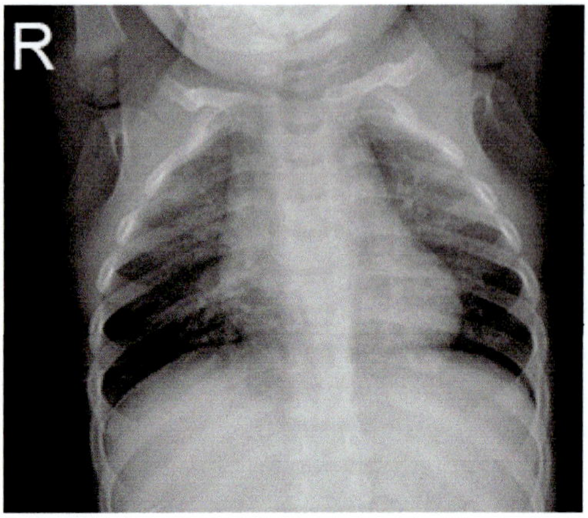

Figure 1: Frontal chest radiograph of a 3-year-old boy shows bilateral perihilar and upper zonal interstitial opacities

Courtesy: Dr Sridhar Gibikote, Christian Medical College, Vellore.

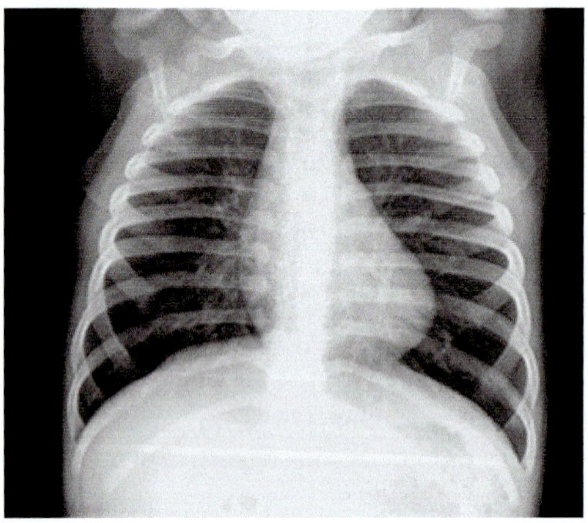

Figure 2: Frontal chest radiograph of a 7-year-old boy shows right perihilar reticulonodular opacities

Courtesy: Dr Sridhar Gibikote, Christian Medical College, Vellore.

Q. What are the various laboratory investigations available for the diagnosis of *M. pneumoniae*?

Various diagnostic tests for *Mycoplasma pneumoniae* are given in table 1.

Q. How should one approach a case of suspected atypical pneumonia?

After a thorough history and physical examination, one may plan the following investigations.

- Routine investigations: hemogram, C-reactive protein, chest X-ray, blood culture/sensitivity, and, blood gas (if indicated)
- Investigations directed at identification of suspected organism.

Treatment

- Evaluation of airway, breathing, and circulation, for need for any support
- Initiation of antibiotic which has a broad coverage against the common causes of atypical pneumonia.

Macrolides are the treatment of choice for atypical pneumonia. Newer macrolides especially clarithromycin and azithromycin have improved activity (in comparison to erythromycin) against *Staphylococcus, Streptococcus,* and *H. influenzae.*

Quinolones also have good activity against atypical organisms. However, they are not routinely used in children. Tetracycline and doxycycline have good efficacy against *M. pneumoniae, C. pneumoniae,* and *Legionella pneumophila*. However, they are not routinely used in pediatric patients because of their toxicity profile (Table 2).

CASE 2

- A 3-month-old male infant was admitted in a private nursing home with complaints of cough, high grade fever, and respiratory distress for the preceding 4 days. At the nursing home, he received ceftriaxone and amoxicillin-clavulanate intravenously for 10 days. He was also nebulized with salbutamol during the initial 3 days of his hospital stay. The child was then referred as the fever and respiratory distress were persisting and his recent chest X-ray showed bilateral patchy infiltrates
- The child was born at 30 weeks gestation and developed respiratory distress syndrome. He had a prolonged neonatal intensive-care unit stay and developed bronchopulmonary dysplasia
- On examination, heart rate was 146/min, respiratory rate 54/min, and temperature 102.6°F. Nasal flaring and retractions were present. Chest auscultation revealed bilateral crepitations.

TABLE 1: **Methods for diagnosing *Mycoplasma* infections**

Method	Specimen	Technique	Comments
Culture of the organism	Respiratory secretions; e.g., throat swab, tracheal aspirate, sputum, and lung biopsy	–	• Gold standard • Not readily available • Report available in 1–3 weeks
Cold hemagglutination	Serum	–	• Rapid test • Simple • Inexpensive • Nonspecific (positivity seen also with CMV and EBV)
Antibody detection	Serum	• Complement fixation test • Indirect hemagglutination • Enzyme-linked immunosorbent assay • Immunofluorescence • Latex agglutination	• Retrospective diagnosis on the basis of rising titers
Antigen detection	Respiratory secretions	• Polymerase chain reaction • Indirect immunofluorescence • Enzyme-linked immunosorbent assay	• Rapid test
	Serum	• Polymerase chain reaction	• Rapid test

CMV, cytomegalovirus; EBV, Epstein-Barr virus; ELISA, enzyme-linked immunosorbent assay.

Note: It may be necessary to combine serology and polymerase chain reaction to achieve maximum sensitivity.

TABLE 2: **Antibiotics useful in atypical pneumonia**

Antibiotic	Dose
Clarithromycin	• 15 mg/kg/day in two divided doses orally (maximum dose is 1 g/day)
Azithromycin	• 10 mg/kg/day once a day orally on day 1 (maximum dose is 500 mg), followed by 5 mg/kg/day once a day orally on day 2 to day 5 (maximum dose is 250 mg)
Roxithromycin	• 5–10 mg/kg/day in two divided doses orally
Erythromycin	• 30–50 mg/kg/day in 3–4 divided doses orally (maximum dose is 2 g/day)
Ciprofloxacin	• 20–30 mg/kg/day in two divided doses orally (maximum dose is 1.5 g/day) • 20–30 mg/kg/day in two divided doses intravenous (maximum dose is 800 mg/day)
Ofloxacin	• 15 mg/kg/day in two divided doses orally
Doxycycline	• 2–5 mg/kg/day in two divided doses orally
Tetracycline	• 20–30 mg/kg/day in four divided doses orally

Q. What are the diagnostic possibilities in this child?

The broad differential diagnosis would be:

- Bronchopneumonia (resistant to β-lactam antibiotics)
- Atypical pneumonia
- Pulmonary tuberculosis.

Subsequently, this child was referred to a tertiary hospital. There, he received meropenem and vancomycin intravenously for 7 days. His blood counts were unremarkable. The blood culture revealed no growth and the tuberculosis work up was negative. However, the child developed severe respiratory distress and required mechanical ventilation.

Q. What do you think is the most probable diagnosis?

Keeping in mind the history of premature birth, respiratory distress syndrome and bronchopulmonary dysplasia, virulent clinical course, nonresponse to β-lactam antibiotics, history of aerosolization, unremarkable blood counts, and routine cultures, the child appears to be suffering from atypical pneumonia probably Legionnaire's disease.

Q. Who are at risk of Legionnaire's disease?

Legionella pneumonia can occur as sporadic infections or as outbreaks (usually associated with hospitals, hotels, office buildings). Historically, epidemics have been linked to cooling towers, air conditioning, hot water tanks, plumbing, and air duct systems.

Legionella infection is rare in otherwise normal children. It is known to occur more commonly in:

- Immunocompromised patients
- Patients with underlying lung disease
- Patients having hospital acquired pneumonia.

The risk factors for nosocomial transmission in neonates are prematurity, congenital heart disease, bronchopulmonary dysplasia, and prolonged steroid therapy.

Q. How is Legionnaire's disease different from other atypical pneumonias?

The course and prognosis of this disease resembles bacterial pneumonia (e.g., pneumococcal pneumonia) rather than atypical pneumonia.

The disease begins with a nonspecific prodrome of headache, myalgia, fatigue, anorexia, malaise, chills, vomiting, and watery diarrhea. The onset may be insidious or acute, but is usually accompanied with high grade fever. This is followed by cough and pleuritic chest pain.

The respiratory examination is usually consistent with a consolidating pneumonia. About one-third of patients may have pleural effusions. Nodular opacities and cavitations may be visible radiographically in immunocompromised patients.

In more severe cases, patients may become progressively ill. Shock, respiratory distress, or both may develop by 5th to 6th day of illness.

Q. What are the extrapulmonary manifestations in Legionnaire's disease?

These are especially seen in the immunocompromised patients. These include neuromuscular (meningoencephalitis, myositis), cardiac (myocarditis), gastrointestinal (hepatitis, pancreatitis), renal (hypophosphatemia, hyponatremia), and hematological abnormalities (thrombocytopenia). However, extrapulmonary manifestations are less common in children as compared to adults.

Q. What are the modalities available for the lab diagnosis of Legionella pneumonia?

Culture of the organism from respiratory secretions is the definitive diagnostic modality. Legionella antigen may be detected in urine specimen early in the course of the disease (by ELISA or solid phase radioimmunoassay), but this method is only established for serogroup 1. Polymerase chain reaction of the serum has also been used for the identification of *Legionella*. Antibody may be detected in the acute phase and convalescent phase by indirect immunofluorescence, but this method is mainly of epidemiological interest. A combination of sputum culture and urine antigen detection may be the best diagnostic method.

CASE 3

- An 8-year-old female child presented to the OPD with complaints of low-grade fever, hoarseness of voice, nonproductive cough, headache, and malaise for 7 days. She developed an acute episode of wheeze on the day of presentation, prompting her to seek medical opinion
- She had been a known case of intermittent asthma for 2 years
- On examination, the child had a heart rate of 102/min and respiratory rate of 42/min with mild intercostal and subcostal retractions and bilateral wheezes on auscultation
- Investigations revealed a total leukocyte count of 9500/µL with 38% neutrophils, 52% lymphocytes, and 8% eosinophils. Chest X-ray revealed bilateral perihilar linear infiltrates and bilateral small effusions.

Q. How will you treat this patient?

Bronchodilator therapy for asthma should be started. The insidious course, unremarkable WBC counts, and perihilar linear infiltrates on chest radiograph are suggestive of atypical pneumonia. Keeping in mind that *C. pneumoniae* is known to trigger wheezes in children with asthma, the patient should be started on macrolides (preferably azithromycin or clarithromycin).

Q. What are the epidemiological and clinical markers suggestive of *C. pneumoniae* infection?

Chlamydophila pneumoniae is a common cause of community acquired pneumonia in the school age children. It is transmitted via respiratory secretions from person to person or through fomites. Concurrent infections with *M. pneumoniae* or *S. pneumoniae* occur frequently.

The infection begins with a nonspecific prodrome of sore throat, malaise, headache, low grade fever, and cough. A significant number of patients develop pneumonia or bronchitis. *Chlamydophila pneumoniae* leads to an immunoglobulin E (IgE)-mediated bronchial reactivity. Hence, it can trigger acute episodes of wheezing in children with asthma.

Q. What are the other manifestations of *C. pneumoniae* infection?

The extrapulmonary complications of *C. pneumoniae* infection include erythema marginatum, reactive arthritis, Guillain-Barré syndrome, meningoencephalitis, myocarditis, and endocarditis. It has been linked to asthma, multiple sclerosis, chronic fatigue syndrome, and atherosclerosis. However, causation has not been confirmed yet.

Q. What are the investigations available to establish *C. pneumoniae* infection?

Isolation of the organism from respiratory secretions remains the gold standard. However, the organism is fastidious and it is not unusual to get negative cultures in the presence of infection.

Serological diagnosis (by complement fixation test, enzyme immunoassay or immunofluorescence test) requires demonstration of a fourfold rise in immunoglobulin G titer or an immunoglobulin M titer greater than 1:16. Polymerase chain reaction in respiratory secretions for detection of microbial antigen is a highly sensitive method. Reliance on a single test for diagnosis is discouraged. A combination of methods should be used.

LEARNING POINTS

- Atypical pneumonia is a common cause of community acquired pneumonia
- It is more common in the age group of 6–18 years but it is being increasingly recognized in younger children
- The clinical spectrum of atypical pneumonia is wide. It may be mild requiring only outpatient department-based treatment or severe enough to require hospitalization and mechanical ventilation
- The radiographic features are nonspecific and include perihilar opacities, reticulonodular infiltrates, segmental/lobar consolidation, and pleural effusion
- Macrolides are the antibiotics of choice in atypical pneumonia.

SUGGESTED READINGS

1. Byington CL, Bradley JS. Pediatric community-acquired pneumonia. In: Cherry JD, Harrison GJ, Kaplan SL, Steinbach WJ, Hotez P, editors. Feigin and Cherry's Textbook of Pediatric Infectious Diseases. 7th ed. Philadelphia: Elsevier Saunders; 2014. p. 283.
2. Salaria M, Singh M. Atypical Pneumonia in children. Indian Pediatr. 2002;39:259-66.
3. Seltz LB, Colvin M, Barton LL. Atypical pneumonias in children. In: Wilmott RW, Bush A, Boat TF, Deterding RR, Ratjen F, Chernick V, editors. Kendig and Chernick's Disorders of Respiratory Tract in Children. 8th ed. Philadelphia: WB Saunders Co.; 2012. p. 493.
4. Thibodeau KP, Viera AJ. Atypical pathogens and challenges in community-acquired pneumonia. Am Fam Physician. 2004;69(7):1699-707.

CHAPTER

23

Fungal Pneumonia

Vinod H Ratageri, Sudhendra R Fattepur

CASE 1

- A 3-year-old girl child with a known case of human immunodeficiency virus (HIV) infection with disseminated tuberculosis on antitubercular therapy for 2 months was presented with fever since 25 days, cough and respiratory distress for 7 days
- On examination, she had oral thrush, generalized lymphadenopathy, and healed skin lesions. Respiratory system revealed bronchial breath sounds on right inter and infrascapular area and bilateral crepitations and rhonchi. Hepatosplenomegaly was noted on abdominal examination. The other system examinations were within normal limits. There was no improvement with initial antibiotic therapy
- Investigations revealed hemoglobin 6.3 g/dL, total leukocyte counts (TLC) were normal, CD4% was 4.80%; chest-X ray revealed ill-defined, irregular haziness seen on right and perihilar region suggestive of consolidation (Fig. 1). Fungal culture of sputum grew-*Aspergillus* spp.

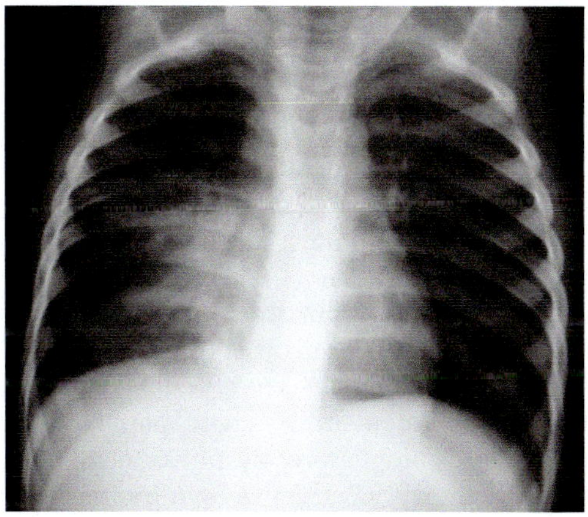

Figure 1: Chest X-ray showing ill-defined irregular haziness on right middle and lower lobe

Q. What is fungal pneumonia? What are the routes of infection?

Fungal pneumonia is defined as an infection of lungs caused by one or more endemic or opportunistic fungi. The routes of fungal infection are by inhalation of spores or conidia, or by the reactivation of a latent infection. Hematogenous dissemination frequently occurs in immunocompromised host.

Q. What are the common fungi which produce pneumonia?

Fungal pneumonia can be caused by one or more endemic or opportunistic fungi.

- Endemic fungal pathogens (e.g., *Histoplasma capsulatum*, *Coccidioides immitis*, *Blastomyces dermatitidis*, *Paracoccidioides brasiliensis*, *Sporothrix schenckii*, and *Cryptococcus neoformans*) can cause infection in healthy hosts and in immunocompromised persons
- Opportunistic fungal organisms (e.g., *Candida* species, *Aspergillus* species, *Mucor* species) tend to cause pneumonia in patients with congenital or acquired defects in the host immune defenses.

Q. What are the predisposing conditions for fungal pneumonia?

The conditions that predispose children to opportunistic fungal infection are given in box 1.

Box 1: Conditions that predispose children to opportunistic fungal infection

Route/source
- Antibiotics
- Burns and other skin problems
- Catheters
- Devices (prosthetic)
- Effects on mucosa
- Fungus isolated previously

Immunodeficiency
- Acquired immuno-deficiency syndrome
- Bone marrow and others
- Cancer
- Drugs
- Endocrine
- Failure of organs

Combination
- Premature neonates
- Intensice care unit

Q. What are the clinical symptoms and signs of fungal pneumonia?

The clinical symptoms and signs of fungal pneumonia are not specific, and are indistinguishable from those associated with respiratory infections of other origins.

Symptoms include fever; cough, usually nonproductive; pleuritic chest pain or dull discomfort; progressive dyspnea; respiratory failure; airway obstructive symptoms from enlarged mediastinal adenopathy in the endemic mycoses; and hemoptysis (in invasive aspergillosis or mucormycosis). In individuals who are neutropenic or immunocompromised, persistent fever (at times without any pulmonary findings) may be an early sign of infection, especially if the fever is unresponsive to broad-spectrum antibiotics.

Clinical signs include temperature elevation, tachycardia, tachypnea, respiratory distress, rales, signs of pulmonary consolidation, and pleural rub.

Q. What are the complications of fungal pneumonia?

Complications of fungal pneumonia include:

- Dissemination to other parts of the body like brain, meninges, skin, liver, spleen, kidneys, adrenals, heart, and eyes
- Blood vessel invasion, which in turn leads to hemoptysis, pulmonary infarction, myocardial infarction, cerebral septic emboli, cerebral infarction, or blindness.

Q. What are the differential diagnoses of fungal pneumonia?

The conditions that can mimic the symptoms or signs of fungal pneumonia are as follows:

- Chlamydial pneumonias
- Eosinophilic pneumonia
- *Pneumocystis jiroveci* pneumonia
- Aspiration pneumonia
- Bacterial pneumonia
- Viral pneumonia
- Cardiogenic pulmonary edema
- Neurogenic pulmonary edema
- Idiopathic pulmonary fibrosis
- Interstitial pulmonary fibrosis (nonidiopathic)
- Tuberculosis.

Q. What are the diagnostics for fungal pneumonia?

Diagnosis of fungal infections is difficult. Standard techniques such as microscopy and culture remain the mainstay of diagnosis.

Nonculture based diagnostic tools, such as galactomannan and β-D-glucan, are of added value for the diagnostic workup of invasive fungal pneumonia. Polymerase chain reaction based assays are also available for detecting various pathogens, including *Aspergillus*, *Histoplasma*, and *Candida* species.

Serological tests play an important role in the diagnosis of infection by *Candida immitis* and histoplasmosis.

Q. What are the radiological hallmarks of fungal pneumonia?

There are a few typical findings on imaging that suggest the diagnosis of fungal pneumonia (Fig. 2).

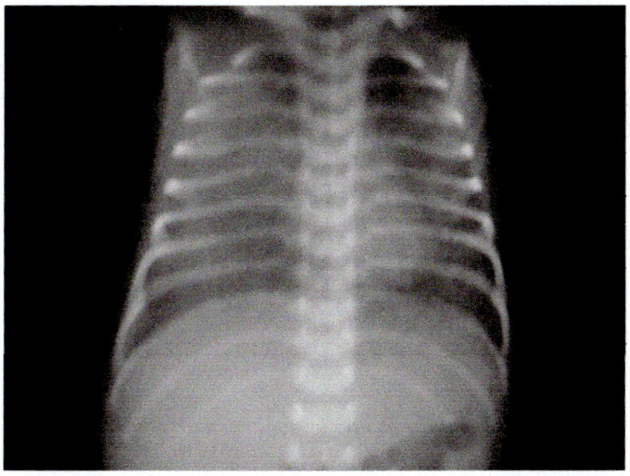

Figure 2: Chest X-rays showing left upper lobe consolidation and lower lobe with cavitation

Halo sign

The halo sign is the computed tomography (CT) finding of a peripheral rim of ground-glass opacity surrounding a pulmonary nodule or mass. The ground-glass opacity represents hemorrhage surrounding infarcted lung and is caused by vascular invasion by the fungus.

Air crescent sign of angioinvasive Aspergillus infection

The air crescent sign is the CT finding of a crescentic collection of air that separates a nodule or mass from the wall of a surrounding cavity. This sign is seen in two types of *Aspergillus* infection: (i) angioinvasive and (ii) mycetoma.

Reverse halo and bird's nest signs

The reverse halo sign is the CT finding of peripheral consolidation surrounding a central area of ground-glass opacity. Associated irregular and intersecting areas of stranding or irregular lines may be present within the area of ground-glass opacity and become evident as the bird's nest sign. These signs are suggestive of invasive fungal infection (e.g., angioinvasive *Aspergillus* infection or mucormycosis) in susceptible patient populations.

Q. How do you manage fungal pneumonia?

Pharmacological therapy is the mainstay of treatment. Amphotericin B is the drug of choice in many cases in the initial therapy. More expensive liposomal preparations of amphotericin B offer equal efficacy with lesser toxicity. In patients with invasive aspergillosis, including pulmonary aspergillosis, voriconazole is the new standard of care, based on its superiority over amphotericin B as primary therapy. Table 1 shows the spectrum of activity of various antifungal agents.

Other antifungal agents used in the treatment of fungal pneumonia are fluconazole, itraconazole, flucytosine, and ketoconazole. Newer antifungal agents, such as the third-generation triazoles or the echinocandins (caspofungin), are more tolerable than amphotericin B or its liposomal preparations are and may even be more effective in first- or second-line treatment.

Table 2 provides data regarding the indications and doses of the antifungal drugs.

TABLE 1: Antifungal agents and their spectrum of activity

Selected fungal species	Amphotericin B products	Fluconazole	Voriconazole	Posaconazole	Echinocandins (caspofungin)
Aspergillus fumigatus	++	–	+++	+++	++
Aspergillus terreus	–	–	+++	+++	++
Aspergillus flavus	++	–	+++	+++	++
Candida albicans	+++	+++	+++	+++	+++
Candida glabrata	++	±	+	+	+++
Candida tropicalis	+++	+++	+++	+++	+++

Continued

Continued

Selected fungal species	Amphotericin B products	Fluconazole	Voriconazole	Posaconazole	Echinocandins (caspofungin)
Cryptococcus neoformans	+++	+++	+++	+++	–
Fusarium species	++ (applies to lipid products)	–	++	++	–
Zygomycetes (e.g., *Absidia, Mucor, Rhizopus*)	+++	–	–	+++	–
Dimorphic fungi	+++	+ +++ *Coccidioides* ± *Sporothrix*	++ – *Sporothrix*	++ + *Sporothrix*	–

TABLE 2: Antifungal agents for treatment of systemic fungal infections

Agent	Route of administration	Dosage per day	Indications	Adverse reactions
Amphotericin B deoxycholate	Intravenous	• 0.25–0.5 mg/kg initially, increased to 0.5–1.5 mg/kg • Dosage for *aspergillosis*: 1.5 mg/kg	• Invasive fungal infections caused by susceptible organisms • Empirical therapy of presumed fungal infections in febrile neutropenic patients	• Infusion-related toxicity • Nephrotoxicity, including hypokalemia
Liposomal amphotericin B	Intravenous	• 3–5 mg/kg • Dosage for aspergillosis: 5–10 mg/kg; likely up to 10 mg/kg	• Invasive fungal infections, refractory or intolerance to conventional amphotericin B	• Fewer infusion-related reactions and nephrotoxicity than amphotericin B deoxycholate
Amphotericin B lipid complex	Intravenous	• 5 mg/kg • Dosage for aspergillosis: 5–10 mg/kg; likely up to 7.5 mg/kg	• Invasive fungal infections; refractory or with intolerance to conventional amphotericin B	• Less nephrotoxicity than amphotericin B deoxycholate
Fluconazole	Oral or intravenous	• Oral: 6 mg/kg once, then 3 mg/kg/day for oropharyngeal or esophageal candidiasis; 6–12 mg/kg/day for invasive fungal infections • Intravenous: 3–6 mg/kg, single dose; up to 12 mg/kg per day for serious infections	• Candida infections • Cryptococcal infections • Antifungal prophylaxis in HSCT patients and neonates	• Rare, serious hepatotoxicity possible • Cytochrome P450 isoenzyme drug interactions

Continued

Continued

Agent	Route of administration	Dosage per day	Indications	Adverse reactions
Itraconazole	Oral or intravenous	• Intravenous, oral: 5–10 mg/kg/day divided into two doses	• Invasive and noninvasive aspergillosis, oropharyngeal and esophageal candidiasis • Blastomycosis • Chronic pulmonary histoplasmosis • Antifungal prophylaxis in HSCT and lung transplant patients	• Elevated liver enzymes • Gastrointestinal intolerance: abdominal pain, vomiting, diarrhea • Cytochrome P450 isoenzyme drug interactions
Voriconazole	Oral or intravenous	• Oral: 8 mg/kg every 12 h for 1 day, then 7 mg/kg every 12 h • Intravenous: 6–8 mg/kg every 12 h for 1 day, then 7 mg/kg every 12 h	• Invasive aspergillosis • Esophageal candidiasis • Refractory infections due to *Scedosporium*, *Angiospermum* and *Fusarium* species	• Main side effects are liver function abnormalities, skin rash, visual disturbances, CYP450 isoenzyme drug interactions
Posaconazole	Oral	• 200 mg four times daily (age ≥13 years)	• Aspergillosis, fusariosis and zygomycosis in patients intolerant/refractory to other agents	• Gastrointestinal symptoms, headache, elevated liver enzymes, cytochrome P450 3A4 enzyme drug interactions
Caspofungin	Intravenous	• 70 mg/m^2 loading, then 50 mg/m^2 once daily	• Candida infections • Invasive aspergillosis in patients refractory/intolerant to other therapy • Empirical therapy in febrile neutropenic • patients	• Liver function abnormalities, fever, headache, rash, gastrointestinal symptoms, anemia
Micafungin	Intravenous	• 4–12 mg/kg once daily (higher doses for children <8 years of age)	• Similar to caspofungin prophylaxis of *Candida* infections in HSCT patients	• Liver function abnormalities, nausea, vomiting
Flucytosine	Oral	• 50–150 mg/kg in four doses	• Combination therapy with amphotericin B for *Candida* and cryptococcal infections	• Gastrointestinal intolerance and bone marrow suppression

HSCT, hematopoietic stem cell transplant; HIV, human immunodeficiency virus.

Q. What is the role of surgical care in fungal pneumonia?

Surgery is indicated in patients with documented invasive aspergillosis who have been treated with antifungal agents but who have residual lesions. When additional immunosuppression is required, the surgery will prevent disease relapse.

Surgery is also indicated as a means to prevent or treat massive bleeding, especially when the lung lesion is contiguous with a large blood vessel.

> **CASE 2**
>
> A 15-year-old female child who with a known case of diabetes mellitus type I presented with history of blurring of vision and decreased movements of right eye for fast 2 days. On further questioning she gave a history of mild to moderate fever with congestion of nose for past 10 days. She also complained of facial pain and blood tinged nasal discharge. On examination, she was found to have black necrotic lesion in the nose. Eye findings included mild proptosis with ophthalmoplegia. Investigations revealed hemoglobin 10 g/dL, TLC 18,600 cells/cmm, P-56%, L-40%, E-4% (leukocytosis) and glycosylated hemoglobin of 9.8%.

Q. How do you diagnose mucormycosis infection?

It is very difficult to diagnose a case of mucormycosis except in rhinocerebral mucormycosis where the typical history is helpful at arriving of the diagnosis. In cases of pulmonary, it presents as consolidation, nodules, cavitary lesions, and air crescent sign as in aspergillosis. A positive culture linked to hyphal identification in cytologic specimens or tissue sections is considered diagnostic. Mere presence of organism or its spores is not diagnostic as they are easily airborne and are contaminants of specimens. The hyphae are typically large (10–30 μm) nonseptate and often twisted or ribbon like and right-angled branching.

Q. In whom mucormycosis usually found and what are the common sites of involvement?

As in other fungal infections, they are commonly encountered in immunocompromised individuals, especially in patients having neutropenia.Other conditions include:

- Uncontrolled diabetic ketoacidosis (DKA) patients—they typically cause rhinocerebral mucormycosis
- Leukemia and other causes of neutropenia—pulmonary/cutaneous/disseminated
- Protein energy malnourished children—gastrointestinal tract (GIT) involvement
- Neonates, especially preterms—cutaneous and GIT causing necrotizing enterocolitis (NEC) like picture
- Burns patients—cutaneous variety
- Other high-risk individuals like patients on desferroxamine, patients receiving antifungals for a long duration without activity against mucorales like fluconazole and voriconazole, and patients suffering from methylmalonic aciduria.

Q. How will you treat mucormycosis?

Antifungal drugs like amphotericin B (lipid formulation) more than 5 mg/kg/day and posaconazole—12 mg/kg/day in 2–4 divided doses. Surgical debridement is a must whenever possible because only drugs may not help

Q. What is the role of prophylactic antifungal therapy?

Prophylactic therapy (suppressive therapy) with amphotericin B is used to prevent recurrence or relapse of coccidioidomycosis, cryptococcosis or histoplasmosis in individuals infected with the HIV who have received adequate treatment for the infection.

Posaconazole is used in the prophylaxis of invasive *Aspergillus* and *Candida* infections in severely immunocompromised patients receiving hematopoietic stem cell transplants who have graft-versus-host disease and in patients with hematologic malignancies who have chemotherapy-induced neutropenia.

Q. Are there any reports of drug resistant fungal pneumonia?

There have been increasing reports of azole resistance in *Aspergillus* species. This could be due to increasing use of these agents for prophylaxis and treatment of fungal infections.

Q. How will you manage refractory or resistant fungal pneumonia?

Caspofungin is the drug used for the treatment of invasive *Aspergillus* infections in patients unresponsive to or unable to receive amphotericin B. Combinations of a triazole with an echinocandin with or without amphotericin B have been anecdotally reported to be effective in some cases of resistant organisms such as *Mucor* or *Zygomycetes* species.

The establishment of neutrophil recovery or engraftment and the reduction of immuno-suppression in certain patients who are at risk for fungal infections are likely to improve the chances of a successful treatment outcome. Granulocyte-macrophage colony-stimulating factor can theoretically augment pulmonary host defenses against *Aspergillus fumigatus* infection.

Q. How do you prevent fungal pneumonia?

Patients undergoing bone marrow transplantation or any period of prolonged neutropenia are advised to avoid activities (e.g., playing in garden) or objects (e.g., potted plants, flowers, fresh fruits and vegetables, uncooked spices) that may unduly cause exposure to spores of *Aspergillus* species or other ubiquitous fungi.

For patients undergoing bone marrow transplantation, solid organ transplantation, or antileukemic chemotherapy, the use of high efficiency particulate air filtration systems in the treatment units may minimize patient risk of exposure to *Aspergillus* spores.

Consider the prophylactic antifungal therapy (i.e., treatment with intranasal or intravenous amphotericin B or its other formulations) in patients at high risk for opportunistic fungal infection, including patients with a history of fungal infection.

Prophylactic posaconazole was shown to be superior to fluconazole in reducing invasive aspergillosis incidence.

LEARNING POINTS

- The incidence of fungal infections is increasing at an alarming rate, may be because of advances in medical and surgical therapy, change in profile of hospitalized patients, severely ill, immunocompromised patient population, and the impact of acquired immunodeficiency syndrome
- Systemic fungal infections can be life-threatening and are associated with high morbidity and mortality
- The most frequently encountered pathogens are *Candida albicans* and *Aspergillus* spp., mucor, however, other fungi such as non-albicans *Candida* spp. are increasingly important
- The most clinical symptoms and signs are not specific
- Diagnosis is difficult; microscopy and culture remain mainstay for diagnosis, nonculture methods, such as galactomannan enzyme assay and polymerase chain reaction, often helpful
- Radiological hallmark for fungal pneumonia are halo, air crescent, and reverse halo signs
- The mainstay of systemic antifungal therapy has been amphotericin B; others are trizoles, echinocandins
- Incidence of fungal infections can be reduced by minimizing risk factors in hospitals.

SUGGESTED READINGS

1. Allen UD. Canadian paediatric society, infectious diseases and immunization committee. antifungal agents for the treatment of systemic fungal infections in children. Paediatr Child Health. 2010;15(9):603-9.
2. American Academy of Pediatrics. Antifungal drugs for systemic fungal infection. In: Pickering LK, Baker CJ, Long SS,

McMillan JA, editors. Red Book 2012 Report of the Committee on Infectious Diseases. 29th ed. Elk Grove Village, IL: American Academy of Pediatrics; 2012. pp. 828-35.
3. Kohler JR, Casadevall A, Perfect J. The spectrum of fungi that infects humans. Cold Spring Harb Perspect Med. 2015;5(1):a019273.
4. Lease ED, Alexander BD. Fungal diagnostics in pneumonia. Semin Respir Crit Care Med. 2011;32(6):663-72.
5. Richardson MD, Jones BL. Therapeutic Guidelines in Systemic Fungal Infection, 3rd edition. London: Current Medical Literature; 2003.
6. Ünal S, Kuýkonmaz B, Tavil B, Elmas SA, Çetinkaya DU, Gümrük F, et al. Early detection of pulmonary fungal infection by CT scan in pediatric ALL patient under chemotherapy or in post-transplantation period with primary complaint of chest pain. Turk J Hematol. 2010;27:34-7.

CHAPTER

24

Pneumocystis jiroveci Pneumonia

Shalini Akunuri, Anupam Jaiswal, Anil K Sapare, Varun Narwal, Ilin Kinimi

CASE 1

- A 2-year-old child presented with complaints of fever for 2 days while on reinduction regimen (oral steroids plus cyclophosphamide) for acute lymphoblastic leukemia. He was started on broad-spectrum antibiotics after his blood samples were drawn. He was afebrile within 24 hours of admission but had persistent dry cough
- His respiratory rate was 40/min and saturation was 95% on room air. Auscultation revealed equal air entry and fine crepitations
- Investigations showed hemoglobin of 11.8 with leucopenia (1190—absolute neutrophil count of 190). Sputum induction was attempted but with poor returns. The child was human immunodeficiency virus (HIV) negative. Bronchoscopy could not be done due to technical issues. Chest X-ray (day 3 of admission) showed a hazy lobar consolidation of the right mid-zone with bilateral perihilar infiltrates and hyperinflated left lung (Fig. 1)
- The child was managed symptomatically with bronchodilators. A computed tomography (CT) thorax (Fig. 2) was ordered (day 4 of admission) which showed bilateral ground-glass nodular attenuation.

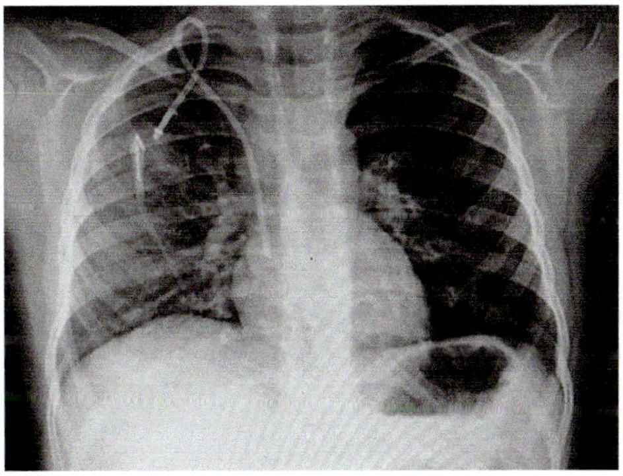

Figure 1: Chest X-ray showing hazy lobar consolidation of the right mid-zone with bilateral perihilar infiltrates and hyperinflated left lung

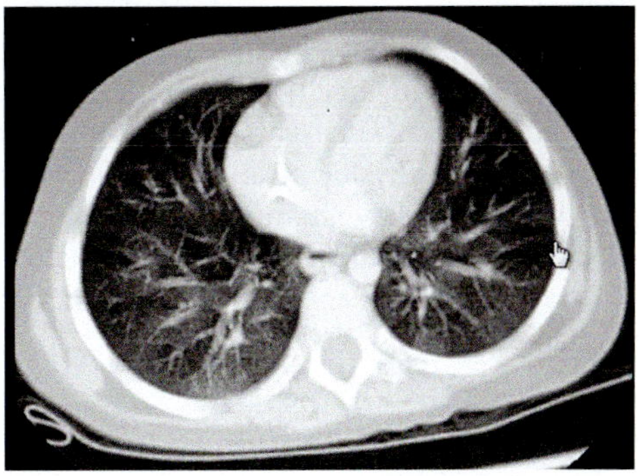

Figure 2: Lung window of computed tomography chest showing bilateral ground-glass nodular attenuation

Q. Did this child have features of *Pneumocystis Jiroveci* pneumonia?

This child had symptoms of lower respiratory tract infection on a background of immunosuppressant treatment, and developed cough after admission, despite being on broad spectrum antibiotics. He was already on co-trimoxazole prophylaxis for *Pneumocystis*. Clinical history and chest X-ray findings were not specific but a possible *Pneumocystis jiroveci* pneumonia (PJP) infection was suspected. High-resolution CT chest provided additional diagnostic pointers.

Q. What is the epidemiology of *Pneumocystis jiroveci* pneumonia?

Pneumocystis jiroveci pneumonia is the most common pulmonary opportunistic infection in patients infected with HIV. It can also present in other immunosuppressed conditions. It is less frequently reported, may be because of failure to diagnose. However, with use of highly active anti-retroviral therapy and PJP prophylaxis, the incidence of PJP has declined dramatically.

Q. What is the pathophysiology of *Pneumocystis jiroveci* pneumonia?

Both cellular immunity and humoral immunity are involved in development of PJP. Once inhaled, the trophic form of this organism attaches to the alveoli. Activated alveolar macrophages without CD4+ cells cannot eradicate these organisms. Subsequently, there is an increased alveolar-capillary permeability with ensuing physiological changes which include hypoxemia with an increased alveolar-arterial oxygen gradient, respiratory alkalosis, impaired diffusing capacity, changes in total lung capacity, and vital capacity.

Q. What is the clinical presentation of *Pneumocystis jiroveci* pneumonia?

The symptoms of PJP are nonspecific and includes: cough (usually nonproductive) (95%), exertional dyspnea (95%), fever (>80%), chest discomfort, weight loss, chills, and rarely hemoptysis. There can be extrapulmonary symptoms also.

Q. What are the important points to be elicited in the history?

Detailed history of symptoms—type of cough (dry cough is predominantly seen in HIV-negative patients), fever, and treatment history (steroids and other immunosuppressive drugs). Duration of therapy with immunosuppressants is important—duration of 12 weeks or more of glucocorticoids is usually associated with PJP. Other points include history of malnutrition, contact history (airborne route of infection), and history of HIV infection.

Q. What are the relevant features in physical examination?

Physical examination findings are nonspecific and include tachypnea, fever, and tachycardia. Chest examination may reveal mild crackles and rhonchi but may be normal in up to 50% of patients. Other findings include cyanosis, nasal flaring, and intercostal retractions in severe cases.

Look also for failure to thrive/signs of malnutrition/thrush.

Q. How will you diagnose *Pneumocystis* pneumonia?

Clinical

Pneumocystis jiroveci pneumonia is suspected on a background of immunosuppression, cancer, transplant, rheumatological disease, and malnutrition with aforementioned clinical features.

Sputum/respiratory secretions

Pneumocystis organisms can be identified by sputum induction (hypertonic saline). Sputum induction is one of the least invasive method for diagnosing PJP, where it is feasible. Sputum induction sensitivity varies from 50% to >90% but specificity is high (99–100%). Expectorated sputum, however, has a poor sensitivity.

Human immunodeficiency disease-associated infection typically leads to a greater alveolar load of organisms and diagnostic yield will be higher.

Bronchoalveolar lavage is the most common invasive procedure used to diagnose PJP, with a yield that exceeds 90%. Bronchoalveolar lavage may be used in patients who cannot cooperate for an induced sputum/sputum findings are negative.

Pneumocystis jiroveci persists in the host for days to weeks after therapy is initiated, hence diagnostic workup can still yield good results even late in the course of illness. In severely ill patients on mechanical ventilation, endotracheal tube aspirates should be attempted for confirmatory diagnosis.

Special stains are required for histopathologic identification of the organism. Cresyl violet, Giemsa, Diff-Quik, and Wright stain are used to detect both the trophozoite and the cyst forms but not the cyst wall. Methenamine silver, toluidine blue, and Gram-Weigert selectively stain the wall of *Pneumocystis* cysts.

Chest radiography

The chest radiographic findings can be normal in patients with early mild disease. Diffuse bilateral infiltrates extending from the perihilar region are visible in most patients with PJP. Less common findings include patchy asymmetric infiltrates, cystic lesions, and pneumatoceles. Pleural effusions and intrathoracic adenopathy are rare.

High-resolution computed tomography

High-resolution CT of chest is helpful when the chest radiography is equivocal. It yields a higher sensitivity in patients with HIV infection. Typically, CT changes include patchy areas of ground-glass attenuation with a background of interlobular septal thickening. However, negative CT scan findings do not rule out PJP.

Q. What is the next step in the management?

All possible bacterial/viral and fungal cultures should be sent to rule out other opportunistic infections. Although histopathologic demonstration of the organism is required for definitive diagnosis, treatment may be initiated before the complete workup in severely ill patients.

Degree of illness is determined by the alveolar-arterial gradient: mild (<35 mmHg), moderate (35–45 mmHg), or severe (>45 mmHg). Severe disease is also indicated by a room air partial pressure of arterial oxygen <70 mmHg.

Q. How will you treat this child?

- Treatment of choice is co-trimoxazole [trimethoprim: 15–20 mg/kg/day in 3–4 divided doses (oral/intravenous)]. Second line agents are pentamidine, dapsone (in combination with pyrimethamine), atovaquone, and clindamycin plus primaquine (after ruling out G6PD). There are a few reports of successful caspofungin administration
- For resistant cases, the combination of clindamycin and primaquine is more effective than intravenous pentamidine
- Treatment of PJP depends on the degree of illness at diagnosis. If no response occurs within the expected time, an appropriate alternative regimen should be used
- The recommended duration of treatment is 21 days in patients with HIV infection and 14 days in others
- The child was initiated on oral co-trimoxazole based on the clinical and chest radiography findings. He showed a dramatic response within 4–5 days and was discharged and is on follow-up for last 2 years.

CASE 2

- A 16-year-old girl presented with history of watery stools associated with dry cough, coryza for 2 weeks, and breathlessness for 1 week, which gradually progressed to orthopnea and intermittent episodes of mild grade fever. She was admitted elsewhere and given parenteral antibiotics. In lieu of clinical deterioration, she was shifted to our hospital
- At admission, she was conscious, oriented, but had respiratory distress. She was afebrile with

saturations of 85% in room air, tachypneic, increased work of breathing, and bilateral crepitations. She also had hepatosplenomegaly. Her initial investigations revealed normal hemoglobin and platelets, total leukocyte count was 8,400 cells/mm^3 (80% neutrophils/10% lymphocytes). Her renal and liver function tests were normal except for a mild elevation of alkaline phosphatase and γ-glutamyl transferase

- Chest roentgenogram showed bilateral extensive reticular nodular opacities with atelectatic changes at bases (Fig. 3)
- She was initiated on broad-spectrum antibiotics, oxygen, and noninvasive ventilator support. However, her hypoxia was unresponsive to broad-spectrum antibiotics. High resolution computed tomography chest showed cystic changes and fibrosis in lower and mid-zones suggestive of PJP. Sputum induction and silver stain of sample was positive for PJP
- She was also found to be HIV-1 positive. Further enquiry revealed that she was diagnosed as HIV positive at 5 years of age, initiated on antiretroviral therapy at 12 years but she had discontinued medications after a year. Her CD4 counts were 26 (3%) and CD8 of 474 (57%). Lactate dehydrogenase was elevated. GeneXpert for *Mycobacterium tuberculosis*/rifampicin was negative.

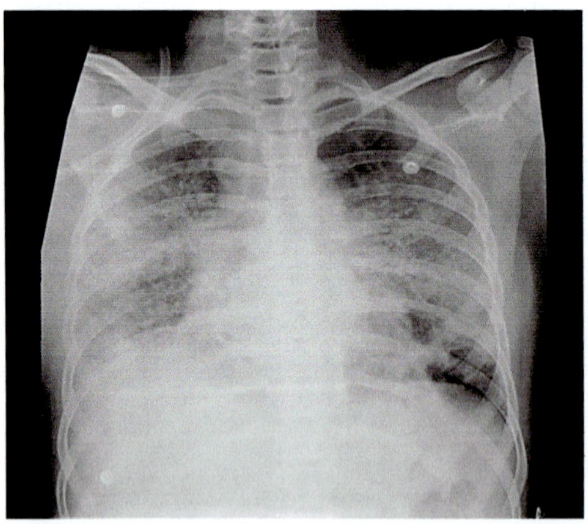

Figure 3: Chest X-ray showing bilateral extensive reticular nodular opacities with atelectatic changes at bases

Q. What are the other laboratory studies to be considered for *Pneumocystis jiroveci* pneumonia?

Lactate dehydrogenase (LDH) levels are usually elevated (>220 U/L) in patients with PJP, particularly those who are infected with HIV. Consistently elevated LDH levels indicate a poor prognosis.

Quantitative polymerase chain reaction may be useful in distinguishing between colonization and active infection, but currently is unavailable for clinical use.

Beta-D-Glucan, a cell-wall component of many fungi, has been shown to be a sensitive test in some trials.

Q. How does *Pneumocystis jiroveci* pneumonia presentation and management differ in human immunodeficiency virus infected versus non-human immunodeficiency virus patient?

Pneumocystis jiroveci pneumonia with HIV infection tends to run a more subacute indolent course and tends to present much later, often after several weeks of symptoms, compared with PJP associated with other immunocompromised conditions.

The dose for HIV infected children aged above 2 months is 3.75–5 mg/kg/dose of trimethoprim (TMP) and 19–25 mg/kg/dose of the sulfamethoxazole (SMX) given intravenously 6 hourly, with each infusion for 1 hour. Duration of treatment is for 21 days. Once the acute symptoms resolve, children with mild/moderate disease who do not have malabsorption or diarrhea can be switched to oral treatment with the same total daily dose.

In patients infected with HIV, the treatment response typically takes longer but usually occurs within the first 8 days. Patients with HIV infection are more prone to recurrence than others.

Q. What is the role of adjunctive corticosteroid therapy?

A short course of corticosteroids, within 72 hours of diagnosis, is recommended in cases of moderate or severe PJP. Microbial clearance can trigger a severe inflammatory response in the lungs that can worsen illness after initiating treatment. Steroids might blunt this response and reduce hypoxemia and respiratory failure. Duration of therapy with corticosteroid is 21 days (prednisolone/equivalent).

Q. What are the extrapulmonary manifestations of *Pneumocystis jiroveci* pneumonia?

Extrapulmonary manifestations are rare, except in patients on aerosolized pentamidine for prophylaxis. They may occur in the absence of lung involvement. *Pneumocystis* infection may present in almost any organ system including central nervous system, bone marrow (pancytopenia), lymphadenopathy, eyes (retinal cotton-wool spots), thyroid (rapidly enlarging thyroid mass), and gastrointestinal tract (loose stools). There have been reports of PJP occurring as part of the immune reconstitution inflammatory syndrome (IRIS).

Treatment of extrapulmonary manifestations is the same as that for PJP.

Q. Are there additional tests to aid in the diagnosis of *Pneumocystis jiroveci* pneumonia?

Pulmonary function tests

A decreased diffusion capacity of carbon monoxide of <75% has a high sensitivity (89–100%) but poor specificity (53%).

Lung biopsy

Open lung biopsy provides the greatest amount of tissue for diagnosis but is reserved for rare cases when bronchoscopy findings are nonconfirmatory.

Q. What is the prognosis of *Pneumocystis* pneumonia?

In patients with HIV infection, mortality rates of 10–20% are reported. *Pneumocystis jiroveci* pneumonia has a worse prognosis in those without HIV infection—mortality rates of 30-50% have been reported in them. Prognosis is worse in patients with concurrent pulmonary disease or who develop pneumothorax and in those requiring mechanical ventilation.

Q. What are the possible differential diagnoses of *Pneumocystis* pneumonia?

They include acute respiratory distress syndrome, *Cytomegalovirus*, lymphocytic interstitial pneumonia, *Mycoplasma* infections, viral pneumonia, pulmonary embolism, legionellosis, tuberculosis, and *Mycobacterium avium* complex infection.

Q. What are the preventive measures for *Pneumocystis jiroveci* pneumonia?

Patients with PJP should not have direct contact with other immunocompromised patients. Smoking cessation is strongly recommended in adolescents with HIV infection.

Q. Which patients require chemoprophylaxis for *Pneumocystis jiroveci* pneumonia??

Patients with an underlying HIV infection, primary immunodeficiency, persistent CD4 count <200/μL, solid organ transplant/hematopoietic stem cell transplant recipients, daily corticosteroid therapy (at least 20 mg daily for at least 1 month), cancer, vasculitides, or collagen vascular disorders and others receiving cytotoxic or immunosuppressive treatments and chemoprophylactic regimens.

Q. What are the drugs used for prophylaxis?

Trimethoprim-sulfamethoxazole is the agent of choice. In patients who cannot tolerate TMP-SMX, other options include dapsone, dapsone plus pyrimethamine, atovaquone, and aerosolized pentamidine.

LEARNING POINTS

- High index of clinical suspicion is required for diagnosis of *Pneumocystis jiroveci* pneumonia
- Treatment must be initiated early in clinically suspected cases
- Normal chest findings or a normal chest X-ray/computed tomography does not rule out *Pneumocystis jiroveci* pneumonia..

SUGGESTED READINGS

1. Bennett NJ, Gilroy SA. 2015. Pneumocystis jiroveci Pneumonia Overview of Pneumocystis jiroveci Pneumonia. [online] Medscape website. Available from: http://emedicine.medscape.com/article/225976-overview. [Accessed February 2016].
2. Kovacs JA, Gill VJ, Meshnick S, Masur H. New insights into transmission, diagnosis, and drug treatment of Pneumocystis carinii pneumonia. JAMA. 2001;286(19):2450-60.
3. McLaughlin GE, Virdee SS, Schleien CL, Holzman BH, Scott GB. Effect of corticosteroids on survival of children with acquired immunodeficiency syndrome and Pneumocystis carinii-related respiratory failure. J Pediatr. 1995;126(5 Pt 1):821-4.
4. Shankar SM, Nania JJ. Management of Pneumocystis jiroveci Pneumonia in Children Receiving Chemotherapy. Pediatric Drugs. 2007;9(5):301-9.
5. Wilkin A, Feinberg J. Pneumocystis carinii Pneumonia: A Clinical Review. Am Fam Physician. 1999;60(6):1699-708, 1713-4.

CHAPTER

25

Recurrent Persistent Pneumonia

Sushil K Kabra

CASE 1

A 19-month-old resident of Bihar presented with cough, fever, breathlessness, and wheezing for 4 days.

Past history: Noisy breathing, recurrent cough, wheeze, and breathlessness since day 25 of life. In addition, he had history of coughing while feeding and occasional vomiting.

No history of infection in other parts of body (pyoderma, diarrhea, oral thrush, ear discharge, etc.), no malabsorption, foreign body aspiration. Required hospitalization four times.

Mother felt that the child continued to have some respiratory difficulty and noisy breathing even when his other symptoms were better.

Family history: No asthma, allergy, sibling death.

Physical examination: He was febrile with temperature of 102°F, with tachycardia and tachypnea (heart rate: 134/min, respiratory rate: 72/min). Capillary refill time was <3 seconds; oxygen saturation in room air was 92%. Examination of chest revealed audible wheeze and lower chest indrawing. Rest of examination was within normal limits.

Investigations suggested mild anemia with polymorphonuclear leukocytosis (hemoglobin: 10.8, total leukocyte count: 15,600, P: 65, L: 35). Nuclear scan for gastroesophageal reflux did not show gastroesophageal reflux. There were multiple X-ray films of chest. There were infiltrates involving different lobes, more commonly seen in right side. Some X-ray films showed clearing as well (Figs 1 and 2).

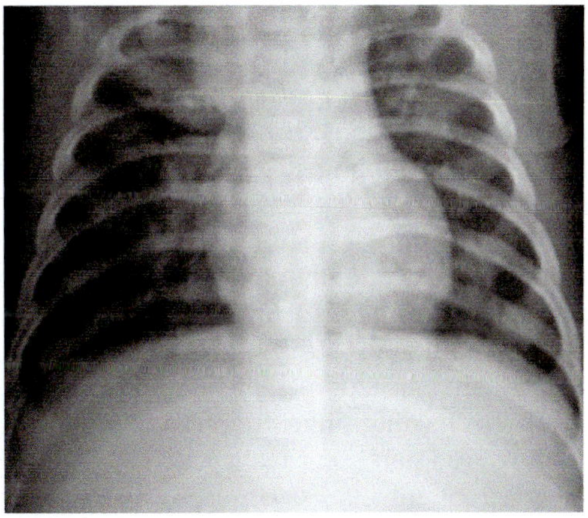

Figure 1: X-ray shows infiltrates in bilateral lung fields

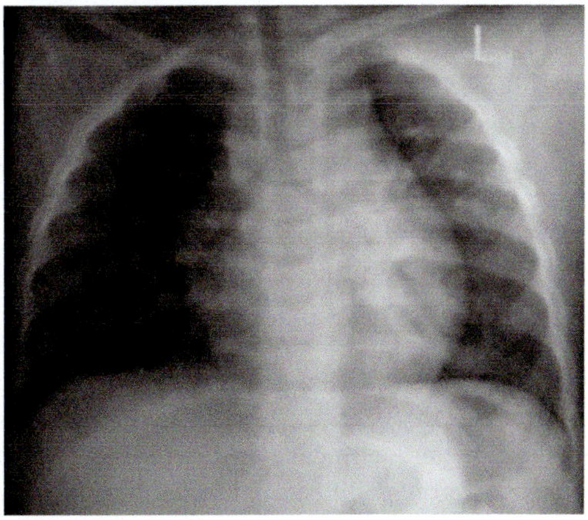

Figure 2: X-ray showing clearance of infiltrates

Q. Is it recurrent pneumonia?

Recurrent pneumonia is defined as two episodes of radiographic documented pneumonia over 1 year or three episodes in any time frame. The child should be symptomatic with abnormal chest X-ray (CXR) and clinical as well as radiographic recovery after episodes of pneumonia.

Present case has recurrent respiratory difficulty (required hospitalization four times) with abnormalities on CXR that shows clearance with treatment, therefore, it may be labeled as recurrent pneumonia.

Q. What additional information should be asked to get a clue for underlying illness?

Causes of recurrent pneumonia can be divided into four major groups: (i) malformations, (ii) recurrent aspirations, (iii) immune deficiency disorders, (iv) impaired airway clearance and others (Box 1).

Malformations manifest during early infancy, and pneumonia may be due to repeated aspirations or impaired airway clearance due to airway obstruction. Clues toward malformation may be early onset, history of feeding difficulty or choking during feeding, and persistent tachypnea even during intercurrent infections. Unresponsive wheeze that is biphasic may suggest fixed (subglottic or tracheal stenosis) or dynamic airway obstruction (laryngotracheomalacia).

Children with recurrent aspirations may present with coughing or choking during feeds. Immediate coughing or choking while feeding suggest aspiration secondary to laryngeal cleft or H type tracheoesophageal fistula. Dysphagia indicates esophageal obstruction. Coughing, choking, or vomiting after few minutes of feeding suggests gastroesophageal reflux.

Defect in airway clearance may manifest with wet cough or expectoration. In addition to wet cough, children with cystic fibrosis (CF) may have clinical features suggestive of malabsorption. Children with primary ciliary dyskinesia (PCD) may have situs inversus in 50%

Box 1: Common causes of recurrent pneumonia

Congenital malformations

- Airways
  - Dynamic obstruction of airways
    - Laryngomalacia
    - Tracheomalacia
    - Bronchomalacia
  - Tracheoesophageal fistulae
  - Pierre Robin syndrome
  - Cleft palate
- Lungs
  - Pulmonary agenesis, hypoplasia
  - Pulmonary sequestration
  - Cystic adenomatoid malformation
  - Congenial lobar emphysema
  - Bronchogenic cyst
  - Neoplasm: benign malignant
- Cardiovascular
    - Congenital heart diseases, especially left to right shunts (ventricular septal defect, atrial septal defect, patent ductus arteriosus)
  - Vascular ring

Aspirations

- Congenital malformations
- Pharyngeal incoordination
- Gastroesophageal reflux disease
- Esophageal obstruction/dysmotility
- Esophageal foreign body
- Esophageal diverticulum
- Neuromuscular disorders (neuropathy/myopathy)

Defects in the clearance of airways secretions

- Primary ciliary dyskinesia
- Cystic fibrosis
- Airway infections and their complications
- Postsurgery (repair of congenital defects)
- Obstruction of airways: Intraluminal growth, foreign body
- External compression of airways due to neoplasm, cysts or lymph nodes

Disorders of local/systemic immunity

- Primary immunodeficiencies
- Acquired immunodeficiencies
- Human immunodeficiency virus infection
- Immunosuppressive therapy
- Malnutrition

and clinical evidence of sinusitis or otitis. The frequency of sinusitis and otitis media increases with advancing age; may not be evident during infancy or early childhood.

Immune deficiency disorders will manifest with recurrent, multisite infections due to usual as well as unusual organisms and course may be prolonged.

In present case, the first episode of pneumonia occurred at age of 25 days, the child has coughing during feeding and occasional vomiting and persistent noisy breathing. This clinical picture gives clue about possibility of underlying malformations in form of airway obstruction with repeated aspiration.

The child had occasional coughing and choking with noisy respiration. Clinical picture suggests a possibility of secondary reflux associated with airway obstruction.

From history of present case, there is no infection in other parts of body. This makes immune deficiency less likely.

In the present case, there is no malabsorption, sinus, or ear problem. Clinically, it is less likely to be CF or PCD.

Q. What investigations should be carried out to confirm cause of recurrent pneumonia?

For children with airway malformation, CXR may give clue for cysts, congenital cystic adenomatoid malformations, or congenital lobar emphysema. If CXR suggests any of these, computed tomography (CT) scan of chest may be done to confirm the diagnosis. If CXR does not give clue for these possibilities, next investigations should be bronchoscopy to look for airway malformations.

For recurrent aspirations due to malformations, CXR/CT scan of chest and bronchoscopy may be useful investigation. Aspiration secondary to gastroesophageal reflux can be confirmed by performing barium swallow, nuclear scan, 24 hours pH esophageal pH studies, or endoscopy.

Diagnosis of CF can be established by documenting sweat chloride of >60 mEq/L on two occasions or two mutations, or abnormal nasal potential difference.

Primary ciliary dyskinesia can be suspected if nasal nitric oxide is less. Diagnosis can be confirmed by documenting ciliary structural abnormalities by electron microscopy. Documentation of abnormal genetic mutation may be available in future.

Workup for immune deficiency disorder includes screening mother and children above 18 months of age for human immunodeficiency virus infection by doing enzyme-linked immunosorbent assay test, immunoglobulin profile, CD4/CD8 counts, and test for phagocytic abnormalities.

Overall assessment based on history, examination, and basic investigations suggest that he may have airway malformation with gastroesophageal reflux leading to recurrent aspiration pneumonia. Therefore, investigations should be bronchoscopy and workup for gastroesophageal reflux.

Case Progression

Cine-esophagogram suggested aspiration of contrast in trachea from above. Bronchoscopy showed grade II laryngeal cleft.

The child was started on nasogastric feeding, within 24 hours respiratory rates decreased to 36/min, noise during breathing disappeared, oxygen saturation improved to 96% in room air. A consultation with ear, nose, and throat surgeon was obtained, child underwent surgery after 7 days and his symptoms improved. Follow-up for 2 years, no more pneumonia.

Discussion

The child was getting recurrent pneumonia with coughing and choking. All clinical manifestations can be explained by laryngeal cleft.

This child was symptomatic since age of 25 days with recurrent pneumonia, coughing and choking during feeds with noisy respiration. Chest X-ray showed infiltrates in multiple lobes that were clearing with treatment. There was no history of multisite infection and no malabsorption. Early age of onset suggests malformation as one of the possibilities. Noisy breathing without malabsorption or multisite infections made it less likely to be immune deficiency or CF.

X-ray film showed infiltrates in multiple lobes without distortion of airways and no space occupying lesions. This suggests a possibility of airway abnormalities. Therefore, a bronchoscopy was performed and diagnosis could be confirmed.

CASE 2

A 4-year-old boy presented with history of recurrent cold, cough, breathlessness, and fever since the age of 1 year. He also passed large foul smelling bulky stools since the age of 6 months. There was no infection in other parts of the body. His appetite was good, but did not gain weight.

Past history: He passed his stools after 3 days of birth after enema. He also had prolonged jaundice during neonatal period.

Family history: There is second degree consanguinity in parents and two siblings died due to pneumonia and malnutrition at 4 and 9 months of age.

Physical examinations: His weight was 10 kg and height 82 cm. He had grade II clubbing and respiratory distress (respiratory rate 52/min, lower chest indrawing and oxygen saturation 94% in room air) and auscultation of chest showed bilateral crepitations. Rest of the examination was within normal limits.

Investigations: Showed normal hemogram. Biochemistry and blood gas analysis revealed hypochloremia, hyponatremia, hypokalemia, and metabolic alkalosis (serum Na^+ 128, K^+ 2.6, Cl^- 84, pH 7.5, and HCO_3 38.

Q. What are the diagnostic possibilities?

Children with recurrent pneumonia and gastrointestinal symptoms may be due to immune deficiency or CF. If stools are watery and respond to antibiotics, it suggests more of infective diarrhea. If stools are suggestive of malabsorption (large bulky foul smelling), it is more likely to be CF.

The child a product of consanguineous marriage, with history of siblings death, having recurrent respiratory problems with malabsorption and hypochloremic metabolic acidosis. The most probable diagnosis is CF.

Q. How to confirm diagnosis of cystic fibrosis?

Diagnosis of CF can be confirmed by either of the following investigations:

- Raised sweat chloride of >60 mEq/L on two occasions
- Identification of two mutations of CF on blood sample
- Demonstration of abnormal nasal potential difference.

Course of patient

Sweat chloride in the patient was 120 and 127 mEq/L on two occasions. Blood for mutations could identify only one delta-F508 mutation.

Q. How to confirm diagnosis when sweat test facility is not available?

Gold standard for making a diagnosis of CF is abnormal test discussed above. If sweat test facility is not available, may try to document hypochloremia, hyponatremia, hypokalemia, alkaline pH, pseudomonas on culture of airway secretions and stool for plenty of fat globules. If two or more than two abnormalities are detected in a setting of recurrent pneumonia and malabsorption, a diagnosis of suspected CF may be made (Flowchart 1). Final diagnosis should be made only after sweat test or mutation analysis.

Q. Can we send mutation studies when sweat test is not available?

There are more than 2,000 mutations for CF identified till now. There is wide variation in prevalence of particular mutation in different population. Testing panel of mutations in Caucasian population may be able to identify more than 90% children with CF. However,

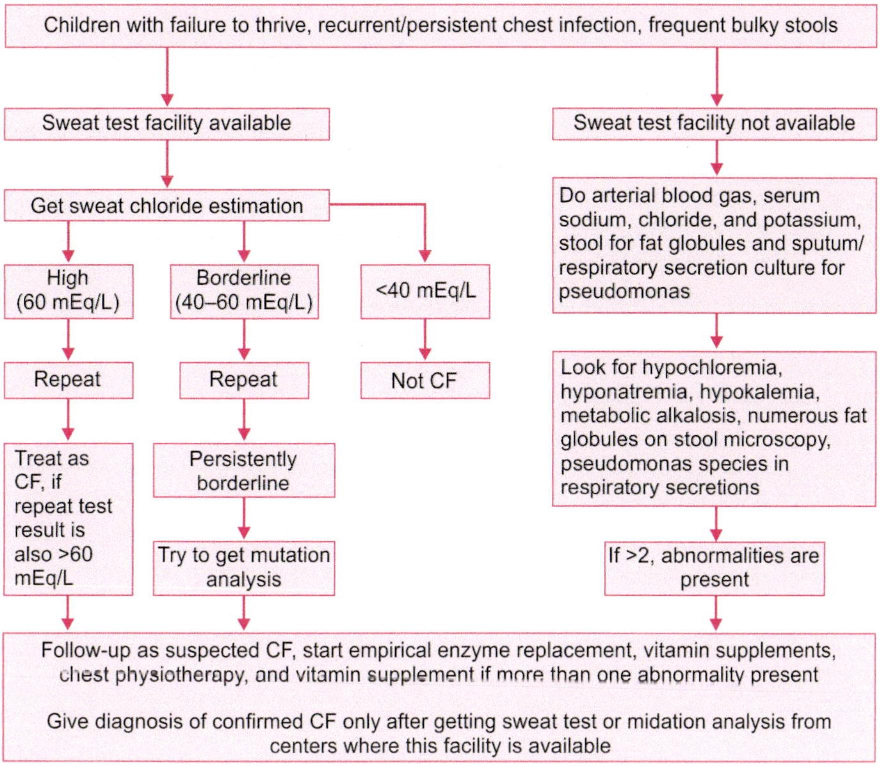

CF, cystic fibrosis.

Flowchart 1: Algorithm for diagnosis of cystic fibrosis when sweat test is not available

Modified from: Kabra SK, Kabra M, Lodha R, Shastri S. Cystic fibrosis in India. Pediatr Pulmonol. 2007;42(12):1087-94.

there is no such panel available for Indian children. Mutations of CF children in India are heterogeneous and varied according to different ethnic background. Panel being used for diagnosis of CF for Caucasian population is not useful for diagnosis of CF in India. Most laboratories in India offer limited number of mutations. Therefore, negative results of mutation studies do not rule out CF. Hence, at present gold standard for making a diagnosis of CF is abnormal sweat test.

Q. If sweat test is gold standard for making a diagnosis of cystic fibrosis, is there any role of doing mutation testing?

Mutation studies in suspected CF may be helpful in following situations:

- Prenatal diagnosis for subsequent pregnancies: Prenatal diagnosis can be performed by identification of mutation or by linkage studies
- Mutation specific drugs: There is search for pharmacologic agents that potentiate CF transmembrane regular protein and improvement in function. The pharmacological agents are mutation specific and may have major role in treatment of CF in future.

LEARNING POINTS

- Recurrent pneumonia is defined as two episodes of radiographic documented pneumonia over 1 year or three episodes in any time frame
- Persistent pneumonia is defined as persistent clinical symptoms with radiological abnormalities for more than 4 weeks

- Common causes can be classified into four groups: malformations, recurrent aspirations, immune deficiency disorders, impaired airway clearance and others
- History and examination give a clue about underlying cause
- Common investigations for identification of underlying cause include: imaging (X ray chest, CT film of chest), contrast studies to document gastroesophageal reflux or H type tracheo-esophageal fistula, work up for primary or secondary immune deficiency, sweat testing for cystic fibrosis
- Treatment depends on cause of underlying illness.

SUGGESTED READINGS

1. Kabra SK, Kabra M, Lodha R, Shastri S. Cystic fibrosis in India. Pediatr Pulmonol. 2007;42:1087-94.
2. Kabra SK, Kabra M, Shastri S, Lodha R. Diagnosing and managing cystic fibrosis in the developing world. Paediatr Respir Rev. 2006;7 Suppl 1:S147-50.
3. Lodha R, Puranik M, Chandra U, Natchu M, Kabra SK. Persistent pneumonia in children. Indian Pediatr. 2003;40(10):967-70.
4. Lodha R, Puranik M, Natchu UC, Kabra SK. Recurrent pneumonia in children: clinical profile and underlying causes. Acta Paediatr. 2002;91:1170-3.

CHAPTER

26

Intrathoracic Tuberculosis

Aparna Mukherjee

CASE 1

A 5-year-old boy presented with cough and fever for the last 2 weeks. He had poor appetite and was not as active as before. He weighed 15 kg, Bacillus Calmette–Guérin (BCG) scar was present, the respiratory rate was 30/min, had no subcostal or intercostal retraction, and air entry was slightly reduced in left mammary region with bronchial breath sound. There was no history of contact with any case of tuberculosis (TB).

Q. What should be the next steps?

Get a tuberculin skin test (TST) and chest X-ray (CXR) done. In case of an CXR suggestive of TB, a trial of antibiotics like oral amoxicillin should be given for 7–10 days and CXR repeated thereafter. If the CXR abnormalities persist, further workup for pulmonary tuberculosis (TB) is warranted. If the child is very sick or antibiotics have already been tried, tuberculosis can be the immediate provisional diagnosis.

Case Progression

Tuberculin skin test showed an induration of 15 mm. Chest X-ray is shown in figure 1.

Q. What other investigations are required to reach to a diagnosis?

Gastric aspirate and induced sputum should be performed on two consecutive days and the samples sent for Ziehl-Neelsen staining for acid fast-bacilli (AFB), liquid mycobacteria growth indicator tube (MGIT) culture and Xpert® MTB/RIF assay, if facilities are available. Induced sputum is feasible and safe even in infants. Gastric lavage can be done on ambulatory basis. If the above does not yield any conclusive results, bronchoalveolar lavage may also be considered. Bacteriological confirmation should be attempted by sending all possible pulmonary samples.

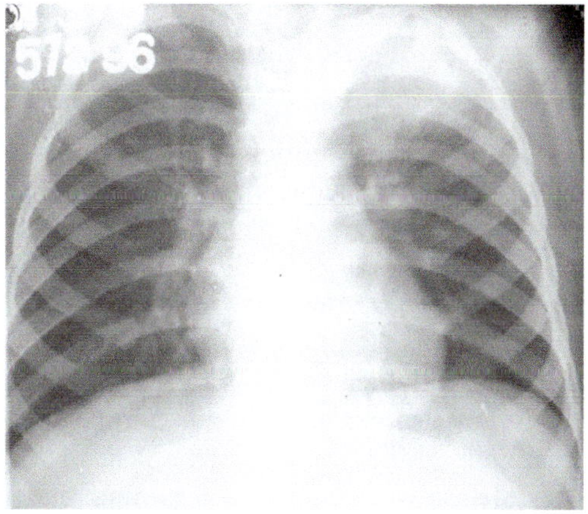

Figure 1: Chest X-ray (posteroanterior view) showing a consolidation in the left upper zone

Contrast-enhanced computed tomography chest may be done if the CXR features are not conclusive.

Q. What are the clinical features suggestive of childhood intrathoracic tuberculosis?

The clinical features suggestive of intrathoracic childhood TB are:

- Cough and/or fever more than 2 weeks, not responding to a course of antibiotic for 7–10 days
- Documented weight loss (>5% of the highest recorded weight in the past 3 months) or not gaining weight
- History of contact with a case of TB in last 2 years.

Q. What is the role of tuberculin skin test or Mantoux test and interferon gamma release assay in the diagnosis of tuberculosis?

An induration of ≥10 mm (≥5 mm in immunocompromised individuals), measured 48–72 hours after intradermal injection of tuberculin 2 TU (PPD RT 23 or equivalent), is considered as a positive TST. A positive TST is indicative of tubercular infection, not disease. In countries like India, with high incidence of TB, a positive TST is only a supportive criterion for diagnosis. Treatment cannot be initiated solely on the basis of positive TST. interferon gamma release assays (IGRAs) are *in vitro* tests for diagnosis of TB infection, performed on a blood sample. In endemic regions, performance of IGRAs and TST is equivalent. In view of higher cost of IGRAs, it is prudent to use TST as an aid in the diagnosis of tubercular infection.

Q. Is there any role of serological diagnosis in pulmonary tuberculosis?

There is no role of any serological diagnosis in the form of antibodies against tubercular antigens in the diagnosis of any type of TB—pulmonary or extrapulmonary. In fact, such tests are currently banned by the Government of India.

Case Progression

After 2 days, Xpert® MTB/RIF assay on induced sputum of this child detected *Mycobacterium tuberculosis*, rifampicin sensitive. Ziehl-Neelsen staining for AFB was negative, MGIT culture was still awaited. What is the diagnosis in this child?

Having a positive Xpert® report confirms the diagnosis of TB. In view of the X-ray findings, the diagnosis is progressive pulmonary TB.

Q. Is there any diagnostic algorithm for childhood intrathoracic tuberculosis?

A suggested diagnostic algorithm is described in flowchart 1.

Q. What treatment should be started?

Category-based anti-TB treatment is applicable for children with TB. In this case, category 1 anti-TB treatment (for new cases) should be started; which includes 2 months of intensive phase with isoniazid, rifampicin, pyrazinamide, and ethambutol followed by 4 months of maintenance phase with isoniazid, rifampicin and ethambutol.

The medications should preferably be given daily on mg/kg body weight basis. Recommended daily doses of the four first-line antitubercular drugs are given in table 1.

Q. How should the child be monitored?

The child should be monitored regularly for improvement in symptoms, weight gain, and any adverse events like hepatitis and rash. In each visit, the dose of the antitubercular drugs should be adjusted according to the current weight of the child.

Q. What should be done if the child develops hepatitis while on antitubercular drugs?

If the child is symptomatic with pain in the abdomen, vomiting or yellowish discoloration of sclera and urine, or if the liver enzymes are deranged (aspartate transaminase/alanine aminotransferase) more than five times the

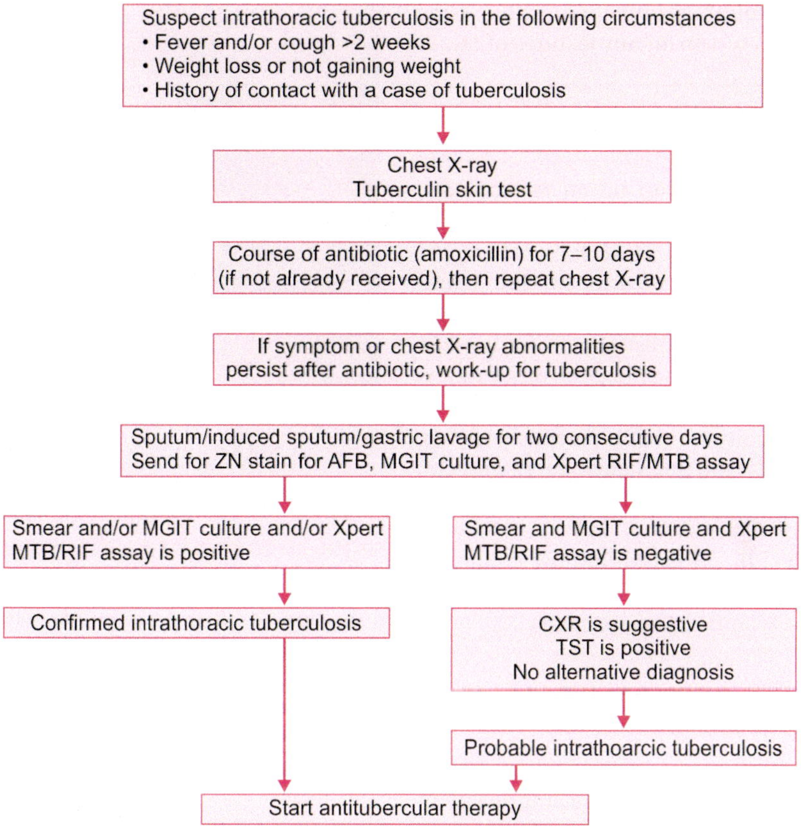

ZN, Ziehl-Neelsen; AFB, acid fast bacilli; MGIT, mycobacteria growth indicator tube; CXR, chest X-ray; TST, tuberculin skin test.

Flowchart 1: Diagnostic algorithm for childhood intrathoracic tuberculosis

TABLE 1: Daily dose and maximum doses of isoniazid, rifampicin, ethambutol, and pyrazinamide in children

Drugs	Dose (range) mg/kg body weight/day	Maximum dose mg/day
Rifampicin	15 (10–20)	600
Isoniazid	10 (7–15)	300
Ethambutol	20–25	1,500
Pyrazinamide	30–35	2,000

upper limit or total bilirubin is raised, the antitubercular drugs should be modified. Isoniazid, rifampicin, and pyrazinamide should be stopped and the modified regimen will contain ethambutol and a fluoroquinolone like ofloxacin. Injectable streptomycin may be added if the disease severity warrants. Once the symptoms are relieved and liver parameters are normalized, the first line antitubercular drugs can be restarted sequentially, increasing every 5–7 days after checking the liver functions. Once the full dose of conventional antitubercular drugs is reached, the modified regimen may be stopped.

Q. What investigations should be done for the family?

Family survey should be done for each child diagnosed with TB; this includes the immediate family members who reside with the child. Family survey should include thorough history taking and clinical examination; chest X-ray may be done to screen for any features of TB.

Q. What is the utility of doing Xpert® MTB/RIF assay?

Xpert® MTB/RIF test is an automated cartridge based nucleic acid amplification test for TB, which can not only detect *M. tuberculosis*, but also detect rifampicin resistance. The World Health Organization (WHO) as of now strongly recommends that this test should be used in children. The main advantage of this assay is the rapid turnover-time, less chance of human error, and ability to simultaneously detect *M. tuberculosis* and resistance to rifampicin. In the meta-analysis published by WHO, the overall pooled sensitivity and specificity of Xpert® MTB/RIF compared against culture as a reference standard in children presumed to have TB was 66 and 98%, respectively.

Q. How is the response to treatment monitored in such a child?

The response to treatment in childhood TB is monitored by clinico-radiological improvement at 2 months and 6 months of anti-TB therapy. If AFB or MGIT is positive at baseline, gastric lavage and induced sputum should be repeated at 2 months for Ziehl-Neelsen staining and MGIT culture.

CASE 2

Parents of a 3-year-old girl were concerned that she did not eat well and did not gain weight, especially since last few months. The girl's grandmother had received anti-TB medications last year for pulmonary TB (sputum positive). On examination BCG scar was present, weight of the child was 9 kg, there was mild pallor and had no other significant findings. Tuberculin skin test showed an induration of 12 mm. Chest X-ray of this child is shown in figure 2.

Q. What can be the differential diagnoses?

The differential diagnosis in this scenario of mediastinal widening includes TB and lymphoma.

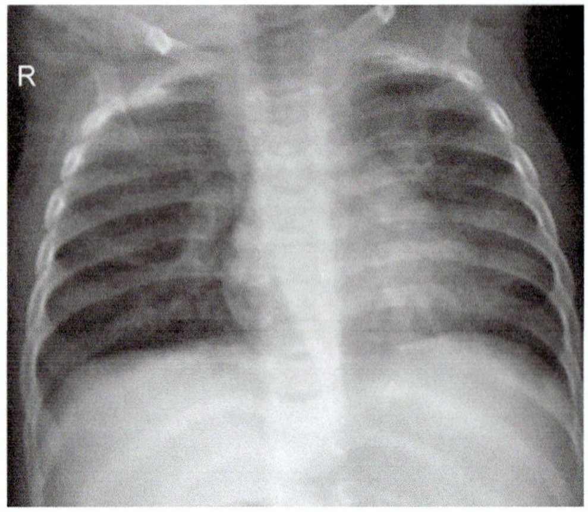

Figure 2: Chest X-ray showing mediastinal widening

Q. What other investigations are required to reach to a diagnosis?

The child underwent gastric lavage and sputum induction for two consecutive days; samples were subjected to Ziehl-Neelsen staining for AFB, culture for *M. tuberculosis* by MGIT culture system, and Xpert® MTB/RIF assay. Every effort should be made to reach to a bacteriological diagnosis.

Contrast-enhanced computed tomography chest may be done in cases where the chest X-ray is not conclusive to look for features suggestive of necrosis in lymph nodes and other signs of active disease.

In cases of mediastinal lymph nodes, CT or ultrasound-guided fine needle aspiration can be done to establish the cytological and microbiological diagnosis. Samples should also be sent for bacteriological confirmation of *M. tuberculosis* as detailed above.

Q. Is ultrasonography useful in diagnosing mediastinal tubercular lymph nodes?

Endobronchial ultrasound (EBUS) is feasible and useful in older children. In case of older children with large hilar or subcarinal lymph nodes, EBUS—transbronchial needle aspiration may be tried to obtain sample for cytological and microbiological diagnosis. This technique is yet to be available widely for diagnosis of TB in children.

Q. In this child, computed tomography showed necrotic mediastinal lymph nodes and fine needle aspiration cytology (from computed tomography-guided aspiration of mediastinal node) showed epithelioid cell granulomas along with acid fast bacilli. A diagnosis of intrathoracic tuberculosis involving mediastinal lymph nodes was made. What treatment should be started?

Category 1 treatment (for new cases) should be started and advised for 6 months. The category-based treatment as advised by Revised National Tuberculosis Control Program is detailed in table 2.

Q. Is there any role of corticosteroids in the treatment of intrathoracic tuberculosis?

Routinely, there is no role of corticosteroids in the management of intrathoracic TB in children. However, in case of superior mediastinal compression syndrome due to mediastinal nodes and endobronchial TB, oral corticosteroids may be used.

Q. What are the usual radiological findings suggestive of intrathoracic tuberculosis?

Radiological features highly suggestive of TB include hilar or paratracheal lymph nodes with or without parenchymal involvement, miliary pattern, and fibrocavitary lesion. Some examples are given in figures 3 to 6.

TABLE 2: Category based treatment for tuberculosis in children (the prefix number denotes the number of months)

Category of treatment	Inclusion criteria	Treatment regimen	
		Intensive phase*	Continuation phase
New cases (category 1)	• New smear positive pulmonary tuberculosis • New smear negative pulmonary tuberculosis • New extrapulmonary tuberculosis	2 HRZE	4HRE**
Previously treated cases (category 2)	• Relapse, failure to respond or treatment after default • Retreatment	2 HRZES + 1 HRZE	5 HRE

H, isoniazid; R, rifampicin; Z, pyrazinamide; E, ethambutol; S, streptomycin

*Intensive phase can be extended by 1 month in case of unsatisfactory response

**Continuation phase to be extended for 10 months in cases of osteoarticular and central nervous system tuberculosis

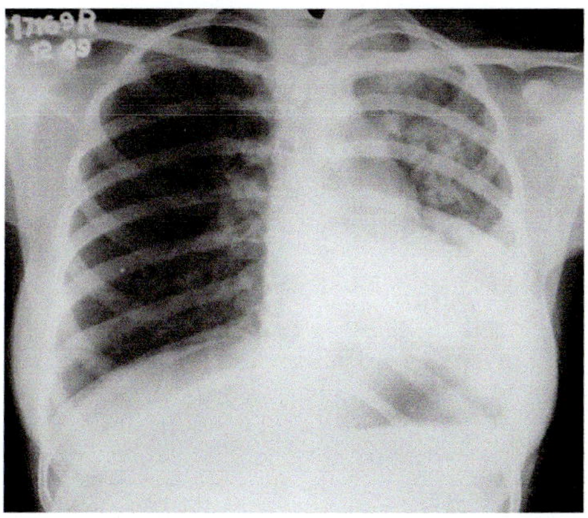

Figure 3: Chest X-ray of a 15-year-old girl with tuberculosis showing consolidation in the left lower and mid zone along with blunting of left costophrenic angle

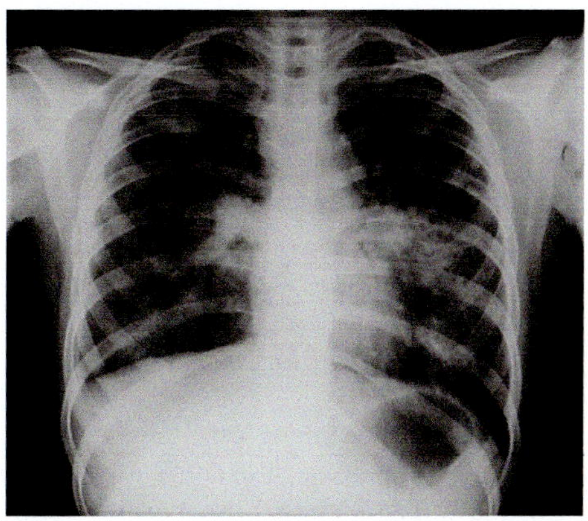

Figure 4: Chest X-ray showing bilateral infiltrates in a child with confirmed tuberculosis

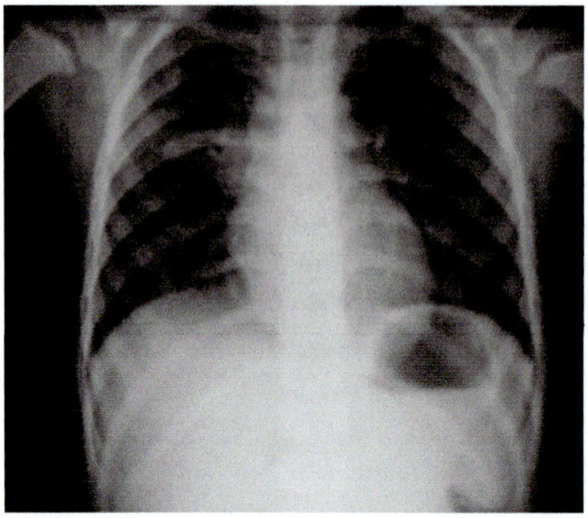

Figure 5: Chest X-ray of a five-year-old with collapse consolidation of the right middle lobe

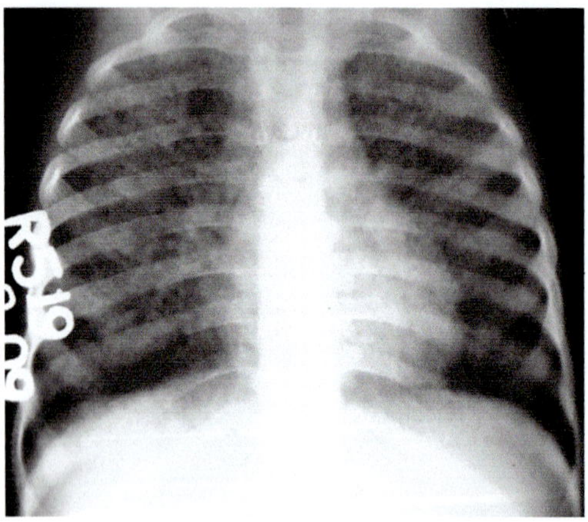

Figure 6: Chest X-ray of a two-and-half-year-old girl with miliary tuberculosis

CASE 3

A 4-year-old boy was brought to the doctor by his mother. His grandfather had developed TB (sputum positive) recently. She wanted to know if her child also needed treatment.

Q. What should be done in such a scenario?

A thorough history taking and clinical examination should be done to exclude any features suggestive of TB. A chest X-ray can be done to rule out any pulmonary involvement. If the child is asymptomatic and has no features of active TB, he should be started on isoniazid preventive therapy.

Q. What is the preventive treatment for tuberculosis?

Isoniazid is prescribed for chemoprophylaxis at a dose of 10 mg/kg of body weight/day, for 6 months.

Tuberculosis preventive therapy or chemoprophylaxis should be provided to:

- All asymptomatic contacts, less than 6 years of age, of an open case of TB (smear positive) after ruling out active disease. Status of BCG vaccination or TST reading does not preclude one from receiving this chemoprophylaxis
- All human immunodeficiency virus infected children with a known exposure to an infectious TB case, but with no active TB disease
- All TST positive children who are receiving immunosuppressive therapy
- A child born to mother who was diagnosed to have TB in pregnancy, after ruling out congenital TB. Bacillus Calmette-Guérin vaccination can be given at birth even if chemoprophylaxis is planned.

LEARNING POINTS

- ☞ Probable intrathoracic tuberculosis is the diagnosis made in children on the basis of suggestive clinico-radiological features
- ☞ All efforts should be made to make bacteriological diagnosis of confirmed intrathoracic tuberculosis by sending samples of sputum/induced sputum/gastric lavage
- ☞ Samples should be sent for Ziehl-Neelsen staining, MGIT culture and Xpert® MTB/RIF assay
- ☞ Category-based treatment should be started in newly diagnosed cases of intrathoracic tuberculosis with 2 months of isoniazid, rifampicin, pyrazinamide, and ethambutol followed by 4 months of isoniazid, rifampicin and ethambutol. (category 1). Category 2 treatment is for relapse, failure to respond, or treatment after default and retreatment
- ☞ The revised doses of isoniazid, rifampicin, and ethambutol should be used, preferably in daily regimen.

SUGGESTED READINGS

1. Kumar A, Gupta D, Nagaraja SB, Singh V, Prasad J; Indian Academy of Pediatrics. Updated national guidelines for pediatric tuberculosis in India, 2012. Indian Pediatr. 2013;50:301-6.
2. Kabra SK, Lodha R, Seth V. Category based treatment of tuberculosis in children. Indian Pediatr. 2004; 41:927-37.
3. World Health Organization. Rapid advice treatment of tuberculosis in children. Geneva, Switzerland: WHO; 2010.
4. World Health Organization. Guidance for national tuberculosis programmes on the management of tuberculosis in children. Geneva, Switzerland: WHO; 2014.
5. World Health Organization. Automated real-time nucleic acid amplification technology for rapid and simultaneous detection of tuberculosis and rifampicin resistance: Xpert MTB/RIF assay for the diagnosis of pulmonary and extrapulmonary TB in adults and children, policy update. Geneva, Switzerland: WHO; 2013.

5 SECTION

Suppurative Lung Diseases

CHAPTER

27

Primary Ciliary Dyskinesia

Umakanth Khatwa, Fei Jamie Dy

CASE 1

A 7-year-old girl who was born full-term was brought to clinic for evaluation of a persistent wet cough and recurrent pneumonia since early infancy. She also had a history of repeated ear and sinus infections.

Past medical history: Glucose 6-phosphatase deficiency.

Family history: Biological parents were first cousins.

Physical examination: Normal vital signs. Measured weight was 16.5 kg (<1st percentile for age). She had 3–4+ tonsillar hypertrophy and dextrocardia with normal heart sounds. Lung examination revealed focally decreased aeration and fine crackles over the left lower lobe. Liver edge was palpable under the left costal margin.

Q. The patient undergoes X-ray and computed tomography imaging of the chest. What do these studies show (Fig. 1)?

Chest X-ray shows situs inversus totalis, and total collapse of the left lower lobe associated with bronchiectasis.

Chest computed tomography (CT) is notable for bronchiectasis—most pronounced in the left lower lobe and associated with chronic volume loss.

Q. Given the history and findings in this patient, what are the main diagnoses that you need to consider and why?

- Primary ciliary dyskinesia (PCD) should be strongly considered in this child who has recurrent otosinopulmonary infections and organ laterality abnormalities
- Immunodeficiency can sometimes coexist with other diagnoses and needs to be evaluated concurrently
- Cystic fibrosis (CF) is a common cause of recurrent sinopulmonary infections and needs to be ruled out.

Q. What is primary ciliary dyskinesia and how common is this disorder?

Primary ciliary dyskinesia is a genetic disorder that is largely inherited in autosomal recessive fashion. It is characterized by chronic lung infections, recurrent rhinosinusitis, middle ear infections associated with hearing loss, and infertility. Kartagener's syndrome is only a subgroup of PCD where the clinical triad of situs inversus, chronic sinusitis, and bronchiectasis occur together. Note that only 40–50% of patients with PCD have situs inversus. Young's syndrome is another subgroup of PCD characterized by sinopulmonary infections and obstructive azoospermia (these patients are infertile).

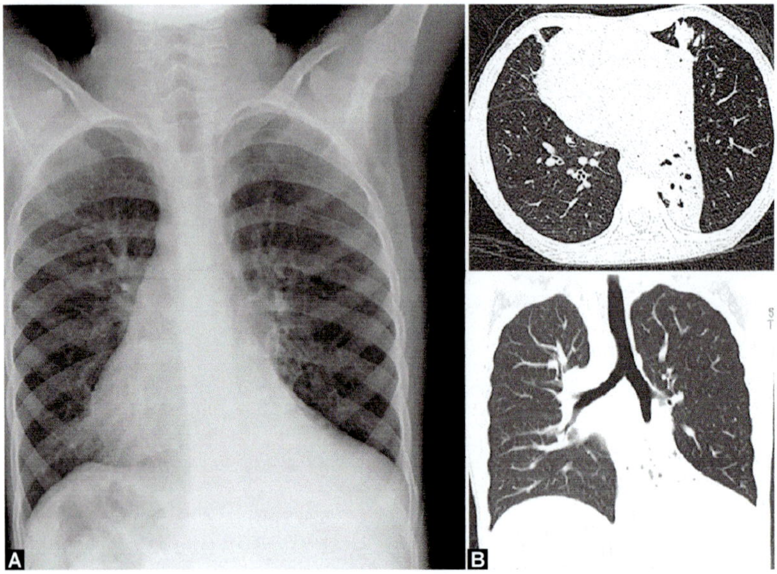

Figure 1: **A,** Chest X-ray and **B,** chest computed tomography with representative axial (top) and coronal (bottom) views

The prevalence of PCD has been estimated around 1:10,000 with higher rates in certain populations that harbor significant consanguinity.

Q. What is the pathogenesis of primary ciliary dyskinesia?

Figure 2 shows the microtubule complex that is the foundation of normal motile cilia. Figure 3

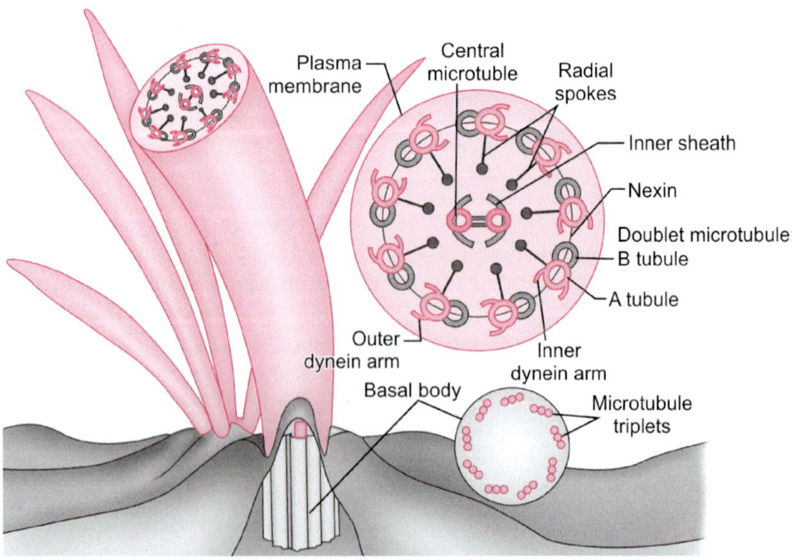

Figure 2: Normal motile cilia (9 + 2) configuration. Motile cilia are composed of highly complex microtubules of α- and β-monomers of tubulin and associated accessory elements

Source: Reprinted with permission of the American Thoracic Society. Copyright ©2015 American Thoracic Society. Knowles MR, Daniels LA, Davis SD, Zariwala MA, Leigh MW. Primary ciliary dyskinesia. Recent advances in diagnostics, genetics, and characterization of clinical disease. Am J Respir Crit Care Med. 2013;188(8):913-22.

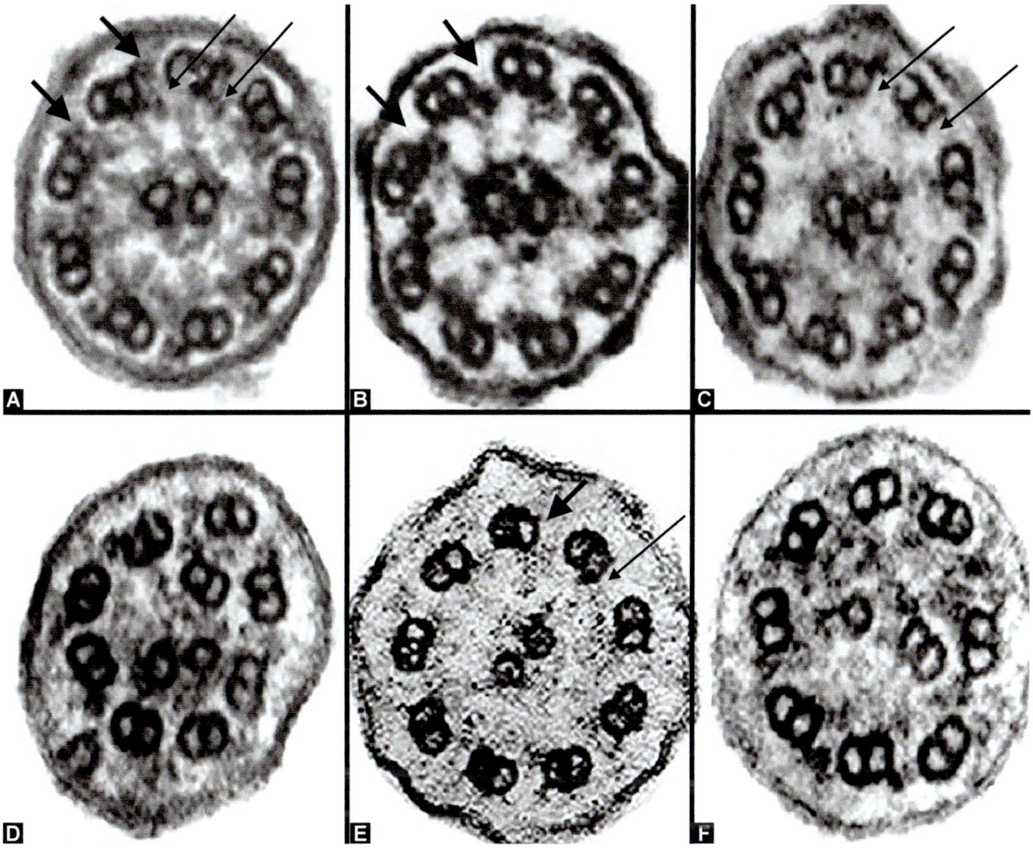

Figure 3: Ciliary ultrastructure by electron micrographs from **A,** normal subject and **B–F,** patients with primary ciliary dyskinesia (PCD). **A,** The 9 + 2 axonemal structure is shown, with thick black arrows showing the outer dynein arm (ODA) and thin black arrows showing the inner dynein arm (IDA). **B,** ODA defect denoted by thick black arrows (*CCDC114* mutations). (C and D) Patient with PCD with *CCDC40* mutations: **C,** IDA defect denoted by thin black arrows and **D,** microtubular disorganization with one outer doublet translocating (disruption of 9 + 2 axonemal structure) into the central region in approximately 10% of cilia. **E,** ODA + IDA defects noted by thick black arrow and thin black arrow. **F,** Central apparatus defect; translocation of outer doublet into central region and loss of one of the central pair (seen in ~5% of cilia with radial spoke head gene mutations)

Source: Reprinted with permission of the American Thoracic Society. Copyright ©2015 American Thoracic Society. Knowles MR, Daniels LA, Davis SD, Zariwala MA, Leigh MW. Primary ciliary dyskinesia. Recent advances in diagnostics, genetics, and characterization of clinical disease. Am J Respir Crit Care Med. 2013;188(8):913-22.

shows the range of structural defects associated with PCD. The most common abnormalities in ciliary ultrastructure are absent or short outer dynein arms, and outer and inner dynein arm defects. Defects in central apparatus and radial spokes are less common. Mutations are also known to affect cytoplasmic proteins that contribute to cilia assembly or protein transport, rather than cilia structure.

Q. What are important clinical factors that raise suspicion for primary ciliary dyskinesia?

The key to this diagnosis always begins with eliciting a detailed clinical history. The classic clinical phenotype is neonatal respiratory distress without apparent cause, early onset chronic rhinorrhea, and recurrent otitis media, sinusitis, and pneumonia. Table 1 describes the important elements of perinatal history and these otosinopulmonary symptoms.

Q. What are important physical findings in children with primary ciliary dyskinesia?

Table 1 highlights aspects of the physical examination which should be noted in suspected or confirmed PCD cases.

Q. How are other organ systems affected in primary ciliary dyskinesia?

Besides motile cilia lining the respiratory system, specialized cilia also exist in the embryonic ventral node (called nodal cilia) and establish the laterality of visceral organs during embryonic development. Therefore, dysfunction of nodal cilia leads to organ laterality defects. These are present in around

TABLE 1: Clinical presentation of primary ciliary dyskinesia

History	
Perinatal events	• Around 85% of infants will experience respiratory distress as early as 12–24 h of life despite term gestation • Tachypnea, increased work of breathing, and upper or middle lobe atelectasis on chest radiographs • Such events are typically misinterpreted as transient tachypnea of the newborn, neonatal pneumonia, or meconium aspiration • All term infants with respiratory distress and dextrocardia should undergo evaluation for primary ciliary dyskinesia (PCD)
Pattern of respiratory symptoms	• Infants develop a persistent, year-round, daily cough early on in life • Cough is usually wet and productive, but may also be dry • Antibiotic therapy can produce partial improvement, but symptom-free periods are unlikely • Recurrent upper and lower airway infections occur in up to 80% of patients by preschool age
Nasal symptoms	• Nasal congestion is perennial and unabating • Chronic rhinosinusitis affects over half of individuals with PCD and nasal polyposis occurs in 15% of patients • Persistent rhinitis may contribute to feeding difficulties in infants • Older children and adults may endorse multiple rounds of antibiotics for sinus infections
Otitis media	• Chronic middle ear infections affect at least 80% of children • Tympanostomy tube placement and conductive hearing loss are frequently reported from a young age (by age 1–2 years)
Physical Examination	
Growth	Underweight, short stature (failure to thrive is common) May be normal
Ear	Chronic middle ear effusion, otorrhea, glue ear, tympanic membrane scarring or perforation, cholesteatoma
Nasopharynx	Nasal turbinate hypertrophy, mucopurulent drainage, nasal polyps
Chest	Intermittent wheezing, coarse rhonchi and/or crackles, barrel chest Heart sounds are typically normal, dextrocardia may be present
Abdomen	May be normal, but situs inversus may be present

half of PCD patients and may be missed without imaging (e.g., intestinal malrotation).

In situs inversus totalis, there is complete mirror-image arrangement of all internal organs, it occurs in about 40–50% of affected individuals. Situs ambiguus or heterotaxy is less common, affecting around 12% of cases. In this condition, normal asymmetry is lost and thoracoabdominal organs are not clearly lateralized across the left-right body axis. Heterotaxy is associated with a 200-fold higher prevalence of cardiovascular abnormalities, as well as immunodeficiency related to asplenia or polysplenia.

Primary ciliary dyskinesia is also linked with male infertility because of reduced sperm motility. Females may be more prone to ectopic pregnancy due to abnormal ciliary function in fallopian tubes.

Q. What specific investigations are used to diagnose primary ciliary dyskinesia?

As other disease entities are ruled out, a panel of tests is often required to confirm the diagnosis of PCD. This is due to the wide spectrum of ciliary defects and the limited scope of individual tests. These tests are complementary to each other and are described in table 2 and flowchart 1. Older tests—such as nasal saccharin testing, radioaerosol mucociliary clearance, ciliary beat frequency, and ciliary waveform analysis

TABLE 2: Recommended diagnostic tests for primary ciliary dyskinesia

Test	Description	Limitations
Ciliary biopsy with electron microscopy (EM)	• Brush biopsy of nasal turbinates or bronchial walls (via bronchoscopy) • Diagnoses up to 70% of primary ciliary dyskinesia (PCD) cases • EM allows visualization of ciliary ultrastructure	• Invasive bronchoscopy with sedation is required to obtain samples • Biopsy yield is variable • Sample processing is labor-intensive and expensive • EM is unable to detect oligociliary defects and PCD mutations that result in normal ciliary ultrastructure (e.g., *DNAH11*) • Results may be confounded by secondary changes in ciliary ultrastructure provoked by infection or pollutants
Nasal nitric oxide (nNO) measurement	• Measured nNO values in PCD patients are only 10–20% of levels measured in healthy controls • If cystic fibrosis has been ruled out, nNO <77nL/min can diagnose PCD with sensitivity of 98% and specificity of >99% • Affords rapid and noninvasive testing, with immediate results	• Less reliable in younger children as testing requires cooperation with blowing into a resistor • Viral respiratory infections, cystic fibrosis, panbronchiolitis and nonatopic sinusitis can produce low nNO measurements (false positive results)
High speed videomicroscopy	• Allows waveform analysis and measurement of cilia beat frequency (normal 8–14 Hz)	• Requires considerable center expertize and sophisticated software for analysis • Viral infections, environmental pollutants, poor sampling and processing can produce false positive results

Continued

Continued

Test	Description	Limitations
Immunofluorescence (IF)	• IF staining detects missing proteins in dynein arms and radial spokes using antibodies against various ciliary structural components • IF testing is not affected by secondary processes	• Sensitivity and specificity still under investigation
Genetic testing	• Mostly autosomal recessive inheritance • 32 genes have been identified to date, and account for up to 65–70% of PCD cases	• Not all genes are tested in commercially-available panels • A negative genetic test does not necessarily rule out PCD

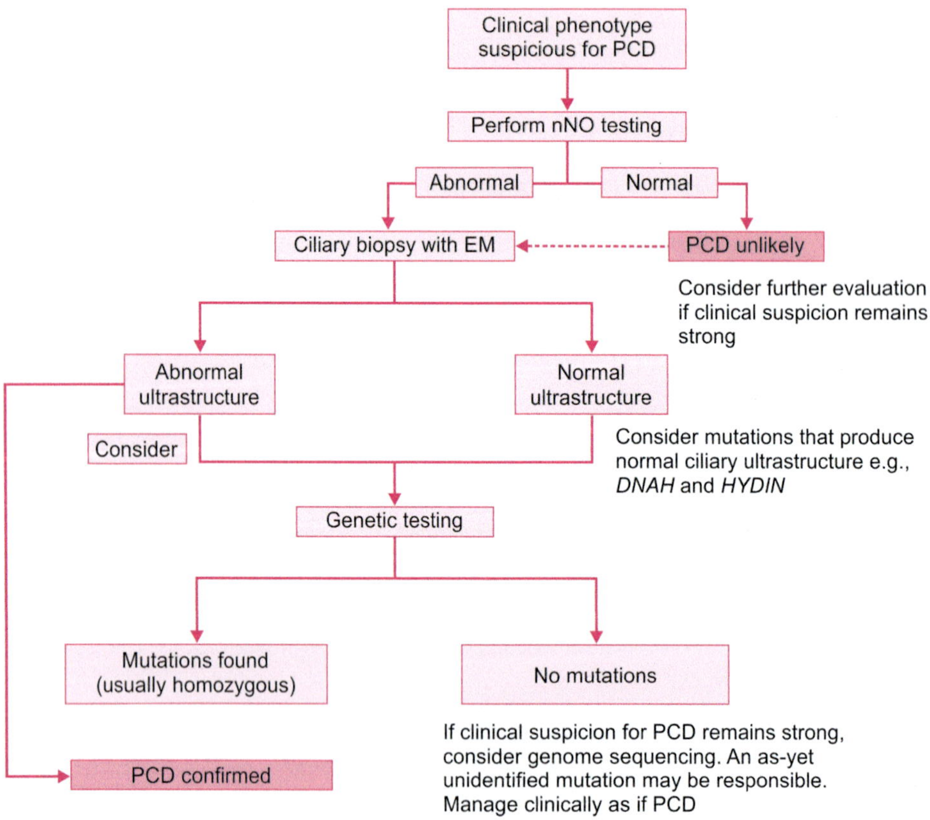

PCD, primary ciliary dyskinesia; nNO, nasal nitric oxide; EM, electron microscopy.

Flowchart 1: Diagnostic algorithm for primary ciliary dyskinesia without high-speed videomicroscopy—are no longer recommended due to the high rate of false positive and negative results.

Q. How is nasal nitric oxide testing performed?

Nitric oxide (NO) is measured using a chemiluminescence analyzer—Sievers 280i nitric oxide analyzer (NOA) or CLD 88 sp. Figure 4 demonstrates the set up for nasal nitric oxide (nNO) testing. Nasal nitric oxide studies should be performed on subjects during clinically stable periods, when they are free of acute upper or lower respiratory illnesses or nasal instrumentation for at least 2 weeks. The nNO concentration is calculated in parts per billion, and then depending on the flow rate of the machine, nNO production is calculated. Nasal nitric oxide production <77 ng/dL is consistent with PCD.

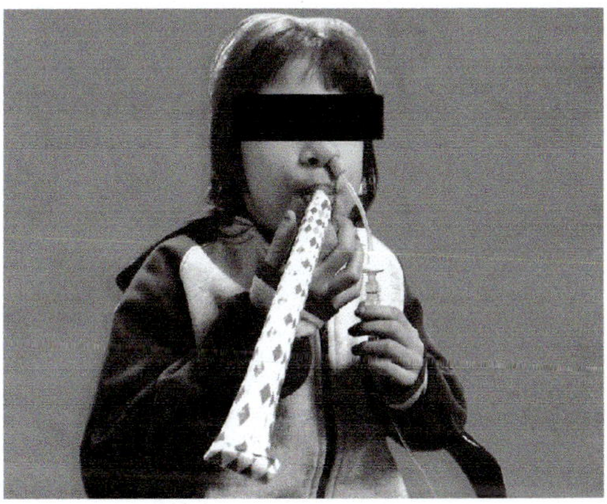

Figure 4: Nasal nitric oxide (nNO) testing. It is measured when subjects achieve palatal closure by exhaling for 20–40 seconds through the mouth into a disposable resistor (a cardboard cylinder with 1 mm opening at distal end or a party favor blowout toy with comparable resistance). Meanwhile nasal gas is aspirated through a line connected to a disposable foam olive that is inserted into one nostril

Q. What is the role of genetic testing in the diagnosis of primary ciliary dyskinesia?

The utility and limitations of genetic testing are described in table 2. The discovery of genes associated with PCD has accelerated in recent years with 32 genes identified to date (Table 3). Almost all are inherited in autosomal recessive fashion.

Q. Is there a cure for primary ciliary dyskinesia?

No curative options exist for PCD at this time. Treatment is supportive and aimed at optimizing nutritive status, hearing, and respiratory health.

Q. What are the principles of management for primary ciliary dyskinesia?

Clinical management is multidisciplinary and should involve otolaryngology, pulmonology,

TABLE 3: Genes associated with primary ciliary dyskinesia

PCD gene	Affected ciliary structure defect	Detectable by		
		Commercial NGS panels	Transmission electron microscopy	Immunofluorescence
NME8	Partial ODA defect	Yes	Yes	Yes
DNAH5 *DNAI1* *DNAI2* *DNAL1*	ODA defect	Yes	Yes	Yes
CCDC114 *CCDC151* *ARMC4*	ODA targeting/docking factor ODA defect	Yes No No	Yes	Yes

Continued

Continued

<table>
<tr><th rowspan="2">PCD gene</th><th rowspan="2">Affected ciliary structure defect</th><th colspan="3">Detectable by</th></tr>
<tr><th>Commercial NGS panels</th><th>Transmission electron microscopy</th><th>Immunofluorescence</th></tr>
<tr><td>CCDC103</td><td rowspan="10">Cytoplasmic dynein arm assembly or transport factor
ODA and IDA defect</td><td>Yes</td><td rowspan="10">Yes</td><td rowspan="10">Yes</td></tr>
<tr><td>DNAAF1</td><td>Yes</td></tr>
<tr><td>DNAAF2</td><td>Yes</td></tr>
<tr><td>DNAAF3</td><td>Yes</td></tr>
<tr><td>LRRC6</td><td>Yes</td></tr>
<tr><td>HEATR2</td><td>Yes</td></tr>
<tr><td>ZMYND10</td><td>No</td></tr>
<tr><td>DYX1C1</td><td>No</td></tr>
<tr><td>SPAG1</td><td>No</td></tr>
<tr><td>C21orf59</td><td>No</td></tr>
<tr><td>RSPH9</td><td rowspan="3">Radial spoke head subunit
May see missing central pair or tubular transposition defect (8 + 1 structure), but often normal</td><td>Yes</td><td rowspan="3">Yes/No</td><td rowspan="3">Yes</td></tr>
<tr><td>RSPH4A</td><td>Yes</td></tr>
<tr><td>RSPH1</td><td>No</td></tr>
<tr><td>CCDC39</td><td rowspan="2">Nexin link/dynein regulatory complex factor
IDA + MTD defect</td><td rowspan="2">Yes</td><td rowspan="2">Yes</td><td rowspan="2">Yes</td></tr>
<tr><td>CCDC40</td></tr>
<tr><td>CCDC164</td><td rowspan="2">Nexin link subunit
Mostly normal</td><td rowspan="2">No</td><td rowspan="2">Rarely</td><td rowspan="2">Yes</td></tr>
<tr><td>CCDC65</td></tr>
<tr><td>DNAH11</td><td>ODA subunit
Normal</td><td>Yes</td><td>No</td><td>No</td></tr>
<tr><td>HYDIN</td><td>Central pair subunit
Normal</td><td>No</td><td>No</td><td>No</td></tr>
<tr><td>CCNO</td><td>Cytoplasmic centriole assembly and docking factor
Oligocilia (residual axoneme normal), may be misinterpreted as secondary ciliary aplasia; basal bodies and rootlets are mislocalized</td><td>No</td><td>Yes/No</td><td>Yes/No</td></tr>
<tr><td>MCIDAS</td><td>Nuclear regulator of CCNO and FOXJ1
Oligocilia (residual axoneme normal), may be misinterpreted as secondary ciliary aplasia</td><td>No</td><td>Yes/No</td><td>Yes/No</td></tr>
<tr><td>RPGR</td><td rowspan="2">Function related to nonmotile cilia; role in motile cilia unknown
Normal</td><td rowspan="2">Yes</td><td rowspan="2">No</td><td rowspan="2">No</td></tr>
<tr><td>OFD1</td></tr>
</table>

PCD, primary ciliary dyskinesia; NGS, next generation sequencing; IDA, inner dynein arm; ODA, outer dynein arm; MTD, microtubule disorganization.

Source: Werner C, Onnebrink JG, Omran H. Diagnosis and management of primary ciliary dyskinesia. Cilia. 2015;4(1):2.

Box 1: Therapies not routinely indicated in primary ciliary dyskinesia

- Inhaled steroids and chronic oral steroids
  - Should be reserved for cases with confirmed reactive airway disease or asthma
  - Consider in cases where patients demonstrate clinical response on bronchodilators and/or have reversible obstructive deficits on spirometry
- Intravenous immunoglobulins
  - Should be reserved for cases where immunodeficiency is confirmed and should not be used empirically
- Anti-tuberculosis treatment
  - Should be reserved for cases where tuberculosis infection is confirmed by sputum AFB stain, culture data and should not be used just based on clinical symptoms, CXR or chest CT findings

AFB, acid-fast bacilli; CXR, chest X-ray; CT, computed tomography.

respiratory therapy, audiology, nutrition, genetic counseling, and social work. Of note, there are several therapies which should not be routinely used for treatment of PCD unless clinically indicated (Box 1).

Otolaryngology management

- Recurrent/chronic otitis media: Antibiotics and tympanostomy tube placement (hearing normalization is reported 80–100% of children with PCD)
- Hearing loss: Regular audiology assessments
- Chronic rhinosinusitis: Daily nasal irrigation with saline, functional endoscopic sinus surgery and nasal polyp removal (occasionally necessary to allow more effective drainage), antibiotics and nasal steroids for acute-on-chronic sinusitis

Respiratory management

The cornerstones of pulmonary care are airway clearance, antimicrobial therapy, and vaccinations.

Airway clearance

- Chest physiotherapy: Manual chest physiotherapy (CPT) and cardiovascular exercise are first line therapies and are strongly recommended. Alternative methods include high frequency chest wall oscillation and oscillatory positive airway pressure devices (such as acapella and flutter)
- Airway hydration and mucolytics: Hypertonic saline (3 or 7% concentration) as well as mucolytics (N-acetylcysteine or dornase alfa) alter mucous rheology and may facilitate clearance. These are well-established therapies in CF but have not been systematically studied in PCD
- Bronchodilators: If there is wheezing and historical response to bronchodilators, inhaled corticosteroids and albuterol can be prescribed to treat reactive airway disease.

Secretion mobilization is impaired while cough clearance is preserved in PCD. Therefore, compared to CF patients, respiratory mucous is easier to expectorate in PCD. A typical airway clearance regimen for baseline health involves nebulized hypertonic saline followed by manual CPT performed twice daily.

Antimicrobial therapy

Acute respiratory exacerbations in PCD manifest as fever, fatigue, worsening of cough, increased sputum production, and work of breathing. Antibiotic choice should be guided by prior respiratory cultures. The most common bacterial pathogens reported in the airways of PCD patients include *Haemophilus influenzae, Streptococcus pneumonia, Moraxella catarrhalis, Staphylococcus aureus,* and *Pseudomonas aeruginosa.*

- Oral antibiotics: At least 2–3 weeks duration for mild exacerbations (based on clinical experience with CF and non-CF bronchiectasis). Amoxicillin with/without clavulanic acid, trimethoprim/sulfamethoxazole, and fluoroquinolones are commonly used
- Intravenous antibiotics: Reserved for severe exacerbations and for cases refractory to

oral therapy. Typical duration of treatment is 2 weeks

- Inhaled antibiotics: Use is extrapolated from studies of non-CF bronchiectasis, where they are suggested to reduce bacterial density in sputum (including *Pseudomonas*) and decrease the risk of acute exacerbations
- Azithromycin: This may be prescribed for its anti-inflammatory and immunomodulatory properties. Azithromycin use has been associated with a reduction in infectious exacerbations in non-CF bronchiectasis patients
- No supporting evidence exists for eradication of *Pseudomonas aeruginosa* and *Burkholderia cepacia*, although such practices are prevalent and seem well-advised.

Preventive care

- Antibiotic prophylaxis: Macrolides, amoxicillin/clavulanic acid, and trimethoprim/sulfamethoxazole are frequently used. However, chronic oral antibiotics should be employed on a case-by-case basis only. Benefit should be weighed against the patient's pattern of exacerbations, their risk of gaining resistant organisms, and potential infection with nontuberculous mycobacteria (which has been linked to chronic macrolide use in cystic fibrosis)
- Vaccinations: Routine immunizations, 23-valent pneumococcal polysaccharide vaccine (for above age 2), annual influenza vaccine (for <6 months), and respiratory syncytial virus antibody prophylaxis for infants.

Surgical intervention

- Lobectomy or segmental wedge resection is considered when bronchiectasis is focally severe and provides a nidus for chronic or recurrent infection, or bleeding
- Lung transplantation is very rarely considered, but has been pursued as a last resort measure in patients with severe lung disease and chronic respiratory failure.

Q. What follow-up is recommended for children with primary ciliary dyskinesia?

Figure 5 outlines clinical and laboratory investigations that should be undertaken at follow-up.

Q. What are the resources available to parents and physicians?

- North America: The PCD foundation is a national collaboration of parents, researchers, and physicians, and connects many specialized PCD centers in North America
- United Kingdom: PCD Family Support Group
- Better Experimental Screening and Treatment for Primary Ciliary Dyskinesia: Funded by the European Union, an international collaboration of PCD experts and patient advocacy groups

Imaging	• Chest X-ray: Every 2-4 years and as needed • Chest CT: Consider baseline study when sedation is not required and as needed
Microbiology	• Sputum culture: At every clinical follow-up • Nontuberculous mycobacterial culture: Every 2 years and/or with clinical decline • Allergic bronchopulmonary aspergillosis testing: With new wheezing and/or with clinical decilne • Bronchoalveolar lavage: If anesthesia risk is acceptable, in the setting of persistent clinical decline despite empiric or tailored intravenous antigiotics
Functional testing	• Pulmonary function tests: At each respiratory follow-up, at least 2-4 times a year • Hearing tests: At the time of diagnosis and as needed

Figure 5: Suggested follow-up for patients with primary ciliary dyskinesia

LEARNING POINTS

- Primary ciliary dyskinesia (PCD) is an autosomal recessive disorder characterized by recurrent otitis media leading to hearing loss, recurrent sinopulmonary infections, and infertility
- Primary ciliary dyskinesia should be on the differential diagnosis for any child with bronchiectasis, recurrent otosinopulmonary infections, and in neonates with unexplained neonatal respiratory distress with dextrocardia
- Cystic fibrosis, immunodeficiency (either primary or concurrent) and infections such as tuberculosis should be ruled out in cases of suspected PCD
- Confirming the diagnosis of PCD may be challenging and, therefore, referral to a specialized center—with the ability to measure nasal nitric oxide and perform ciliary biopsies—is recommended
- Genetic testing is expensive and can diagnose up to two-thirds of cases of PCD only. At the same time, normal ciliary ultrastructure seen on biopsy samples does not necessarily rule out this disorder in patients who have the typical clinical phenotype as up to 10–15% of cases of PCD can have normal ciliary ultrastructure (e.g., *DNAH11* mutation).

SUGGESTED READINGS

1. Burgess A, Lucas JS, Mitchison HM, Moya E, Williamson M, Hogg C, et al. Diagnosis and management of primary ciliary dyskinesia. Arch Dis Child. 2014;99(9):850-6.
2. Knowles MR, Daniels LA, Davis SD, Zariwala MA, Leigh MW. Primary ciliary dyskinesia. Recent advances in diagnostics, genetics, and characterization of clinical disease. Am J Respir Crit Care Med. 2013;188(8):913-22.
3. Lucas JS, Leigh MW. Diagnosis of primary ciliary dyskinesia: searching for a gold standard. Eur Respir J. 2014;44(6):1418-22.
4. Werner C, Onnebrink JG, Omran H. Diagnosis and management of primary ciliary dyskinesia. Cilia. 2015;4(1):2.

CHAPTER 28

Cystic Fibrosis

Esra Caylan, Sankaran Krishnan

CASE 1

A 10-month-old male with a history of failure to thrive (FTT) and chronic cough was brought in for evaluation of chronic cough.

Birth history: Term, born to a 21-year-old mother without any risk factors. Had delayed meconium passage (at 3rd day of life) and discharged home on 4th day of life.

Past medical history: Cough since 2 months of age, required hospitalization once for respiratory distress, diagnosed with bronchiolitis. History of poor growth, formula fed, had frequent loose greasy stools, on 10th percentile for weight and 50% for height.

Family history: Not significant.

Laboratory findings: Newborn screening—negative, sweat chloride levels are pending.

Q. Does he have cystic fibrosis?

Cystic fibrosis (CF) is the most common fatal inherited disorder among Caucasians. However, it is described in all ethnicities and races. Cystic fibrosis is an autosomal recessive disorder caused by mutations in the cystic fibrosis transmembrane regulator (*CFTR*) gene located on chromosome number 7. Cystic fibrosis transmembrane regulator is a cyclic adenosine monophosphate regulated chloride channel found in mucosal epithelial cells in the airways, pancreatic ducts, biliary tree, intestines, vas deferens, and sweat glands. Cystic fibrosis is diagnosed with elevated sweat chloride (over 60 mEq/L) or genetic testing (presence of two mutations in the *CFTR* gene).

Q. What are the salient points on history?

- Birth history: Meconium ileus
- Chronic cough, frequent pneumonias, bronchiolitis
- Failure to thrive
- Signs of malabsorption: Loose, greasy stools
- Signs of vitamin deficiencies (fat soluble vitamins: A, D, E, and K) (Table 1).

Q. What is the differential diagnosis?

Cystic fibrosis is a complex disorder, affecting multiple organ systems with different levels of severity. A patient can manifest with multiple organ systems involvement or can have symptoms specific to one system.

For pulmonary manifestations, differential diagnosis include asthma, bronchiolitis, allergic bronchopulmonary aspergillosis, bronchiectasis, and primary ciliary dyskinesia. The latter can present with recurrent sinusitis and bronchiectasis along with FTT. For gastro-

TABLE 1: Clinical manifestations of cystic fibrosis

Respiratory	Gastrointestinal	Upper airway	Other
• Chronic productive cough • Lower airway bacterial colonization • Hypoxemia • Bronchiectasis • Hemoptysis • Pulmonary hypertension	• Protein and fat malabsorption • Malnutrition/failure to thrive • Meconium ileus • Distal intestinal obstruction syndrome • Focal biliary cirrhosis • Rectal prolapse • Recurrent pancreatitis	• Chronic pansinusitis • Nasal polyposis	• Diabetes mellitus • Digital clubbing • Hyponatremic dehydration • Hypochloremic alkalosis • Vitamin deficiencies • Male infertility

CASE 2

A 12-year-old female with history of severe asthma, not well controlled on combination therapy (inhaled corticosteroid with long-acting β-agonist) referred by the pediatrician to the pulmonology clinic for further evaluation.

Past history: Child adopted at the age of 5 years, no previous history available. History of multiple hospitalizations for asthma exacerbations and pneumonias, several documented on chest X-rays; as treated with standard antibiotics. No cultures available. No history of allergies.

Family history: Sibling (brother) with severe, persistent asthma.

Physical examination: Well-developed girl. On auscultation—good aeration bilaterally with bilateral crackles. No wheeze.

Laboratory findings: Spirometry revealed mild, reversible, obstructive lung disease. Mantoux test (purified protein derivative) was negative. Chest X-ray demonstrates thickened bronchial walls and no focal infiltrates. Immunologic workup and nasal ciliary biopsy were negative. Sweat test was positive with a chloride of 68 mEq/L.

intestinal manifestations, differential diagnosis includes celiac disease, nutritional deficiencies for FTT, and other causes for acute pancreatitis.

Q. What additional investigations would you consider?

Sweat chloride test is the gold standard for diagnosis of CF. The test is performed with the method of quantitative pilocarpine iontophoresis. It involves stimulation of sweat gland with pilocarpine and collecting, weighing sweat and measuring, chloride. See table 2 for cutoff values. Any patient with indeterminate or high levels should be referred to a CF center for further evaluation and follow-up.

TABLE 2: Cutoff values for sweat chloride concentration for diagnosis of cystic fibrosis

	Normal	Indeterminate	Cystic fibrosis
Infants (<6 months)	<30	30–60	>60
Older children and adults	<40	40–60	>60

This patient had a positive sweat test with a chloride of 68 mEq/L. Cystic fibrosis can also be diagnosed with deoxyribonucleic acid analysis to identify specific *CFTR* mutations. There are >1,800 mutations described in the *CFTR* gene. Based on the effect on *CFTR*, mutations are classified into six groups (Table 3). Class I, II, and III mutations are associated with severe progressive pulmonary disease and pancreatic insufficiency, while class IV–VI mutations tend to have milder disease.

The patient described in case 2 had two mutations that were identified as *delF508* (class 2 mutation) and R117H (class 4 mutation).

Q. What are the manifestations of cystic fibrosis?

- Lung disease: Progressive obstructive lung disease is the most common manifestation of CF. Lung disease starts with thickening

TABLE 3: Six classes of cystic fibrosis mutations

Class I	Premature stop codon/alteration of RNA results in failure to synthesis full length CFTR protein
Class II	Improper folding resulting in defective cellular processing and delivery of CFTR protein to cell surface
Class III	Impaired opening of CFTR chloride channel
Class IV	Structural defect in the CFTR channel that reduces the passage of ions
Class V	Errors in RNA splicing, lead to reduced quantity of functional CFTR
Class VI	Increased cell surface turnover and degradation of CFTR

RNA, ribonucleic acid; CFTR, cystic fibrosis transmembrane regulator; CF, cystic fibrosis.

CASE 3

A 13-year-old female with history of cystic fibrosis and pancreatic insufficiency, presented with chronic cough for 1 month, increased sputum production, decreased appetite, and 2 kg weight loss. Her symptoms did not improve with 2 weeks of oral antibiotics (ciprofloxacin). She had a history of *Pseudomonas aeruginosa* positive in sputum cultures several times in the past. She denied any fever, vomiting, or sick contacts.

Past medical history: Cystic fibrosis diagnosed at 1 year of age with positive sweat test, three previous hospitalizations for pulmonary exacerbations.

Physical examination: Tired looking, and on auscultation—decreased aeration at the bases with diffuse bilateral crackles.

Laboratory findings: Elevated white blood cells count. Normal electrolytes. Worsening obstruction on spirometry with no response to inhaled bronchodilator. Chest X-ray with bilateral increased bronchial markings, predominantly on the right side—possible early bronchiectasis.

of airway mucus, leading to colonization of airways with pathogenic bacteria. This chronic infection and inflammation causes endobronchial destruction and subsequent destruction of lung parenchyma. Most common pathologic bacteria found in CF patients' airways are *Pseudomonas aeruginosa, Staphylococcus aureus,* and *Haemophilus influenzae.* Multidrug resistant organisms are common in later life due to repeated administration of antibiotics. Colonization with Burkholderia cepacia is associated with a poor prognosis. Rare pulmonary complications of CF include hemoptysis and spontaneous pneumothorax

- Pancreatic disease: Most CF patients have some degree of pancreatic insufficiency. Pancreatic ducts get obstructed with thickened secretions and results in decreased secretion of pancreatic enzymes. Some may have recurrent episodes of pancreatitis. Patients with pancreatic insufficiency usually present with signs of fat malabsorption and malnutrition such as frequent, greasy, foul-smelling stools, abdominal distension, cramping, and poor weight gain. Patients may also have fat soluble vitamin (vitamin A, D, E, and K) deficiencies

  Cystic fibrosis patients are also at risk of developing CF-related diabetes in later life as a result of destruction of exocrine pancreas
- Intestinal disease: Thickened intestinal secretions due to malfunctioning *CFTR* channels can cause intestinal obstruction. In newborn period, this may manifest as meconium ileus when affected infants fail to pass meconium for first few days of life. Later in life, the same mechanism can cause distal intestinal obstruction syndrome for CF patients when loose stool becomes thick and accumulates in the distal intestine. Rectal prolapse is a rare complication of CF
- Hepatobiliary disease: Thickened biliary secretions can cause decreased mobility of secretions and gallbladder disease with or without gallstones. Almost one-third of CF patients will develop liver dysfunction; rarely progress to cirrhosis and liver failure
- Upper airway disease: Most patients will present with recurrent sinusitis and opacification of sinuses in CT. Nasal polyps are more common in CF patients than in the general population.

Q. What are the treatment options?

- Pulmonary therapies: Parenteral antibiotics are the mainstay of treatment for pulmonary exacerbations. Cystic fibrosis patients should have sputum or deep throat cultures at any exacerbation and also on a regular basis to guide appropriate antibiotic selection. Cystic fibrosis patients tend to demonstrate altered pharmacokinetics for medications and often require higher than normal dosing for weight regimens. Antibiotic choices should cover Gram-negative pathogens like *Pseudomonas, Stenotrophomonas,* and *Escherichia coli,* as well as *S. aureus.* Long-term prophylactic antibiotic use is an option for some CF patients, especially patients those with chronic *Pseudomonas* colonization, some regimens include inhaled tobramycin or aztreonam, and thrice weekly azithromycin. Airway clearance therapies (ACT) are a key element to protect and improve lung function in CF patients. Pharmacological interventions include aerosolized dornase-α (Pulmozyme), hypertonic saline (7%), and inhaled mannitol. Mechanical interventions include manual chest physiotherapy, high-frequency chest wall oscillators (the Vest), hand-held vibratory expiration appliances (Acapella, Flutter), and aerosolized broncho-dilators. It is essential to incorporate an ACT regimen in the daily routine of treatment, not just during exacerbations, but rather on a daily basis to prevent mucus adherence and infection cycles
- Metabolic: Pancreatic enzymes replacement prior to meals (and snacks) is essential to promote fat absorption and maintain calorie intake. Several products are available for this purpose containing varying amounts of lipase and other pancreatic enzymes. The dosing is based on response and is customized in each patient depending on the stool pattern and weight gain. Cystic fibrosis patients also need higher calorie intake, including nutritional supplements if calorie intake is suboptimal. High fat/calorie diet is recommended with adequate pancreatic enzyme replacement. Sometimes, a gastrostomy tube placement is necessary for supplemental feeds in case weight gain remains an issue. Vitamins A, D, E, and K (fat soluble vitamins) supplementation is also recommended for CF patients
- Genetic treatments: Over the past 2–3 years, genetic treatments in the form of *CFTR* potentiators and correctors are available for some patients with specific mutations for CF. Ivacaftor (Kalydeco) is a genetic treatment available for patients with the *G551D, R117H,* and certain other mutations. In such patients, oral administration of Kalydeco corrects the defect in *CFTR* and can restore near normal function. Recently, a combination of ivacaftor and lumacaftor (Orkambi) was approved for use in patients homozygous for the *delF508* mutation (the most common mutation in Caucasians), in whom it improves lung function by modifying *CFTR.*

LEARNING POINTS

- Cystic fibrosis is diagnosed with elevated sweat chloride (over 60 mEq/L) or genetic testing (presence of two mutations in the *CFTR* gene)
- Recurrent respiratory tract infections and gastrointestinal symptoms are common clinical manifestations of cystic fibrosis (CF)
- Based on the effect on CFTR, mutations in CF are classified into six groups
- Antibiotics, chest physiotherapy, inhaled medi-cations, and pancreatic enzymes replacement are the mainstay for management
- Over the past 2–3 years, genetic treatments in the form of *CFTR* potentiators and correctors are available for some patients with specific mutations for CF.

SUGGESTED READINGS

1. Farrell P, Rosenstein B, White TB, Accurso FJ, Castellani C, Cutting GR, et al. Guidelines for cystic fibrosis in newborns through older adults: Cystic Fibrosis Foundation consensus report. J Pediatr. 2008;153(2):S4-S14.
2. Montgomery G, Howenstine M. Cystic fibrosis. Pediatr Rev. 2009;30(8):302-9.
3. Rowe S, Miller S, Sorscher EJ. Cystic fibrosis. N Engl J Med. 2005;352(19);1992-2001.
4. Stoltz DA, Meyerholz DK, Welsh MJ. Origins of cystic fibrosis lung disease. N Engl J Med. 2015;372:351-62.

CHAPTER 29

Non-Cystic Fibrosis Bronchiectasis in Children

Ajay Kumar

CASE 1

A 6-year-old girl was brought to the chest clinic with complaints of cough, wheezing, breathlessness, sneezing, repeated nasal discharge, fever, and expectoration off and on for 1 year.

Past history: She was admitted for post-measles pneumonia 10 months back. She was discharged on antitubercular drugs which she stopped after 3 months without doctor's advice (details not available). She also gave history of nebulization occasionally and ear discharge 1 month back.

Physical examination: Weight—15.0 kg [<–2 standard deviation (SD)], height—102 cm (<–2 SD), Bacillus Calmette-Guérin (BCG) scar present, no respiratory distress, grade 1 clubbing present, no lymphadenopathy, generalized crepitations and rhonchi on chest auscultation, rest systemic examination normal.

Q. What is bronchiectasis and what are the causes of non-cystic fibrosis bronchiectasis in children?

Bronchiectasis is dilatation of conducting airways and it is characterized clinically by chronic wet cough, airway hyperreactivity, recurrent chest infections, and failure to thrive. The causes of non-cystic fibrosis bronchiectasis in children are given in box 1.

Box 1: Causes of non-cystic fibrosis bronchiectasis in children*

- Congenital airway malformation—tracheomalacia, bronchomalacia, etc.
- Recurrent aspiration—tracheoesophageal fistula, gastroesophageal reflux
- Postinfectious—after severe lower respiratory tract infection: tuberculosis, pertussis, measles, and severe viral pneumonia
- Neuromuscular weakness
- Airway obstruction (intraluminal or external compression)—foreign body, granulation tissue, lymph node, tumor, vascular ring
- Allergic bronchopulmonary aspergillosis
- Immune deficiencies—both primary and secondary
- Interstitial lung disease
- Bronchiolitis obliterans (postviral, posttransplant)
- Yellow nail lymphedema syndrome
- Marfan syndrome
- Usher syndrome
- Alpha-1 trypsin deficiency
- Primary ciliary dyskinesia
- Eosinophilic lung disease
- Idiopathic

*Not in order of incidence or prevalence

Q. What is differential diagnosis for case 1?

The child has cough, cold with breathlessness, wheezing, crepitations, and clubbing. It suggests obstructive airway disease with suppuration. Differential diagnosis will include asthma with allergic bronchopulmonary aspergillosis (ABPA), postinfectious bronchiectasis, and possibly reactivation of tuberculosis (Table 1).

Q. What investigations should be done to confirm diagnosis?

Investigations should be directed toward the etiologies suspected based on history and examination. Diagnostic possibilities in case 1 are reactivation of tuberculosis, postinfectious bronchiectasis, and allergic bronchopulmonary aspergillosis. For tuberculosis, investigations include Mantoux test, gastric aspirates/induced sputum examination for smear, and culture for *Mycobacterium tuberculosis*. A repeat X-ray should be done after a course of antibiotics to see clearance of chest X-ray findings.

For allergic bronchopulmonary aspergillosis, chest X-ray may show fleeting shadows, peripheral blood eosinophilia, sputum may be positive for *Aspergillus*, raised serum total and specific immunoglobulin E against *Aspergillus*, and positive skin test for *Aspergillus*. Computed tomography (CT) chest may show bronchiectasis.

Postinfectious bronchiectasis may be confirmed by bronchiectasis on chest X-ray and CT chest and ruling out other causes of bronchiectasis (Table 2). Based on investigations as given in table 2, final diagnosis of case 1 is bronchiectasis, possibly postinfectious.

Q. How to manage this child?

Treatment of bronchiectasis may be medical and/or surgical. Most patients can be managed with medical treatment.

Medical treatment

Medical treatment includes the followings:

- General measures: To ensure adequate nutritional intake and appropriate immunization against common respiratory pathogens. Commonly available vaccines that should be administered to children with bronchiectasis are BCG, DPT (diphtheria, pertussis, and tetanus), measles, *Haemophilus influenza* type b (HiB), influenza, and pneumococcal.
- Airway clearance: For effective airway clearance, maintain good hydration, bronchodilators (if wheezing), and inhaled corticosteroids (if reactive airway disease). Chest physiotherapy (choose a method/device acceptable to family and child). If sputum is very sticky and difficult to clear, nebulized hypertonic saline (3/5%) may be

TABLE 1: Differential diagnosis of case 1

Disease	Points in favor	Points against
Tuberculosis (reactivation)	• History of measles and inadequate antituberculosis treatment with poor growth • Chest X-ray showing patchy opacity bilateral	• Mantoux test negative, • Bacille Calmette-Guérin scar present • No lymphadenopathy • Clubbing present
Allergic bronchopulmonary aspergillosis	• Clinical signs and symptoms suggestive of obstructive airway disease • History of getting nebulized medications • Clubbing present • Chest X-ray—patchy opacity bilateral	• No eosinophilia • No family history of asthma • No exposure of allergen
Postinfectious bronchiectasis	• History of measles, clubbing with wet cough	–

TABLE 2: Investigations and their interpretation in case 1

Investigation	Result	Interpretation
Repeat chest X-ray	Patchy opacity persist	Possibility of tuberculosis (TB), allergic bronchopulmonary aspergillosis (ABPA), or resistant bacterial infection
Gastric aspirate for acid-fast bacilli (AFB)—day 1 and 2	Negative for AFB—both	Reactivation of TB less likely
Serum immunoglobulin E (IgE) level	40 IU/mL (normal for age, for ABPA >1,000 IU/mL)	Increased in asthma and ABPA
Aspergillus specific IgE level	0.06 kU/L (normal for age)	Increased in ABPA
Skin test for *Aspergillus* species	Negative for common *Aspergillus* species	ABPA ruled out
High resolution computerized tomography chest	Cystic bronchiectasis right upper lobe with mediastinal and hilar lymphadenopathy	Bronchiectasis
Sweat chloride test	20 mEq/L (normal <40 mEq/L, positive >60 mEq/L on two occasions)	Cystic fibrosis ruled out
Bronchoscopy and brochoalveolar lavage analysis	Bronchoscopy: Normal. Bronchoalveolar lavage negative for AFB, bacteria and fungus. GeneXpert negative for *Mycobacterium tuberculosis* (MTB)	TB less likely

administered before doing physiotherapy. There is no role of mucolytic agents like bromhexin and ambroxol. In children with cystic fibrosis, mucolytic agent like deoxyribonuclease may be considered

- Antibiotics: For pulmonary exacerbations, appropriate antibiotics should be administered based on sputum culture. Role of inhaled antibiotics in non-cystic fibrosis bronchiectasis is still evolving. If a child is chronically colonized with pseudomonas, long-term inhaled antibiotics (tobramycin/colistin) may be considered. Oral co-trimoxazole prophylaxis may be considered in children having recurrent respiratory exacerbations
- Monitoring: Children with bronchiectasis should be monitored regularly every 3–6 months. On each visit, the following should be monitored:
    - History of respiratory symptoms
    - Physical examination
    - Spirometry in older children
    - Sputum culture for bacterial pathogens and other pathogens (if indicated)
- Specific treatment: Depending on underlying illness, appropriate specific treatment may be considered. Conditions requiring specific treatment include ABPA, panhypogammaglobulinemia, airway compression, gastroesophageal reflux, etc.

Surgical treatment

Majority of the children can be managed with medical treatment. Surgery is indicated only in localized disease that is not getting controlled with medical treatment or has life-threatening bleed. If there are some correctable abnormalities (congenital or acquired), surgical intervention is helpful.

For index case

Diagnosis is bronchiectasis, possibly post-infectious. Management will be medical as described above.

CASE 2

A 10-year-old girl was brought to the chest clinic with complaints of cough, wheezing, breathlessness, fever and recurrent pneumonia since the age of 1 month. He was was hospitalized 6–7 times in the last 3 years due to chest infection. He was investigated by local doctor and investigation reports were as follows:

- Hemoglobin: 12.1 g/dL
- Total leukocyte count: 11,700/mm^3 (P45 L55)
- Erythrocyte sedimentation rate: 15 mm in first hour
- Mantoux test: Negative (8 mm x 6 mm)
- Chest X-ray: Bilateral hyperinflation
- Gastric aspirate for acid-fast bacilli (D1 and 2) was negative and contrast-enhanced computed tomography chest shows bronchiectasis with bronchial wall irregularity and centrilobular nodule in tree and bud patterns with bilateral lung and mediastinal lymphadenopathy.

Past history: No history of contact with tuberculosis. No history of cough or choking during feeding.

Family history: Family history revealed nothing relevant.

Physical examination: The patient was conscious. Weight—21.0 kg [<–2 standard deviation (SD)], height—130 cm (<–1 SD). Bacillus Calmette-Guérin scar present, no respiratory distress, no pallor, no cyanosis, grade 2 clubbing present, insignificant cervical lymphadenopathy (<1 cm), generalized crepitations and rhonchi present on chest auscultation, tenderness over maxillary sinus present.

Other systemic examination was normal. SpO$_2$—85% in room air, forced expiratory volume in 1 second—65% of expected, and forced vital capacity—62% of expected.

Q. What is differential diagnosis for this patient?

The differential diagnosis for this patient include immunodeficiency, cystic fibrosis, primary ciliary dyskinesia (PCD), and recurrent aspiration. Details are given in table 3.

TABLE 3: Differential diagnosis for case 2

Disease	Points in favor	Points against
Immunodeficiency	• Early age of onset of sign/symptoms • Repeated chest infection • Repeated hospitalization • Clubbing • Under nutrition	• No family history of similar illness, sibling death • No history of infection in other parts of body
Cystic fibrosis	• Early age of onset of sign/symptoms • Repeated chest infection • Repeated hospitalization • Clubbing • Under nutrition	• No history of obvious malabsorption • No other contributory history in form of similar illness in sibling, consanguinity, etc.
Primary ciliary dyskinesia	• Early age of onset of sign/symptoms • Repeated chest infection • Repeated hospitalization • Clubbing, under nutrition • Maxillary sinus tenderness present	• No other contributory history
Repeated aspiration secondary to gastroesophageal reflux	• Early age of onset of sign/symptoms • Repeated chest infection • Repeated hospitalization • Under nutrition	• No history of cough or choking during feeding

Q. How to confirm diagnosis in this patient?

This patient has recurrent pneumonia with evidence of sinusitis. Therefore, investigations should be planned to to rule out primary ciliary dyskinesia, sweat test, and immunoglobulin profile. Diagnosis of PCD can be suspected by documenting low fractional excretion of nitric oxide (FENO) or nasal nitric oxide. The later is more specific. Diagnosis can be confirmed by demonstration of structural abnormalities in ciliary structure by doing electron microscopy of nasal mucosal scrapping. Diagnosis of cystic fibrosis can be established by documenting higher sweat chloride values of >60 mEq/L on two occasions. For humoral immune deficiency, serum immunoglobulins can be performed.

In index case

Fractional excretion of nitric oxide was 5 ppm, sweat chloride test was 23 mEq/L, and serum immunoglobulin (Ig) profile was within normal limits (IgA: 312 IU/mL, IgG: 1,531 IU/mL, IgM: 117 IU/mL). Based on recurrent pneumonia with sinusitis and low FENO, a probable diagnosis of PCD was made.

Q. What should be the treatment for this patient?

Since diagnosis is primary ciliary dyskinesia, there is no cure for illness. Treatment will include supportive care in form of nutrition, immunization, and airway clearance with antibiotics for pulmonary exacerbations.

LEARNING POINTS

- Bronchiectasis is not an uncommon condition in pediatric population
- Cystic fibrosis is the most common cause of bronchiectasis in developed countries, while in developing countries non-cystic fibrosis etiologies are more common
- High resolution computed tomography chest is the gold standard noninvasive method to diagnose bronchiectasis
- In Indian children, common causes of non-cystic fibrosis bronchiectasis are postinfectious, PCD, and allergic bronchopulmonary aspergillosis
- In one-third cases, cause of non-cystic fibrosis bronchiectasis is not identified
- Medical treatment (chest physiotherapy, bronchodilator, inhaled corticosteroids,, antibiotic during acute exacerbations, etc.) is mainstay of treatment.

SUGGESTED READINGS

1. Kabra SK. Suppurative lung diseases. In: Kabra SK, Lodha R, editors. Essential Pediatric Pulmonology. 2nd ed. New Delhi: Nobele Vision; 2010. pp. 106-10.
2. Kumar A, Lodha R, Kumar P, Kabra SK. Non-cystic fibrosis bronchiectasis in children: clinical profile, etiology and outcome. Indian Pediatr. 2015;52(1):35-7.
3. Redding GJ, Chang AB. Bronchiectasis and chronic suppurative lung disease. In: Wilmott RW, Bush A, Boat TF, Deterding RR, Ratjen F, Chernick V, editors. Kendig and Chernick's Disorders of the Respiratory Tract in Children, 8th edition. Philadelphia: Elsevier Saunders; 2012. pp. 473-88.

CHAPTER

30

Lung Abscess

Jasmeet K Wadhwa

CASE 1

A 5-year-old child admitted in ward with complaints of fever and cough for 3 weeks preceded by symptoms of cold and cough. Fever was high grade, spikes two to three times in a day associated with loss of appetite. Cough was productive in nature with no diurnal variation. No significant past or family history of tuberculosis. The child had respiratory rate of 26/min, heart rate of 110 beats/min. On inspection chest was normal, on auscultation there was decreased air entry at inframammary and infra-axillary region with bronchial breath sound and fine crepitations. On blood investigation, leukocyte count of 26,000/mm^3, 64% neutrophils, 24% lymphocytes, and hemoglobin of 10.6 g/dL. On peripheral smear examination, there were band cells and toxic granules. Mantoux skin test for tuberculosis was negative. Chest X-ray shows right middle zone opacity with air fluid level (Fig. 1).

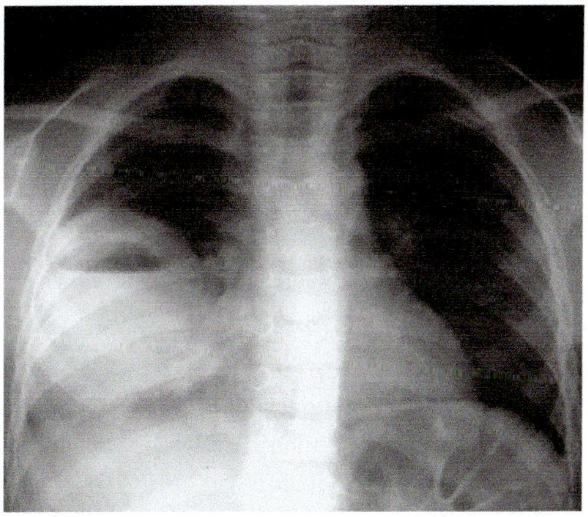

Figure 1: Chest X-ray showing right middle zone opacity with air fluid level

Q. What is the possible diagnosis?

The child is symptomatic for 3 weeks having high fever, cough, and anorexia with localized pathology on right side. There is no significant past or family history of tuberculosis or any other chronic illness. There is leukocytosis and shift to left in peripheral smear suggesting bacterial infection. Possible diagnosis is lung parenchymal lesion—a primary lung abscess or necrotizing pneumonia.

Q. What is the etiology of lung abscess?

Lung abscess is defined as necrosis of the pulmonary parenchyma caused by microbial infection. It is most commonly seen in children beyond infancy. Lung abscesses can be classified as acute or chronic based upon the duration of symptoms. Symptoms present for >4 weeks are considered as chronic. Lung abscess may be primary or secondary. Abscesses in healthy patients with no underlying illness are usually considered primary. Secondary lung abscess occurs in patient with underlying illness causing repeated aspirations, preexisting bulla, lung cyst, bronchogenic neoplasm or any systemic disease that compromises immune defenses.

Q. What are the predisposing factors for development of lung abscess?

Factors predisposing children to develop lung abscess due to endogenous aerobic and anaerobic bacteria flora are given in box 1.

Box 1: Predisposing risk factors for development of lung abscess

- Lesions causing aspiration and airway obstruction
    - Condition causing abnormal pulmonary drainage: Congenital sequestration of lung, lobar emphysema, bronchiectasis, pneumatocele
    - Obstruction due to aspirated foreign body
    - Prolonged gastroesophageal reflux and nasogastric tube feedings
    - Depressed cough reflex due to neurological disease or neuromuscular disorders causing oropharyngeal incoordination
    - Congenital or acquired tracheoesophageal malformation
    - Extended endotracheal intubation and prolonged tracheostomy.
- Change in oropharyngeal flora
    - Poor oral hygiene, gingivitis, and periodontitis (prolonged anticonvulsants)
    - Long-term hospitalization, use of prolonged antibiotics, and oral colonization with hospital flora
- Impaired immunological and other defenses
    - Genetic disorders (Down's syndrome or cystic fibrosis)
    - Congenital ciliary dysfunction
    - Congenital or acquired humoral or cellular immunity

Q. What are the pathogens causing lung abscess?

Common aerobic or anaerobic organisms responsible for development of lung abscess are given in box 2.

Box 2: Organism responsible for development of lung abscess

- Aerobic and facultative bacteria
    - Gram-positive cocci
        - *Streptococcus pneumoniae*
        - Group A β-hemolytic streptococci
        - *Staphylococcus aureus* and *S. epidermidis*
    - Gram-negative bacilli
        - *Proteus* spp.
        - *Klebsiella pneumonia*
        - *Pseudomonas* spp.
        - *Escherichia coli*
- Anaerobic bacteria
    - *Peptostreptococcus* spp.
    - *Fusobacterium* spp.
    - *Bacteroides* spp.
    - *Clostridium* spp.
    - *Bacteroides fragilis*

Q. What are the other relevant points to be considered on history and physical examination of this child so as to support the diagnosis?

History

Detail history regarding type and character of cough. In lung abscess, there is wet cough, mucoid, purulent, or blood stained according to the underlying illness along with high fever, malaise, anorexia, weight loss, and dyspnea. There can be history suggestive of recurrent aspiration, foreign body inhalation, recurrent boils, chest pain, loose motions, or infection of the skin, mucous membrane, and dentition.

Physical examination

Look for any signs of gingivitis, periodontal disease, or skin infections in general physical examination. There can be mild tachypnea with or without chest retraction. Chest inspection is generally normal. Clinical findings of concomitant consolidation or pleural effusion may be present (decreased breath sounds/ dullness to percussion/bronchial breath sounds/coarse inspiratory crackles) on the affected site. The examination findings also vary depending on the causative organisms, the severity, and extent of the disease.

CASE 2

A 3-year-old boy presented with fever for 15 days and cough for 3 days. No previous history of recurrent cough or chest infections, hemoptysis, foreign body aspiration, or any systemic symptoms. On examination, he was febrile 103°F, respiratory rate 40/min, heart rate 106/min, and blood pressure 90/60 mmHg. No cyanosis, clubbing, or lymphadenopathy. His oxygen saturation was 92% in room air. His weight was 11 kg, height 85 cm. Chest examination showed decrease tactile fremitus, dullness on percussion, and decreased breath sounds at right infra scapular and axillary areas. Other systems examinations were unremarkable.

Investigations: Hemoglobin 11.1 g/dL, total lymphocyte count (TLC) 31,700/mm^3, neutrophils 74%, lymphocytes 26%, platelets 700,000/mm^3, erythrocyte sedimentation rate (ESR) 60 mm, C-reactive protein (CRP) 178, blood culture sterile. Chest X-ray showed homogenous opacity in right middle and lower zones (Fig. 2). Computed tomography (CT) scan of chest showed multiple cysts with air fluid levels and a large cyst measuring 9 × 7 cm having multiple septations suggestive of congenital cystic adenomatoid malformation with lung abscess (Fig. 3).

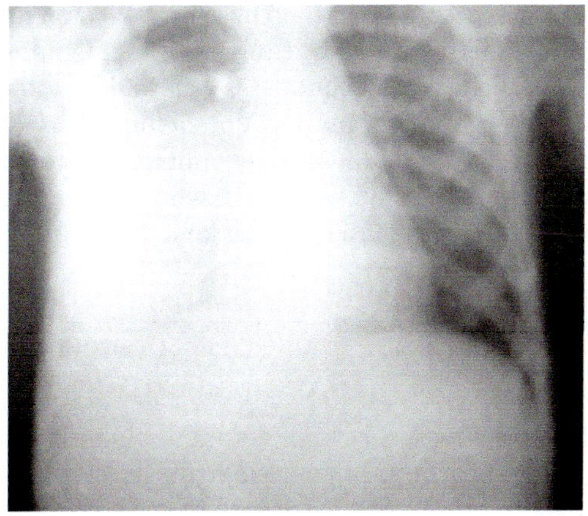

Figure 2: Homogenous opacity on right middle and lower zone

Q. What is the diagnosis in the above case?

The child is having secondary lung abscess with underlying congenital cystic adenomatoid lung malformation.

Q. What are the imaging studies needed to diagnose lung abscess?

Chest X-ray is the most important modality to diagnose lung abscess. It shows homogenous opacities with areas of breakdown and sometimes an air fluid level. Lung abscesses can

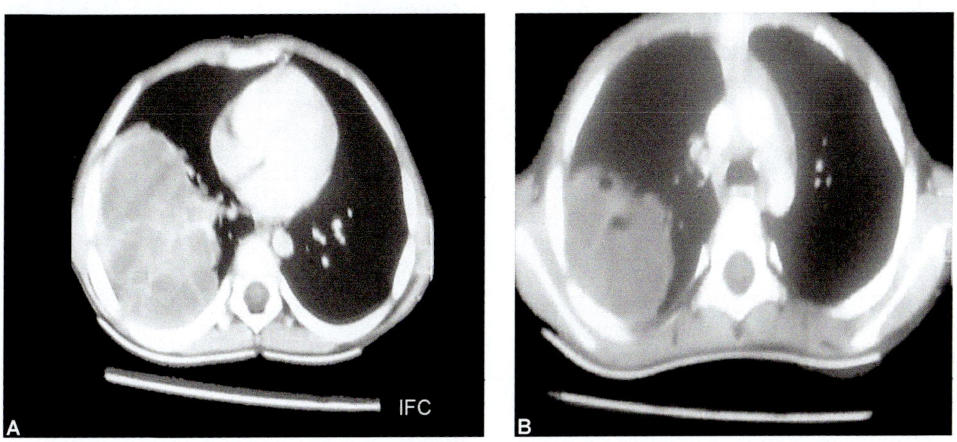

Figure 3: Computed tomography scan chest showing multiple cysts and air fluid level involving right lower lobe

vary in size and wall thickness by 2–20 cm and 5–15 mm, respectively. Computed tomography scan of chest with contrast is required to know the extent and communication of lung abscess. It is useful in identifying concomitant empyema or underlying illness such as congenital cyst, sequestration of lung, or lung infarction.

Q. What can be the differential diagnosis in the above case and how to differentiate them on imaging studies?

Lung abscess can mimic round pneumonia, infected hydatid cyst, tuberculosis, sequestration of lung, cystic adenomatoid lung malformation, bronchogenic cyst, metastasis lung, cavitating pneumoconiosis, or localized empyema.

Lung abscesses due to aspiration on chest X-ray is generally single, with irregular walls with or without air fluid levels, mostly on dependent areas of lung (posterior segment of right upper lobe or superior segment of lower lobe or both), necrotizing pneumonia due to *Staphylococcus aureus* are small, multiple, and thick walled having ragged inner lining with no lobar predilection. In tuberculosis, there are smooth, thick-walled abscess involving upper lobes and apical segment of lower lobes with or without fibrosis or consolidation. Lung abscess in sequestrated lung can be thick or thin walled with surrounding pneumonia. Bronchogenic cyst has lower lobe predilection with surrounding pneumonia. Pulmonary infarctions are at lower lobes, thick walled with shaggy inner lining.

CASE 3

A 2.5-year-old male child admitted with complaints of high fever, cough, and decreased appetite for 2 weeks, received oral antibiotics with no relief. In past history, the child got operated for patent ductus arteriosus at 1 year of age. On admission, the child weight of 13 kg, height 90 cm, febrile with respiratory rate of 50/min, and heart rate of 160/min. On auscultation, there were decreased respiratory sounds with fine crepitation on right supramammary and infrascapular regions. On investigations, total leukocyte counts was 30,400/mm^3 with 70% polymorphs, ESR 130 mm/h, CRP 150 ng/mL, chest X-ray showed right upper zone opacity consistent with lobar pneumonia. The child was started on appropriate parenteral antibiotics with a diagnosis of right upper lobe pneumonia. Chest X-ray was taken on the third day of antibiotics as fever was persisting. It showed a cavity with an air-fluid level in right upper zone (Fig. 4). Based on these findings, appropriate antibiotics with proper dosages against anaerobic and *S. aureus* were started. After 48 hours, CT chest was done that showed cavitary lesion measuring 5 x 6 cm in diameter with an air fluid level in right upper zone consistent with lung abscess (Fig. 5). After 10 days of antibiotics, TLC count, ESR, and CRP decreased markedly, however high fever persisted. A repeat chest X-ray showed increase in the diameters of abscess cavity so percutaneous drainage under CT guidance was performed. Around 70 mL purulent material was drained from the abscess cavity. As there was an air leak due to a fistula formation between the abscess cavity and bronchus, drainage tube was kept in place for 16 days. On the 16th day of percutaneous drainage, air leakage healed and the child improved considerably. Intravenous antibiotics were continued for appropriate duration without a need for further intervention.

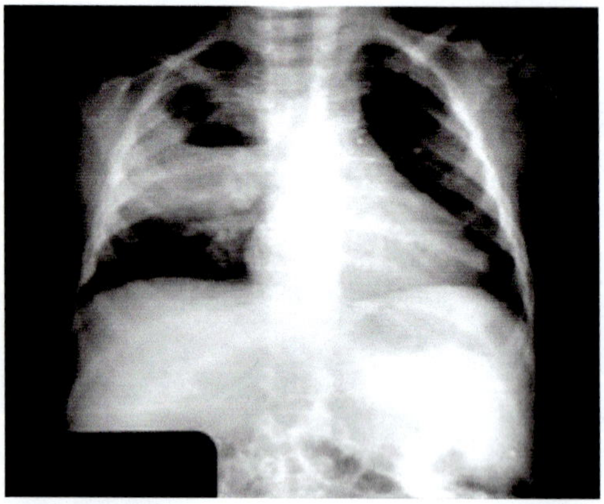

Figure 4: Chest X-ray showing right upper zone cavity with an air fluid level

Q. What are the other investigations required in management of lung abscess?

Blood investigations show leukocytosis with shift to left except when symptoms are there for >4 weeks or the child is on prior antibiotic

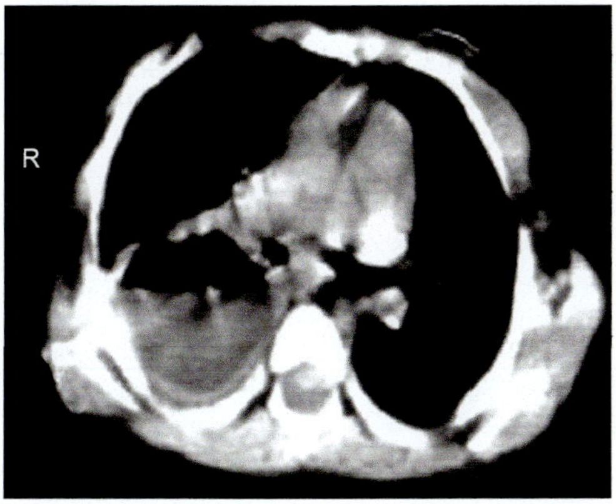

Figure 5: Computed tomography chest showing right lung abscess with air fluid level

therapy. There may be raised levels of CRP and ESR. Blood culture sensitivity is helpful if there is septicemia or blood borne abscess. Hydatid serology is needed if hydatid cyst is suspected. Investigations according to underlying illness, such as immunoglobulin profile, human immunodeficiency virus, and sweat test can be performed. Other than blood, sputum specimen can be cultured from material obtained by drainage with bronchoscopy or by transtracheal or percutaneous aspiration.

Q. What is the treatment of lung abscess?

The mainstay of treatment is conservative with prolonged antibiotics therapy. No treatment recommendation has been issued by major societies, specifically for lung abscess. As it is difficult to isolate the offending organism, treatment is most of the time empirical or according to age and underlying or associated illness. Course of antibiotics is preferably for 4–6 weeks depending on clinical and radiological response. Other modalities include effective physiotherapy for pus drainage, ultrasound, or CT guided insertion of percutaneous placed pigtail catheter in cases not responsive to medical treatment or for rapid defervescence of fever and symptoms and to shorten the period of intravenous antibiotics and hospitalization as done in the above case.

Q. What are the antibiotic regimens to be followed for treatment?

Initial choice of antimicrobial therapy is generally empirical as it is difficult to isolate organism from the pus or abscess. For primary lung abscess, it is recommended to use antibiotics against most common aerobes such as *Streptococcus pneumoniae*, Gram-negative bacilli, or *S. aureus*. If there is secondary cause due to aspiration then anaerobic coverage should be added to the regime as given in table 1.

TABLE 1: Antibiotic therapy against organisms causing lung abscess

Organisms	Antibiotics
Streptococcus pneumoniae/Klebsiella spp./*Haemophilus influenzae/ Pseudomonas aeruginosa*	Penicillin G 250,000–400,000 units/kg in four divided doses or amoxycillin-clavulanic acid 75–100 mg/kg/day in three divided doses + third-generation cephalosporin ceftriaxone/cefotaxime 75–100 mg/kg in two divided doses or amikacin 10–15 mg/kg/day in two divided doses
Anaerobes	Cloxacillin 100 -200 mg/kg in 3 -4 divided doses or Vancomycin 10 mg/kg IV every 3 -4 divided doses or Linezolid 10 -15 mg/kg in three divided doses
Staphylococcus aureus	Cloxacillin 100–200 mg/kg in 3–4 div. doses Or vancomycin 10 mg/kg IV every 3–4 div. doses Or linezolid 10–15 mg/kg in three div. doses
Case of aspiration in immunocompetent host, suspected organism, and anaerobes and methicillin resistant *Staphylococcus aureus*	Clindamycin, or ticarcillin + clavulanate combination, or carbapenems, plus vancomycin/linezolid
Immunocompromised host (suspected fungal infection)	Add antifungals (amphotericin B/ itraconazole)

Q. What are the indications for surgical intervention in lung abscess?

When there is persistence of fever and toxicity after 7–10 days of appropriate intravenous antimicrobial therapy or when the abscess is >4 cm diameter—causing mediastinal shift or airways compression, surgical intervention in the form of ultrasound or CT guided percutaneous tube drainage or needle aspiration of abscess is required. Procedure like lobectomy or pneumonectomy are rarely required in cases like congenital lung malformation or suspected neoplasm

Q. What course is expected after antibiotics in the above cases?

Appropriate antibiotic therapy with or without surgical intervention subsides fever in 7 days. Complete clinical resolution is achieved in 2–3 weeks. Radiological improvement starts after 2 weeks, may completely resolve in 4 weeks or persist longer in few cases.

Complications are rare if medical treatment is appropriate. Rarely, in secondary lung abscess, there can be spontaneous rupture of abscess in other part of lung, i.e., bronchopleural fistula, empyema, or cerebral abscess

Q. What are the complications and prognosis of lung abscess?

Primary lung abscess has rare complications with good prognosis as seen in case 1. Secondary lung abscess can have complications like fistula communicating with pleural cavity or bronchus as seen in case 3, spread of infection to other lung segments, bronchiectasis, empyema, and bacteremia with metastatic infection such as brain abscess.

LEARNING POINTS

- Lung abscess in children is rare nowadays, seen in children with unresponsive bacterial pneumonia
- Lung abscess can be primary or secondary with recurrent aspirations, tuberculosis, or malformations (sequestration lung or cyst) as the most common predisposing factors
- Chest X-ray in erect position diagnose majority of lung abscess. Ultrasound or computed tomography guided percutaneous aspiration is needed in few unresponsive cases so as to decrease complications and rapid defervescence of signs and symptoms
- Effective treatment includes appropriate antibiotics for 4–6 weeks, chest physiotherapy, and nutritional rehabilitation.

SUGGESTED READINGS

1 Brook I. Lung abscess and pulmonary infections due to anaerobic bacteria. In: Chernick V, Boat TF, Wilmott RW, Bush A, editors Kendig's Disorder of the Respiratory tract in Children, 7th edition. Philadelphia: Elsevier; 2006. pp. 478-84.

2 Chen SJ, Yen CC, Tang RB, Chin TW. Pediatric lung abscess: a retrospective review of 23 cases. J Microbiol Immunol Infect. 2004;37(1):45-9.

3 Huang LM, Chan PC, Wu PS, Chang PY, Yang TT, Lu CY, et al. Clinical management and outcome of childhood lung abscess: a 16-year experience. J Microbiol Immunol Infect. 2005;38(3):183-8.

4 Puligandla PS, Laberge JM. Respiratory infections: pneumonia, lung abscess, and empyema. Semin Pediatr Surg. 2008; 17(1):42-52.

6

SECTION

Childhood Interstitial Lung Diseases

CHAPTER

31

Pulmonary Hemorrhage

Saptharishi Lalgudi Ganesan, Pankaj C Vaidya

CASE 1

A 4-year-old boy was brought with complaints of altered blood in his sputum. There was also history of fever, cough, and rapid breathing for the last 9 days. Prior to this, he was healthy and asymptomatic.

Physical examination: Vital signs were normal for age with no tachypnea. Anthropometry was normal for age. Pallor was present. No icterus, cyanosis, clubbing, or lymphadenopathy. Examination of nasopharynx and oral cavity was normal.

Systemic examination: Respiratory system examination revealed mediastinal shift to the right with decreased air entry in the right lower zones. There were crepitations in the right inframammary and infra-axillary regions.

Radiology: There was evidence of collapse-consolidation of the right middle lobe with a pneumatocele in the right lower zone (Fig. 1).

Q. What is hemoptysis?

Hemoptysis is defined as expectoration of blood or blood-tinged sputum from the lower respiratory tract. Unlike in adults, all cases of pulmonary hemorrhage may not manifest with hemoptysis as children tend to swallow their sputum. "Pseudohemoptysis" and "factitious hemoptysis" are close mimickers of true pulmonary hemorrhage.

Q. Does this child truly have pulmonary hemorrhage?

Pulmonary hemorrhage and hemoptysis are relatively uncommon in children. The first step in the management of any child with pulmonary hemorrhage is to confirm that the blood is indeed pulmonary in origin. It is not uncommon for bleeding from the upper airway or gastrointestinal tract to be mistaken for "true" pulmonary hemorrhage in children. In this context, the index case could have bled from nose, infected tonsils, adenoids, or the upper gastrointestinal tract.

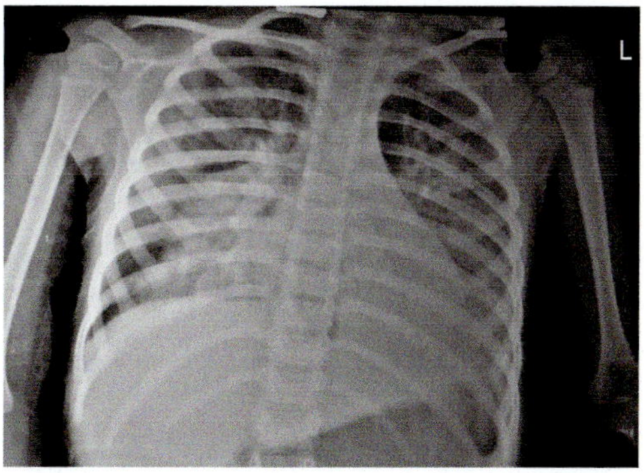

Figure 1: Chest radiograph of case 1 showing bilateral consolidation more prominent in the right middle lobe with breakdown

The history of altered blood, vomiting, and presence of hepatic or gastric disease would suggest hematemesis. Blood in hematemesis will be nonfrothy, brownish-black in color, and acidic pH, whereas true hemoptysis will be frothy, bright red in color, and alkaline pH. Children tend to swallow the blood and hence may present with altered blood in vomitus, whereas actually, they may be having pulmonary hemorrhage.

Q. What clues on physical examination should one actively look for?

A thorough examination of the oral cavity and nasopharynx may help identify a factitious hemoptysis. Once pulmonary hemorrhage is suspected, the first step in physical examination is to look for clues to a chronic pathology. Failure to thrive, significant pallor, or clubbing could be a clue to an underlying chronic etiology such as tuberculosis, cystic fibrosis, bronchiectasis, congenital, as well as acquired cardiac diseases. One should also look for rash, serositis, sinusitis, etc. that could point toward autoimmune etiologies such as systemic lupus erythematosus (SLE) or Wegener's granulomatosis. Abnormal chest examination findings, such as localized wheeze or crepitations or decreased breath sounds, could be valuable clues.

Q. How useful is chest radiography in a child with suspected pulmonary hemorrhage?

In a child with suspected pulmonary hemorrhage, chest radiography is a routine and most often the first investigation. However, a normal radiograph does not rule out pulmonary hemorrhage. Unilateral air trapping may suggest a missed foreign body aspiration. As in the index case, localized chest infiltrates may suggest a focal consolidation or bronchiectasis as the cause of pulmonary hemorrhage. One may find hilar lymphadenopathy or pleural effusion as clues to underlying tuberculosis. Abnormal cardiac shadows or straightening of left heart border can point to a cardiac pathology such as mitral stenosis.

Q. So, what is the cause of hemoptysis in this child and how should one manage it?

The cause here appears to be a lower respiratory tract infection, as history, examination, and investigations point toward a lobar pneumonia, probably necrotizing in nature. This child should be initially started on parenteral antibiotics and observed. If there is no recurrence of pulmonary hemorrhage, no further evaluation may be required. If there is recurrence of bleeding, a bronchoscopy may be needed.

CASE 2

An 8-year-old girl being treated for pulmonary tuberculosis with appropriate antitubercular therapy for the last 2 weeks was wheeled into emergency with history of sudden onset breathing difficulty and a large amount of fresh blood in the sputum.

Physical examination: The child had significant tachycardia and tachypnea with cyanosis and feeble pulses. On 100% oxygen via nonrebreathing mask, her oxygen saturation was around 90%. Her blood pressure was 74/50 mmHg with feeble pulses and cold, clammy skin. On auscultation, there was no air entry in the right lung with crepitations on the left side.

Radiology: She was too unwell to be transported for a chest radiograph.

Q. What is massive hemoptysis?

Bleeding of >8 mL/kg or 200 mL/day is considered massive. However, any child with significant blood in sputum and acute cardiovascular or respiratory compromise should be considered to have massive hemoptysis. Radiologically, involvement (opacification) of two or more lobes may be considered massive.

Q. What is the difference in the management of children with minor and massive hemoptysis?

In contrast to children with minor hemoptysis, these children require airway stabilization, maintenance of adequate oxygenation, control of bleeding, and shock resuscitation. In children with massive hemoptysis, stabilization of the child takes precedence over diagnostic considerations. Irrespective of the etiology, a child with massive hemoptysis and respiratory failure needs intubation, as in the index case. Sometimes selective intubation of the good lung may be even more beneficial. Intravenous fluid boluses followed by blood transfusion will be required to treat cardiovascular collapse and prevent cardiac arrest; however, it must be emphasized that most deaths occur due to asphyxiation and not exsanguination.

Q. What would be the subsequent management in such children?

After the initial resuscitation, these children require urgent fiber-optic bronchoscopy through an existing endotracheal tube, at the bedside in the intensive care unit. Immediate bronchoscopy seems to be the current consensus. If flexible bronchoscopy is not available or feasible or does not identify the site, rigid bronchoscopy may be considered. Both flexible and rigid bronchoscopies have their advantages and disadvantages. Though the ability to clear clots or secretions and maintain a reliable airway can be advantageous, the need for general anesthesia for rigid bronchoscopy is a disadvantage. After the bleeding site is localized, topical vasoconstrictors, fibrin glues, neodymium-doped yttrium aluminium garnet laser, carbon dioxide laser, endoscopic balloon occlusion, etc. may be used to control the bleed. Sidman et al. have reported the use of pulmonary lavage with epinephrine washes (1:10,000 solution) quite successfully.

One could also consider selective embolization of bronchial arteries to stop the bleeding; however, this involves shifting the unstable child to the intervention radiology suite. Emergency bronchial arteriography may help identify the bleeder and selective, targeted embolization will control hemorrhage in nearly three fourths of the cases.

Q. When is surgical management considered?

When embolization and other medical therapies fail, surgery is considered. Surgery may be offered only to those who are stable enough to tolerate general anesthesia and pulmonary resection if needed. Segmentectomy or lobectomy could be especially useful in localized pathology such as bronchiectasis and can effectively control the bleeding.

Q. After the bleeding is controlled, what should be the subsequent approach?

In this case scenario, due to the underlying pulmonary tuberculosis, rupture of a Rasmussen's aneurysm (arterial bleeding) seems to be the most probable cause for such a massive, life-threatening pulmonary hemorrhage. Otherwise, in any child with massive pulmonary hemorrhage, after the acute resuscitation phase, the following laboratory investigations are required: complete blood count, coagulation studies, urinalysis, chest radiograph, sputum test for bacterial, fungal and mycobacterial etiologies, high resolution computed tomography chest with or without contrast, lung biopsy [in suspected diffuse alveolar hemorrhage (DAH)], echocardiography, and ventilation-perfusion studies.

Q. What are the common etiologies for pulmonary hemorrhage in children?

The causes can be classified based on a pathophysiological or epidemiological approach.

TABLE 1: Etiologies for pulmonary hemorrhage in children

Common	Uncommon
• Foreign-body aspiration • Cystic fibrosis • Bronchiectasis • Tuberculosis	• Trauma—accidental/ deliberate • Tracheotomy-related trauma • Congenital cardiac diseases • Pulmonary hypertension • Pulmonary embolism
Rare	**Very rare**
• Tumors ○ Adenoma ○ Carcinoid • A-V fistula • Primary hematologic bleeding diseases • Bleeding in immuno-compromised children • Celiac disease	• Pulmonary-renal syndromes ○ Goodpasture's syndrome ○ Systemic lupus erythematosus ○ Wegener's granulomatosis ○ Microscopic polyangiitis ○ Henoch-Schonlein purpura • Idiopathic pulmonary hemosiderosis • Factitious hemoptysis

Adapted from: Godfrey S. Pulmonary hemorrhage/hemoptysis in children. Pediatr Pulmonol. 2004;37(6):476-84.

Table 1 puts together the causes based on their incidence. The pathophysiological approach based on whether the hemorrhage is diffuse or focal has been outlined in flowcharts 1 and 2.

CASE 3

A 4-year-old boy, symptomatic since 2 years of age in the form of fever, recurrent episodes of cough—nonparoxysmal, associated with streaks of blood in mucus and dyspnea on exertion which was progressive.

Past medical history: Not significant.

Family history: No history of contact with tuberculosis.

Physical examination: Vitals—suggestive of tachypnea and tachycardia, severe pallor, grade 2 clubbing. Respiratory system examination revealed bilateral fine crepitations and wheeze.

Radiology: Chest radiography demonstrates bilateral symmetric reticular opacities with relative sparing of apices and pulmonary artery prominence (Fig. 2).

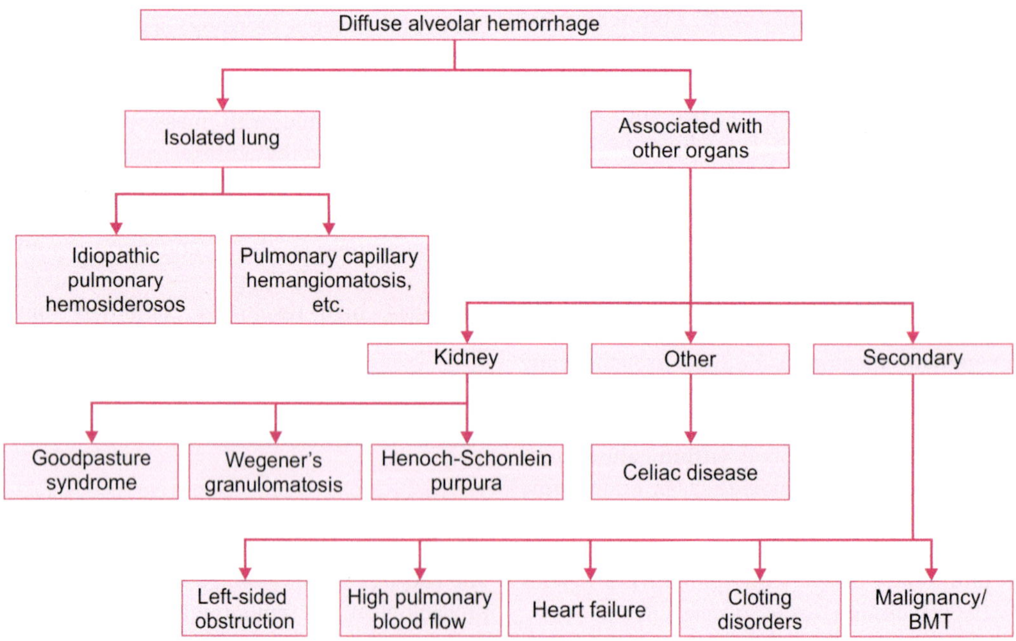

BMT, bone marrow transplant.

Flowchart 1: Diffuse pulmonary hemorrhage—etiologies

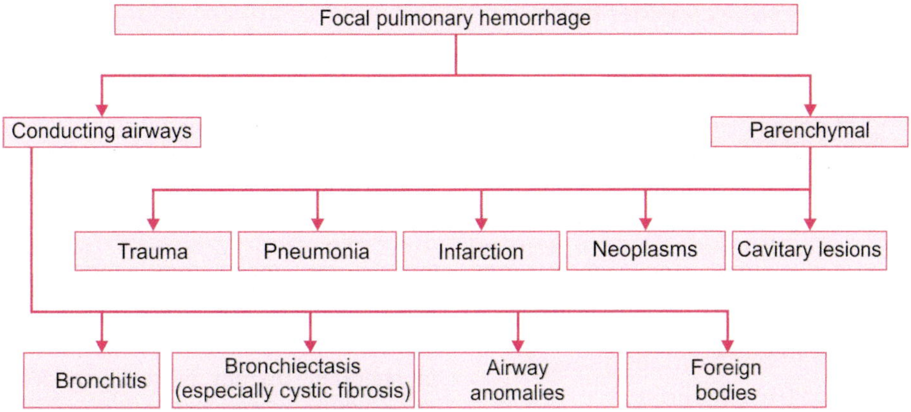

Flowchart 2: Focal pulmonary hemorrhage—etiologies

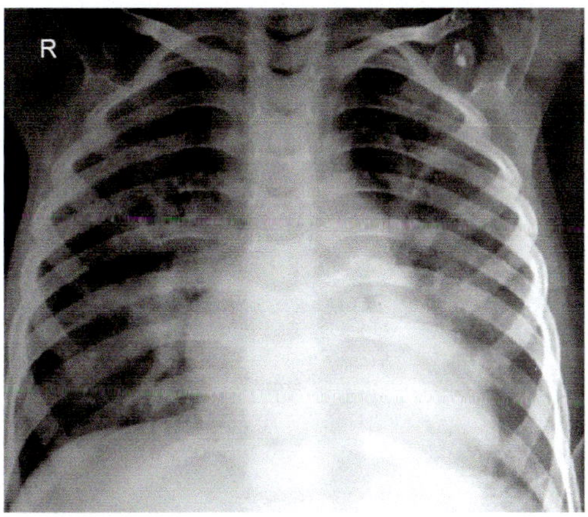

Figure 2: Chest radiograph of case 3 showing bilateral symmetric reticular opacities with relative sparing of apices and pulmonary artery prominence

Q. What would be the clinical possibility in such a case?

It is most likely diffuse alveolar hemorrhage. Diffuse alveolar hemorrhage is a condition in which there is flooding of alveoli with blood usually at multiple sites. The diagnosis of DAH relies on clinical, laboratory, radiological, and pathologic features. It usually presents with hemoptysis, anemia, hypoxemic respiratory failure, and diffuse alveolar infiltrates. The diagnosis can be confirmed by the observation of accumulation of hemosiderin-laden macrophages in the alveolar spaces by doing a gastric or bronchoalveolar lavage. Diffuse alveolar hemorrhage is most commonly of two types—with vasculitis or capillaritis and bland variety without any capillaritis. Idiopathic pulmonary hemosiderosis (IPH), a subtype of DAH, is usually a diagnosis of exclusion, when no underlying etiology is found. It is to be remembered that DAH is a medical emergency and requires thorough evaluation under the guidance of a pediatric pulmonologist.

Q. What should be the plan for further evaluation of such a child?

After a careful history taking and detailed physical evaluation looking for the clues of systemic vasculitic illnesses, basic laboratory investigations, namely complete blood count, liver and renal function tests, and urine analysis, should be done. In all these children, it is important to screen for autoantibodies such as antineutrophil antibody, antiglomerular basement membrane antibodies, serum anti-neutrophil cytoplasmic antibody, antiphospholipid antibody, and tissue transglutaminase. Total immunoglobulin E and C3/C4 levels may be obtained when there is a clinical suspicion of Churg-Strauss syndrome and SLE, respectively.

Early bronchoscopy and BAL is usually required to confirm the suspicion of a DAH. The primary purpose is to confirm alveolar hemorrhage and rule out infections by sending BAL samples for routine bacterial, viral, mycobacterial, and fungal cultures.

Q. When should one consider the diagnosis of idiopathic pulmonary hemosiderosis?

The triad of anemia (iron deficiency), hemoptysis, and multiple bilateral infiltrates on chest radiographs characterize pulmonary hemosiderosis. The diagnosis of IPH is made when there is evidence of chronic or recurrent DAH and when exhaustive evaluations for secondary etiologies have negative results.

Q. What should be the management strategy for diffuse alveolar hemorrhage in children?

Supportive treatment measures

Oxygen, volume resuscitation, blood and blood products, and control of super-added infections is always important. Treat coexisting wheeze with bronchodilators and infection with antibiotics.

Definitive treatment measures

Immunosuppressants are the mainstay of therapy. Corticosteroids are the drug of choice—usually prednisolone. In the acute stages, intravenous pulse therapy is useful. Later, it can be shifted to oral therapy which has to be gradually tapered. Cyclophosphamide is useful in children with SLE, Wegener's and antiglomerular basement membrane diseases. Azathioprine, rituximab, etanercept, mycophenolate mofetil, etc. are being used for various causes of DAH in children. Therapy is best provided under the guidance of a pediatric immunology team. Plasmapheresis is the treatment of choice in Goodpasture syndrome.

To treat IPH, the regimen given in flowchart 3 may be followed. Treat each acute exacerbation with oral steroids 1-2 mg/kg/day for 1-2 months then taper off slowly as mentioned flowchart 3.

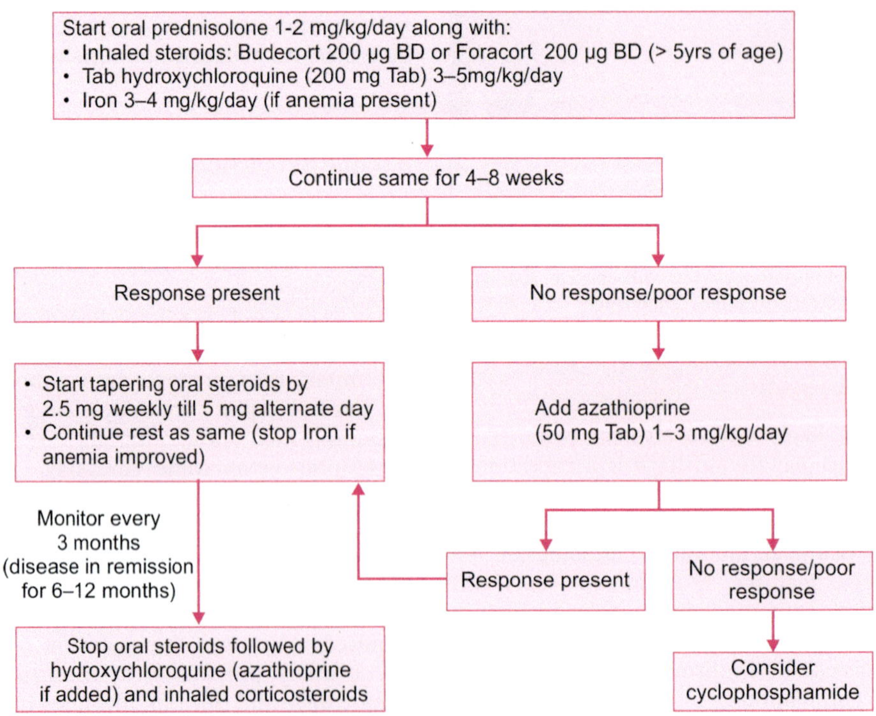

Flowchart 3: Regimen for treatment of idiopathic pulmonary hemosiderosis

LEARNING POINTS

- Always differentiate hematemesis and spurious or pseudohemoptysis from true hemoptysis before proceeding with any further evaluation
- A thorough physical examination and chest radiography may give valuable clues (fairly specific) but possess poor sensitivity
- In a child with massive hemoptysis, stabilization of airway and hemodynamics takes precedence over any diagnostic investigation. Poststabilization, child must undergo a flexible fiber-optic bronchoscopy
- A systematic diagnostic approach based on diffuse or focal pathology may be useful. The diffuse alveolar hemorrhage group may be vasculitic or nonvasculitic. All these children must be screened for autoantibodies
- The treatment for diffuse alveolar hemorrhage/ idiopathic pulmonary hemosiderosis consists of supportive care with immunomodulation. Steroids are the mainstay of therapy. A treatment algorithm is suggested.

SUGGESTED READINGS

1. Gaude GS. Hemoptysis in children. Indian Pediatrics. 2010;47: 245-54.
2. Godfrey S. Pulmonary hemorrhage/hemoptysis in children. Pediatr Pulmonol. 2004;37:476-84.
3. Pachner RW, Bidwell JB. Hemoptysis: diagnosis and management. Am Fam Physician. 2005;72:1253-60.
4. Sarthi M. Pulmonary hemorrhage and idiopathic pulmonary hemosiderosis. In: Kabra SK, Lodha R, editors Essential Pediatric Pulmonology. 2nd ed. New Delhi: Noble Vision; 2010. pp. 255-60.
5. Vece TJ, De Guzman MM, Langston C, Fan LL. Diffuse alveolar hemorrhage in children. In: Wilmott RW, Andrew B, Chernick V, Boat TF, Ratjen F, Deterding RR, editors. Kendig and Chernick's Disorders of the Respiratory Tract in Children. 8th ed. Philadelphia: Elsevier Saunders; 2012. pp. 848-57.

CHAPTER

32

Cow Milk Protein Allergy

Poonam Mehta

CASE 1

A 16-month-old child presented with history of loose stools for last 10 months. Since the onset, he had 4–6 greenish loose stools which were nongreasy and not foul smelling. They were associated with colicky abdominal pain and vomiting. He also had atopic dermatitis.

Birth history: The baby was born full term by normal vaginal delivery with birth weight of 3 kg.

Past history: The baby was apparently well till 6 months of age.

Family history: The father had nasal allergy.

Examination: The child was thin, pale, and irritable. Weight 6 kg and length 80 cm. Nasal examination was essentially normal except turbinate hypertrophy.

Q. What are differential diagnoses for this child?

Child presented with features of chronic diarrhea, vomiting with colicky abdominal pain with atopic dermatitis, and family history of allergic diathesis. The onset of symptoms is 6 months correlating with period of weaning. Child also had failure to thrive. Differential diagnosis can be celiac disease, lactose intolerance, immunodeficiency, metabolic disorders, infections, cow milk protein allergy (CMPA), and surgical causes related to gastrointestinal tract.

Q. What are the most important points to elicit in his history and physical examination to get clue for diagnosis?

The following details in history may help in getting a clue for underlying illness:

- Exclusive breastfeeding duration
- Timing of introduction of top milk
- Family history of atopic dermatitis
- Symptoms pertaining to other systems
- How quickly symptoms appear after ingestion of cow milk?
- How long symptoms last?
- Severity of symptoms?
- Perioral lesions that may appear or worsen on contact with milk.

Physical examination

The following findings on examination may help to reach to diagnosis of underlying illness:

- Anthropometry (weight/height)
- Skin exam: Urticaria, rash
- Anemia
- Features of atopy in form of wheezing, nasal turbinate hypertrophy
- Dermographism.

Findings in index case

On asking the following questions, the duration of exclusive breastfeeding was 6 months, cow milk was added in diet at the age of 6 months. Symptoms appeared within 4 weeks of addition of cow milk. Severity of diarrhea and vomiting was such that the child required admission twice in the last 8 months and dehydration correction. Parents also gave history of rash on the skin due to spilling of milk. Child did not have multisystem infections including oral thrush, skin infections. Child also has failure to thrive. All the symptoms or signs point toward CMPA as the most preferred diagnosis.

Q. What is cow milk protein allergy?

It is an immune mediated reaction to proteins in milk. Milk contains caseins [α (s1)-casein, α (s2)-casein, β-casein and κ-caseins] and serum (whey) proteins [α-lactoalbumin, β-lactoglobulin, bovine lactoferrin, bovine sero albumin, and bovine immunoglobulin], in proportions of 80 and 20%, respectively. The predominant milk allergens are caseins, β-lactoglobulin, and α-lactoglobulin.

Q. What are the types of cow milk protein allergy?

Cow milk protein allergy is of two types:

1. Immunoglobulin E (IgE) mediated: Accounts for 54% of all the cases. It is due to type 1 hypersensitivity immune response to one or more milk proteins. Onset of symptoms is acute (symptoms usually appear within few minutes after ingestion of cow milk protein and almost always within an hour). On investigations, these patients will have positive skin prick test and positive serum specific IgE for cow milk protein
2. Non-IgE mediated: Accounts for almost 46% of total cases. It is due to delayed hypersensitivity (type 4) immune response. Presentation is protean and is usually delayed and often due to chronic exposure to cow milk protein during infancy. Occasionally, may present with severe form of allergic reaction. The skin prick test and the serum specific IgE to cow milk protein is usually negative and the only reliable test is strict elimination diet.

Q. Which age group is most commonly affected?

Usually, cow milk allergy can affect all ages but most prevalent in infancy. It affects 2–7% of formula fed infants and 0.5% of exclusively fed infants.

Q. How does cow milk allergy manifest?

Common clinical manifestations of CMPA are given in table 1.

TABLE 1: Common symptoms and signs of immunoglobulin E and non-immunoglobulin E mediated cow milk protein allergy

IgE mediated	Non-IgE mediated
Skin manifestations (50–70%)	
• Atopic dermatitis • Urticaria • Erythema/pruritus • Swelling of lips and eyes (angioedema)	• Contact rash • Atopic dermatitis • Erythema/pruritus
Gastrointestinal reactions (50–60%)	
• Nausea/vomiting • Abdominal colic • Diarrhea • Dysphagia • Angioedema of lips and tongue	• Failure to thrive • Anorexia • Occult blood/blood in stool • Early satiety • Refusal to feeds • Gastroesophageal reflux disease • Dyspepsia • Transient enteropathy • Protein-losing enteropathy • Perianal rash • Constipation
Respiratory reactions (20–30%)	
• Allergic rhinitis • Rhinoconjunctivitis • Chronic cough/ wheezing • Laryngeal edema • Asthma	• Pulmonary hemosiderosis • Other reactions: Food dependent exercise-induced asthma
Others	
• Systemic anaphylaxis • Iron deficiency anemia	

IgE, immunoglobulin E.

Q. How to confirm diagnosis of cow milk protein allergy?

No single laboratory test or combinations of tests are diagnostic of CMPA. Hence, diagnosis of CMPA still is based on well-defined food elimination and challenges procedures including double-blind placebo-controlled food challenges in children older than 2–3 years. As oral challenge is time consuming, relatively expensive, and not always without a risk for the patient, quantification of specific IgE to cow milk protein has been suggested as an alternative to oral challenge in diagnosis of CMPA. There is no significant relationship between quantification of specific IgE and the challenge threshold dose in food allergic children. Casein-specific IgE is superior to whole milk extract. The diagnostic algorithm is shown below in flowchart 1.

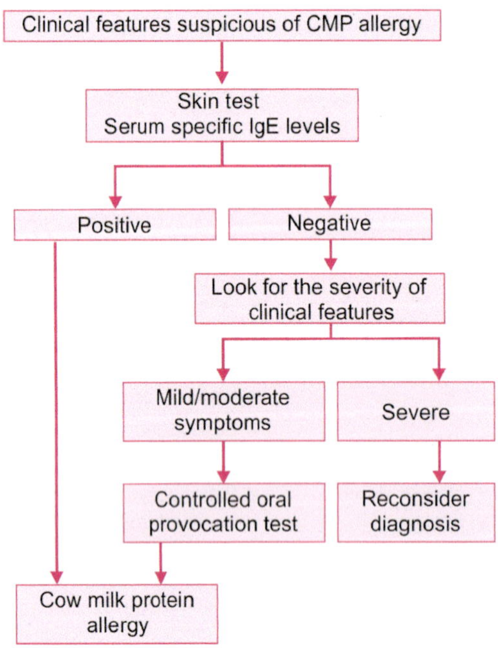

CMP, cow milk protein; IgE, immunoglobulin E.

Flowchart 1: Algorithm for diagnosis of cow milk protein allergy

Findings in index case

The skin prick test showed a wheal of 6 mm and IgE level against specific cow milk protein is 10 kU/L

Q. How to interpret results of skin prick tests and immunoglobulin E levels (radioallergosorbent test) for cow milk protein allergy?

A positive reading is suggested by a wheal measuring 3 mm or more in size. This test is positive in IgE-mediated CMPA. In clinical practice, a value of 0.35kU/L is taken as positive cutoff point for IgE levels. Casein-specific IgE is considered superior to whole milk extract as well as the other proteins and a cutoff of 6.6 kU/L has a 100% specificity.

Q. What is the sensitivity and specificity of skin prick test?

The sensitivity of skin testing is highly variable (50–100%) depending on the age of patient and type of extract used. Specificity of test is 38% with a negative predictive value of 97% and positive predictive value of 56%.

Q. What is the role of skin prick test and radioallergosorbent test in diagnosis of cow milk protein allergy?

Skin prick test and radioallergosorbent test (RAST) are helpful in diagnosis as well as prognosis in patient with cow milk allergy. Children with negative RAST and skin prick test at the diagnosis become tolerant to the offending protein at a younger age. Negative test also reduces the risk of severe acute reaction during challenge.

Q. As this child is on top feed, how to manage this child?

The management of CMPA allergy depends on age of patients, feeding whether on exclusive breast feeding/top feed and severity of symptoms. Management algorithms for formula fed children is provided in flowcharts 2 and 3.

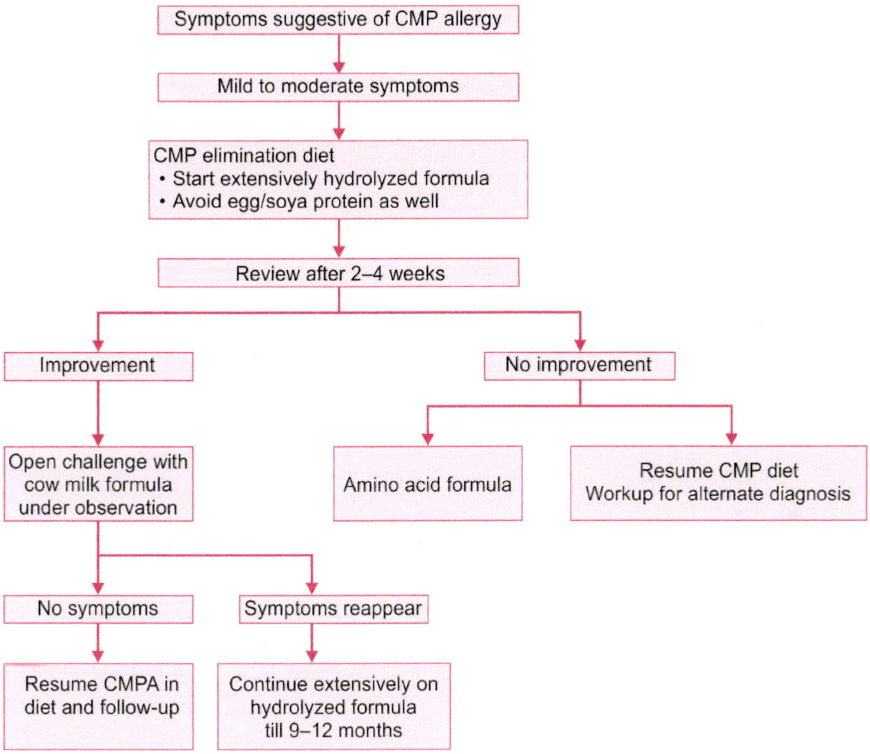

CMPA, cow milk protein allergy; CMP, cow milk protein.

Flowchart 2: Management algorithm for children with mild to moderate symptoms of cow milk protein allergy on formula feeds

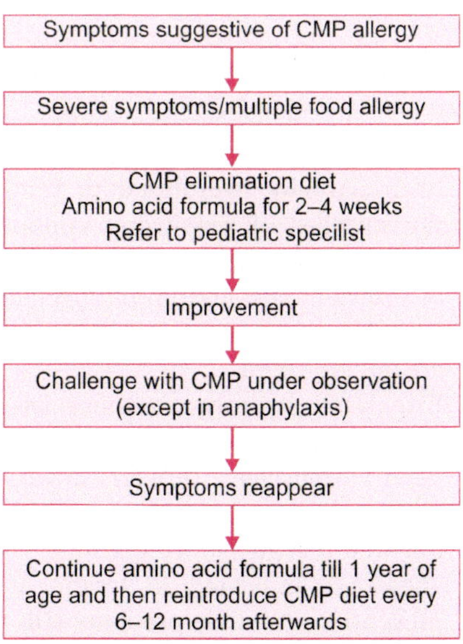

Flowchart 3: Management algorithm for children with severe symptoms of cow milk protein allergy on formula feeds

CASE 2

An otherwise well thriving 5-week-old breastfeed infant presented with frequent loose stools, irritability, and perianal redness. As physical examination was otherwise unremarkable and stool examination and culture were negative, infant was referred for pediatric gastroenterologist opinion. Food protein-induced proctocolitis was suspected.

Q. How to approach this case?

In this case, the baby is on exclusive breastfeed, the management is different from earlier case as shown in flowchart 4.

Q. Does she have to avoid other food products in addition to cow milk protein containing products?

Adverse reactions to other foods have been reported in 41–75% of children with CMPA. The

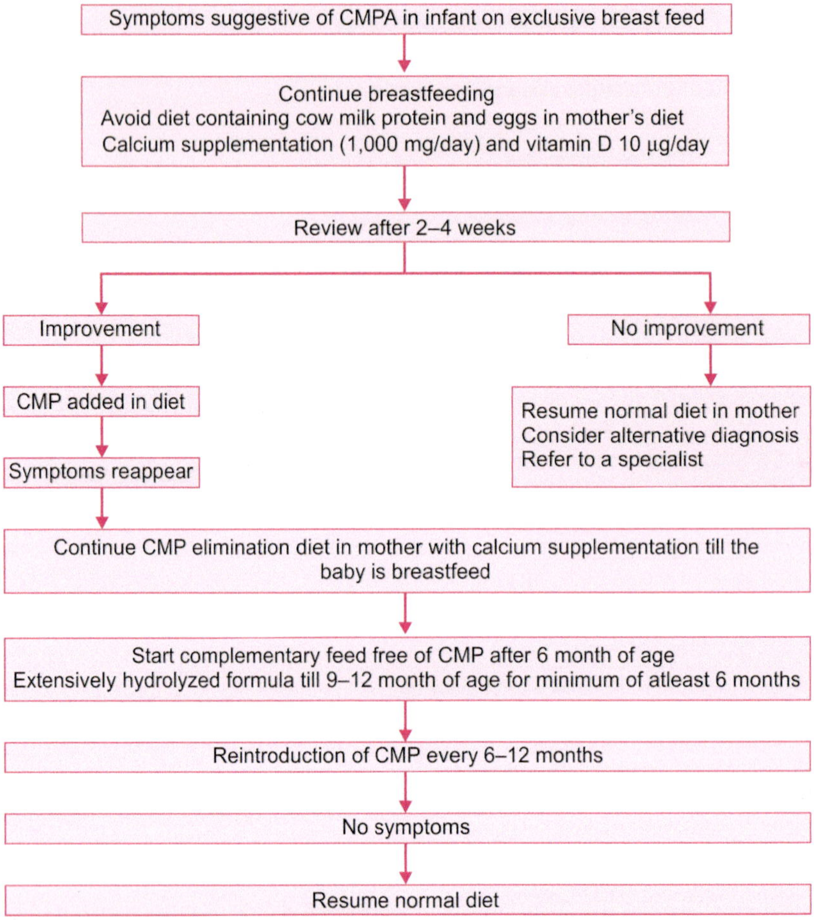

CMPA, cow milk protein allergy; CMP, cow milk protein.

Flowchart 4: Management algorithm for infant with cow milk protein allergy on exclusive breastfeed

most frequent reactions are against egg, soya, peanut, fish, etc. Hence, these food products should be avoided during cow milk protein elimination diet.

Q. What is the alternative diet a mother can give in child with cow milk protein allergy?

Alternative formulas that can be used in children with CMPA are as follows:

- Cow milk formulas are hydrolyzed in order to remove the allergenic epitopes
  - Partially hydrolyzed: These formulas contain cow's milk proteins that have been partially hydrolyzed to minimize the number of sensitizing epitopes in milk protein, however, retaining peptides of sufficient size and immunogenicity to stimulate oral tolerance. Nowadays, these are not indicated
  - Extensively hydrolyzed: These formulas contain cow's milk proteins that have been extensively broken down into smaller peptides (<1,500 kDa) that are not well recognized by immune system. These are indicated in treatment and prevention. The only problem with these formulas is their less palatability

- Amino acid formulas: These formulas have been developed to overcome the hypersensitivity that can result from the residual proteins in extensively hydrolyzed formula. These are indicated in treatment, not in prevention. These are of first choice in infants with severe cow milk protein reaction
- Partially hydrolyzed rice protein formulas
- Soya-based formulas
- Extensive nondairy soya and meat (pig collagen) protein hydrolysate.

Q. What is the current status on soy-based formulas in patient with cow milk protein allergy?

These formulas were used earlier due to lesser cost and superior palatability. However, it has been seen that up to 14% of children and infants with IgE-mediated allergy also react with soya. Approximately 70% of infants with CMPA below 1-year age reacted to soy. Therefore, soya milk should not be recommended to infants and young children whereas can be tolerated by older children.

Q. Mother is confused and asks whether she can give milk from other mammals. What should be the answer for this mother?

Goat and sheep milk are not recommended due to cross reactivity with cow milk protein. Milk from nonbovid mammals like donkey, mare, and camel show less casein protein homology and may be tolerated by some patients although milk of this kind is not currently available. Till date, milk from other mammals is not recommended.

Q. Mother wants to know whether extensively heated milk can be an option in children with cow milk protein allergy. What is the answer to her query?

Heat treatment denatures most of the whey protein in cow's milk whereas casein proteins are not destroyed. Hence, those patients who are sensitized to whey protein can tolerate, however, those sensitized to casein (more common) do not tolerate extensively heated milk.

Q. Mother is concerned whether this disease persists for life. How to prognosticate the mother regarding the disease?

The overall prognosis of patient with CMPA is good with total recovery of 45–56% at 1 year, 60–77% at 2 years, 84–87% at 3 years, and approximately 90–95% at 5–10 years of age.

Q. How can we prevent development of cow milk protein allergy??

Exclusive breastfeeding for at least 6 months in infants with high risk of allergy. If breastfeeding is not possible, an adapted cow milk formula is advised.

LEARNING POINTS

- Cow's milk allergy affects 2–3% of children, and 0.5% of purely breastfed infants
- Most patients develop symptoms before 1 month of age often within 1 week of introduction of cow milk protein-based formula
- Most patients with milk allergy will outgrow it [immunoglobulin E (IgE) mediated by 5 years of age and non-IgE mediated by 3 years of age]
- Diagnostic criteria for cow's milk allergy
  - Temporal association between occurrence of symptoms and milk ingestion
  - Involvement of multiple organ systems affected. Most commonly the skin, gastrointestinal tract, and respiratory system, particularly if symptoms of allergic diathesis are present

- Family history of atopy
- Exclusion of lactose intolerance
- Positive allergy tests—skin prick tests, specific IgE testing, eosinophilia
- Failure to respond to other treatments including exclusion of functional causes

- Infants on formula fed can be treated with extensively hydrolyzed formula, however, should be started on amino acid formula in case of no improvement
- Milk from other mammals is not recommended
- Infants with severe symptoms and multiple food allergies should be started directly on amino acid formulas
- Soya milk is not recommended for infants less than 1 year of age
- Patients with severe symptoms, multiple food allergies, and faltering growth which improve on exclusion diet, should be referred to a specialist
- No role of addition of prebiotics and probiotics in hypoallergenic formulas.

SUGGESTED READINGS

1. Brueton M, Vandenplas Y, Dupont C, Hill D, Isolauri E, Koletzko S, et al. Guidelines for the diagnosis and management of cow's milk protein allergy in infants. Arch Dis Child. 2007;92(10):902-8.
2. De Greef E, Vandenplas Y, Devreker T. Treatment of cow's milk protein allergy. Pediatr Gastroenterol Hepatol Nutr. 2014;17(1):1-5.
3. Martorell-Aragonés A, Echeverría-Zudaire L, Alonso-Lebrero E, Boné-Calvo J, Martín-Muñoz MF, Nevot-Falcó S, et al.; Food allergy committee of SEICAP (Spanish Society of Pediatric Allergy, Asthma and Clinical Immunology). Position document: IgE-mediated cow's milk allergy. Allergol Immunopathol (Madr). 2015;43(5):507-26.
4. Host A, Halken S. Cow's milk allergy: where have we come from and where are we going? Endocrine Metab Immune Disord Drug Targets. 2014;14(1):2-8.
5. Ludman S, Shah N, Fox AT. Managing cow milk allergy in children. BMJ. 2013;347:f5424.

CHAPTER

33

Hypersensitivity Pneumonitis

Prahalad Kumar A

CASE 1

A 10-year-old boy child presented with sudden onset of fever, cough, and myalgia since 6 hours. There was no history of wheeze. Six hours before the onset of symptom, the child was playing with parrots in the garden.

Past history: There were history of similar episodes since the age of 6 years; each episode was precipitated on exposure to birds.

Family history: There was no family history of asthma or atopy.

Birth history: The baby was born full term by normal vaginal delivery with average birth weight. Growth and development were normal and had received primary and booster immunization.

Examination: The child was in respiratory distress. There was no clubbing and cyanosis. On chest auscultation, bilateral diffuse crackles were present. Oxygen saturation was 60% in room air and 90% with 5 liter of oxygen. Arterial blood gas analysis revealed hypoxia (PaO_2 of 60 with 5 liter of oxygen). Laboratory results revealed leukocytosis with neutrophilia, elevated C-reactive protein and erythrocyte sedimentation rate (ESR). The chest radiograph showed bilateral reticulonodular infiltrates, more in the basal regions.

Q. What are the differential diagnoses for this child?

Since the symptoms are confiding to the respiratory system and triggered on exposure to birds, the differential diagnoses in this case could be asthma, hypersensitivity pneumonitis, and allergic bronchopulmonary aspergillosis.

Q. What are the most important points to elicit in his history and physical examination to get clue for diagnosis of hypersensitivity pneumonitis?

The following details in history may help in getting a clue for diagnosis:

- The onset is often sudden and on exposure to particular antigens like bird droppings, molds, and in the absence of other triggering factors in asthma like dust or smoke
- The symptoms mimic flu-like illness
- Respiratory system examination may reveal crackles rather than wheeze.

Q. What is hypersensitivity pneumonitis?

Hypersensitivity pneumonitis or extrinsic allergic alveolitis is a non-immunoglobulin E immunologically mediated diffuse inflammatory disease of the pulmonary interstitium caused by inhalation of variety of antigens. Antigens are typically of animal or vegetable origin and 1–5 μm in size and deposit in the alveoli. The disease has been mainly reported in adults with occupational exposure to antigens. Whereas cases reported in children typically involve avian and fungal antigens resulting from exposure to birds and molds.

Hypersensitivity pneumonitis also known as extrinsic allergic alveolitis was originally described by Ramazzini in 1793 in his book called *Diseases of the Workers*, what is now called farmers lung. The first pediatric case was reported by Stiehm and coworkers in 1967. There has been a case report on an infant as young as 10 weeks old (so far 119 cases have been reported in children.

Q. What is the etiology of hypersensitivity pneumonitis?

Numerous organic and inorganic antigens can cause hypersensitivity pneumonitis. Avian and animal products—pigeon droppings, fungal products—mold and hay, and certain chemicals like toluene diisocyanate (e.g., in spray paint and glue) are some of the triggering agents for hypersensitivity pneumonitis.

Q. What is the pathophysiology in hypersensitivity pneumonitis?

The pathophysiology of hypersensitivity pneumonitis is not fully understood. After a sensitized subject inhales the antigen, immune complexes are formed with precipitating antibodies (type 3 reaction of Gell and Coombs) and the complement cascade is activated. This leads to transient neutrophilic alveolitis that is responsible for the acute respiratory symptoms. This event is followed by influx of activated CD8 cells that is followed by an increase of CD4 cells. Activated macrophages produce pro-inflammatory cytokines such as tumor necrosis factor-α, interleukin-1, and interleukin-8. This lymphocyte reaction (type 4 of Gell and Coombs) is also associated with granulomatous inflammation of the distal airways and alveoli.

Q. What are the clinical manifestations of hypersensitivity pneumonitis?

The mean age of presentation is 9.7 years and there is 1.4:1 male to female ratio. Seventy seven percent of reported pediatric cases are caused by exposure to bird antigens (pigeons, parrots, doves, and others) and 22 % are caused by exposure to molds (*Aspergillus, Penicillium,* and others).

The disease manifests in three clinical forms—(i) acute, (ii) subacute, and (iii) chronic forms.

Acute hypersensitivity pneumonitis

Presents 4–6 hours after an intense exposure to antigen, patients develop flu-like illness associated with fever, chills, cough, myalgia, and malaise. Physical examination reveals an ill appearing child with dyspnea and bibasilar crackles.

If not reexposed to antigen, symptoms usually subside by 24 hours. Laboratory results reveal leukocytosis with neutrophilia, elevated C-reactive protein, and ESR.

The chest radiograph reveals bilateral reticulonodular infiltrates more evident in the lower lung zones. High resolution computed tomography of the chest shows ground glass appearance and poorly defined centrilobular nodules. Pulmonary function test reveals hypoxemia and restrictive lung disease pattern. Treatment of acute form consists of avoidance of the offending antigen. In severe cases, corticosteroids may be helpful.

Subacute hypersensitivity pneumonitis

It is the result of repeated low dose exposure to an antigen and is even more challenging to diagnose; systemic symptoms comprise of low-grade fever, arthralgia, myalgia, fatigue, and respiratory symptoms; signs include cough, exertional dyspnea, crackles, and rhonchi. Chest X-ray and high-resolution computed tomography will show micronodular infiltrates and areas of mild fibrosis. Pulmonary function test shows evidence of restrictive lung disease. Laboratory studies show elevated C-reactive protein and ESR and lymphocytosis with a normal CD4/CD8 ratio.

Chronic hypersensitivity pneumonitis

It is characterized by progressive cough, dyspnea on exertion, anorexia, weight loss, and malaise. Physical examination shows clubbing and respiratory system examination shows crackles. Chest imaging shows diffuse infiltrates, patchy ground glass opacities, and centrilobular nodules. In advanced lung disease, honeycombing may be seen.

Q. How do we confirm the diagnosis of hypersensitivity pneumonitis?

The diagnosis is mainly clinical. In addition to the above typical clinical manifestation, chest X-ray will show bilateral reticulonodular infiltrates more evident in the lower lung zones. High resolution computed tomography of the chest shows ground glass appearance and poorly defined centrilobular nodules. Pulmonary function test reveals restrictive lung disease pattern. Allergic skin test may be a useful test to find out the triggering antigen.

Q. What is the treatment for hypersensitivity pneumonitis?

Antigen avoidance remains the mainstay of treatment. A short course of steroid will be useful for acute condition. For chronic disease, corticosteroids may be required for few weeks to few months.

Q. What is the prognosis of hypersensitivity pneumonitis?

Overall prognosis for acute hypersensitivity pneumonitis is excellent if diagnosed early and repeated exposures to particular antigens are avoided.

LEARNING POINTS

- Hypersensitivity pneumonitis or extrinsic allergic alveolitis is a non-immunoglobulin E immunologically mediated diffuse inflammatory disease of the pulmonary interstitium caused by inhalation of variety of antigens
- Hypersensitivity pneumonitis may present as acute, subacute, and chronic forms
- It is characterized by neutrophilic response in laboratory tests and restrictive pattern on pulmonary function tests. Imaging typically reveals interstitial pattern
- Antigen avoidance is best therapy with or without steroids.

Acknowledgment

The author sincerely thank the head of the institution (Indira Gandhi Institute of Child Health, Bangalore), all the faculty, and postgraduates for giving their valuable input in the preparation of this chapter.

SUGGESTED READINGS

1. Elias J, Fishman A, Fishman J, Grippi M, Senior R, Pack A. Pulmonary Diseases and Disorders. 4th ed. Beijing: McGraw-Hill; 2008. pp. 1161-72.
2. Lacasse Y, Girard M, Cormier Y. Recent advances in hypersensitivity pneumonitis. Chest. 2012;142(1):208-17.
3. McSharry C, Anderson K, Bourke SJ, Boyd G. Takes your breaths away-the immunology of allergic alveolitis. Clin Exp Immunol. 2002;128(1):3-9.
4. Ohshimo S, Bonella F, Guzman J, Costabel U. Hypersensitivity pneumonitis. Immunol Allergy Clin N Am. 2012;32(4):537-56.
5. Patel AM, Ryer JH, Reed CE. Hypersensitivity pneumonitis: current concepts and future questions. J Allerg Clinic Immunol. 2001;108(5):661-70.

Chapter

34

Eosinophilic Lung Diseases

Subramanya N K, Vidya K

CASE 1

A 12-year-old girl diagnosed as atopic asthma was evaluated. She was found to be regular on inhalation therapy. Complete blood count (CBC) showed total count of 12,500 cells/mm^3. Differential count showed neutrophils (N) 59, lymphocytes (L) 25, monocytes (M) 05, eosinophils (E) 09, and basophils (B) 01. Chest X-ray unremarkable. Absolute eosinophil count 800/mm^3. Stool examination was ordered and no ova or cysts were found. Empirical deworming was done.

Q. How will you interpret the laboratory values and will you give diethylcarbamazine in this case?

Children with atopic asthma can have mild to moderate eosinophilia. Unless there is marked eosinophilia at this stage, there is no need to order tests to evaluate eosinophilia. Treatment with diethylcarbamazine (DEC) is not necessary. Asthmatic children can have eosinophilic or neutrophilic inflammation. The subset of asthmatic children with predominant eosinophilic inflammation will respond to inhalational steroids well.

CASE 2

A 15-year-old girl with breathlessness and wheezing was evaluated; CBC showed total count 10,500 cells/mm^3. Differential count showed N 53, L 25, E 15, M 05, and B 02. Chest X-ray unremarkable. Absolute eosinophil count 3,500/mm^3.

Q. What are eosinophilic lung diseases? What are the differential diagnoses or the other conditions that should be considered when there is peripheral eosinophilia and respiratory symptoms?

Unlike the previous case, the eosinophil counts in this girl are very high. She is likely to be having eosinophilic lung disease.

The eosinophilic lung diseases are a heterogeneous group of disorders characterized by pulmonary infiltrates associated with peripheral and/or tissue eosinophilia. A large number of lung diseases have peripheral blood eosinophilia; with the advent of bronchoscopy, eosinophilia is often demonstrated in bronchoalveolar lavage (BAL) or in lung biopsy. The rapid expansion in the understanding of eosinophil cell biology and biochemistry, including the role of cytokines and mediators, has improved the management and outcome of eosinophilic lung diseases. Some diseases affect lung parenchyma, others lung vasculature or both. While some diseases are mild and self-limiting, a few others have a poor outcome.

Q. What is the role of eosinophil and what are the normal laboratory values?

A quick recap of the basics regarding eosinophil and normal laboratory values will be useful in approaching eosinophilic lung diseases. The word "EOS" mean "dawn". Eosinophil is a two lobed polymorphonuclear leukocyte with 12–15 µm diameter. These are produced by bone marrow and regulated by interleukin-3 (IL-3) (IL3) predominantly, also by IL-5, granulocyte macrophage colony stimulating factor with involvement of Th2 lymphocytes. The granules in eosinophils stain red with eosin that contain mainly major basic protein, histamine, eosinophil chemotactic protein, platelet activating factor, and leukotrienes. Functions of eosinophils include host defense against parasites and fungi, modulator of inflammation, and tissue destroyer.

Eosinophils are more abundant in tissues than in blood. Hence, blood eosinophil numbers do not necessarily indicate the extent of eosinophilic involvement in affected tissues. Eosinophils are most numerous in tissues with a mucosal epithelial interface within the environment, such as the respiratory, gastrointestinal, and lower genitourinary tracts. Eosinophils are not present in the lungs of healthy people, therefore, their presence in tissue or BAL fluid (>5% of differential count) identifies a pathologic process. The normal values of eosinophil in peripheral blood and BAL are given in table 1.

TABLE 1: Normal values of eosinophil in peripheral blood and bronchoalveolar lavage

Eosinophil count normal	50–250 cells/mm^3
Eosinophilia: • Mild • Moderate • Severe	 • 500–1,500 cells/mm^3 • 1,500–5,000 cells/mm^3 • >5,000 cells/mm^3
Bronchoscopy BAL eosinophils	Normally <2%
BAL eosinophils: Percentage rather than absolute number is more important	Increased • >5%: Idiopathic, drug related, PCP, ILD, parasitic infestations • >20%: Primary pulmonary eosinophilic syndromes

PCP, *Pneumocystis carinii*; ILD, interstitial lung disease; BAL, bronchoalveolar lavage.

Q. How do we classify eosinophilic lung diseases?

There is currently no ideal classification of eosinophilic lung diseases given the diversity of clinical presentations. The classification focuses on the etiology (primary/secondary), severity (benign/severe), duration (acute/chronic), and the clinical presentation as respiratory or multisystem disease (Tables 2 and 3).

The findings are consistent with eosinophilic lung disease. Serial X-ray or a close follow-up can solve this case to be benign self-limiting or progressive disease. This child turned out be Loeffler's syndrome and showed improvement over 10 days with steroids.

TABLE 2: Classification of eosinophilic lung diseases (depending on the etiology)

Primary	Secondary
• Simple pulmonary eosinophilia (Loeffler's syndrome) • Acute eosinophilic pneumonia • Chronic eosinophilic pneumonia • Idiopathic hyper-eosinophilic syndrome	• Tropical pulmonary eosinophilia • Pulmonary eosinophilia with asthma • Poly arteritis nodosa • Churg-Strauss syndrome • Allergic bron-chopulmonary aspergillosis • Drug induced

TABLE 3: Classification of eosinophilic lung diseases by severity

Benign	Loeffler's syndrome
Intermediate	Eosinophilic pneumonia
Severe	Hypersensitivity angitis, polyarteritis nodosa

CASE 3

A 9-year-old boy presented with difficulty in breathing for 2 weeks. The CBC showed 12% eosinophil and his X-ray chest revealed diffuse infiltrates on right side (Fig. 1). How will you proceed?

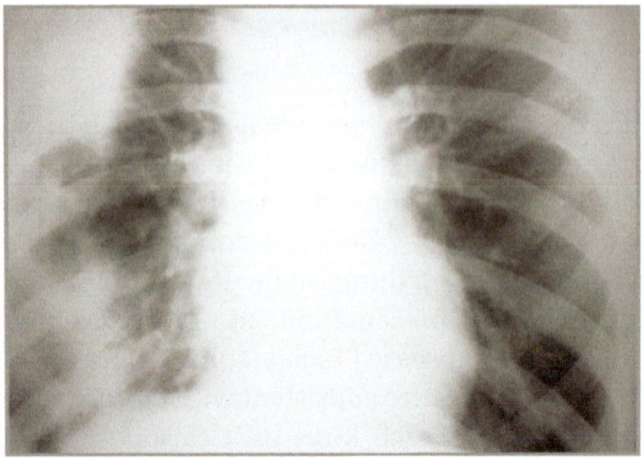

Figure 1: Chest X-ray showing diffuse infiltrates on right side

Q. What is Loeffler's syndrome?

In 1932, Loeffler first described a clinical syndrome characterized by mild respiratory symptoms, peripheral blood eosinophilia, and transient migratory pulmonary infiltrates. This condition can be seen at any age. Table 4 summarizes the main features of Loeffler's syndrome.

TABLE 4: **Summary of Loeffler's syndrome**

Etiology	• Immune hypersensitivity parasites: ○ *Ascaris lumbricoides, Ancyclostoma duodenale, Strongyloides stercoralis* • Drug induced (penicillin, nitrofurantoin, minocycline) • Idiopathic
Clinical features	• Low grade fever, nonproductive cough, dyspnea • Respiratory manifestations are self-limiting and typically resolve in 1–2 weeks
Treatment	• Systemic corticosteroids like prednisolone 0.5–2 mg/kg/day • The dose of steroids needs to be tapered to maintenance dose within first few weeks • In conditions caused due to parasitic infection, antihelminthic drugs should be given

Q. What are differential diagnoses of case 3?

Acute and chronic eosinophilic pneumonia are due to variety of fungi, toxic inhalation, and drugs. Clinical features are breathlessness, fever, and cough. Computed tomography scan chest will show ground glass opacification. Acute eosinophilic pneumonia is characterized by hypoxemia which requires immediate intervention with methyl prednisolone. Prednisolone, antifungal therapy, and avoidance of offenders like drugs and toxins form the mainstay of the therapy depending on etiology.

Idiopathic hypereosinophilic syndrome

Idiopathic hypereosinophilic syndrome is not a single entity but constellation of leukoproliferative disorders characterized by sustained overproduction of eosinophils. The three original diagnostic criteria are shown in box 1.

Box 1: Three original diagnostic criteria

- Eosinophilia in excess of 1,500/μL for longer than 6 months
- Lack of parasitic, allergic/other etiology, absence of other eosinophilic syndromes
- Signs and symptoms of organ involvement with persisting or sustained eosinophilia

Idiopathic hypereosinophilic syndrome is characterized by cough, dyspnea, and fatigue. In some cases, myeloproliferative features are demonstrable like anemia, splenomegaly, and increased B12 levels. A course of prednisolone is useful.

CASE 4

An 18-year-old teenager presented with wheezing, and dyspnea. She was diagnosed initially as asthma; later on developed skin rashes, myalgia, joint pains, and hematuria. Peripheral blood showed marked eosinophilia. How do you approach?

This teenager is likely to be having multisystem disease. Detailed history of travel, worm infestation, and drug intake is required. Secondary eosinophilic lung diseases are possibility. The differential diagnoses include:

- Tropical pulmonary eosinophilia: It is generally caused by filarial worm, is endemic in tropics and subtropics, and endemic in India. The diagnosis is established by cough worsening at night, eosinophilia >3,300/mm^3 in children living in endemic area. The chest X-ray shows infiltrates and erythrocyte sedimentation rate is elevated. The symptoms improve with administration of DEC
- Churg-Strauss syndrome: Churg-Strauss syndrome an allergic granulomatous angitis is rare syndrome that affects small- to medium-sized arteries and veins. It is a systemic disorder characterized by asthma, transient pulmonary infiltrates, hyper eosinophilia, and systemic vasculitis as evidenced by multiorgan, multisystem features involving heart, nervous system, skin, and gastrointestinal system. The etiology is autoimmune and steroids form the mainstay of treatment
- Allergic bronchopulmonary aspergillosis: This occurs in children with asthma and cystic fibrosis and is discussed in detail in a separate chapter.

Q. How to approach parasite-induced lung diseases? Is stool examination helpful?

Many parasites cause pulmonary infiltrates with blood or alveolar eosinophilia. A travel history is important. Patients infected with one parasite are at risk for multiple parasites. Therefore, failure of pulmonary symptoms or eosinophilia to resolve despite treatment should prompt a search for additional parasites. The magnitude of eosinophilia depends on the parasite load and host response. Serology and stool examination may help to find out the helminth responsible for pulmonary manifestation. Inability to demonstrate the ova or cyst in stool examination does not exclude the clinical diagnosis. Antihelminthic drugs are given depending on the suspected worm. The response to treatment may be prolonged as even dead parasites remain as antigenic source for eosinophilia.

Q. What is drug-induced eosinophilic lung disease?

History of drug intake with pulmonary findings and eosinophilia that improves after cessation of the drug gives the diagnosis. Some drugs like nitrofurantion, penicillin, sulfonamide, amiodarone, and thiazides are commonly associated with eosinophilic lung diseases. Rarely, antimalarials, antitubercular drugs, cephalosporins, and tetracycline are responsible for manifestations. The cessation of drug, followed by steroids can alleviate the symptoms.

LEARNING POINTS

- Eosinophilic lung diseases are heterogeneous and the pulmonary manifestations with peripheral eosinophilia are the hall mark of the diseases
- The spectrum of presentations can be acute or chronic, primary (idiopathic) or secondary, self-limiting or progressive, and pulmonary and/or multisystem involvement
- A detailed history of travel, past history, treatment, and exposure can give the clue to etiology
- Ascertain the diagnosis before starting steroids as the findings revert with treatment.

SUGGESTED READINGS

1. Bush A, Wilmott RW, Boat TF, Deterding RR, Ratjen F, Chernick V, editors. Kendig and Chernick's Disorders of the Respiratory Tract in Children. 8th ed. Philadelphia: Saunders; 2012.
2. Geme JS, Kliegma RM, Stanton BM, Schor NF, Behrman RE, editors. Nelson Textbook of Pediatrics. 19th ed. Philadelphia: Saunders; 2011.
3. Longo DL, Kasper DL, Jameson JL, Fauci AS, Hauser SL, Loscalzo J, editors. Harrison's Principles of Internal Medicine. 18th ed. McGraw-Hill Professional; 2011.

CHAPTER

35

Pulmonary Alveolar Proteinosis in Children

Balasubramanian Sundaram

CASE 1

A 4-month-old male infant presented with breathlessness and poor feeding noticed from 2 weeks of age with a birth weight of 3 kg. Immediate neonatal period was uneventful. The infant was exclusively breastfed and had increasing breathlessness with chest retractions without cyanosis. There had been some occasional cough and the mother had noticed that he had been feeding less recently. On examination, he was dusky (oxygen saturation of 87%). The nails appeared to show early clubbing. Respiratory findings included tachypnea (62/min) with marked intercostal retractions and bilateral scattered crackles, particularly in the lower lobes. Repeat X-ray chest showed increased bronchovascular markings on both sides with features of bilateral hyperinflation and cardiac size arterial blood gas revealed features of hypoxia with mild metabolic acidosis (well compensated). Echocardiography study did not reveal any abnormality.

The infant required 2 liter of oxygen supplementation to maintain oxygen saturation and was feeding at the breasts with difficulty.

Q. What are the diagnostic possibilities?

A provisional diagnosis of primary lung disease possibly interstitial lung disease (ILD) was made because of chronic respiratory with hypoxia without noisy breathing or significant cough. Absence of fever and extrapulmonary manifestations made infection or immunodeficiency an unlikely diagnosis. Airway diseases are unlikely because of the absence of noisy breathing and significant cough. Cyanotic congenital heart disease as a possible diagnosis is unlikely due to the absence of murmurs or abnormal heart sounds, or cardiomegaly. Aspiration syndromes are unlikely due to absence of choking episodes or frequent vomiting. The onset of symptoms in the neonatal period makes a congenital disorder as the most likely diagnosis.

Q. What is the role of high resolution computerized tomography in the diagnostic workup?

High-resolution computerized tomography (HRCT) is more sensitive than chest X-ray for diagnosing ILD in childhood and more precise for assessing the extent of disease severity. High resolution computerized tomography in ILD may show hyperinflation, mosaic pattern, air trapping, ground glass opacities, consolidation, linear or reticular opacities, and nodulocystic lesions. Ground glass opacities, consolidation, septal thickening, and crazy paving are frequently observed in pulmonary alveolar proteinosis (PAP). In the case under discussion, HRCT scan of thorax showed diffuse interstitial and alveolar infiltrates bilaterally suggesting a diagnosis of ILD.

Q. What is the role of bronchoalveolar lavage in diagnosis of interstitial lung disease?

Flexible bronchoscopy with bronchoalveolar lavage (BAL) is an important procedure in the diagnostic workup, which is a first step in ruling out causes such as infection or airway anomalies. Pulmonary hemorrhage syndromes, PAP, pulmonary histiocytosis, sarcoidosis, Niemann-Pick disease, and aspiration are diagnoses which can be picked up by BAL cytology. Presence of lipid laden macrophages is a specific clue to diagnosis of aspiration.

Microbiological diagnosis of infections such as tuberculosis, pneumocystis pneumonia, etc. may be made from BAL specimens.

In the case cited, BAL was carried out. Bacterial cultures were negative and acidfast bacilli and fungal smears were negative. Bronchoalveolar lavage fluid stained with periodic acid-Schiff (PAS) showed extracellular positive proteinaceous material and lipid-laden macrophages, suggesting the diagnosis of PAP. The infant died of progressive respiratory failure in a week's time.

CASE 2

A 5-year-old female child who had progressive breathlessness from 3 years of age was presented at he clinic. The breathlessness which was initially present only on exertion like walking fast progressed to dyspnea at rest. Her cousin had died at 3 years of age due to a similar illness. She weighed 12 kg at 3 years and had lost weight slowly over the last 2 years. She was born after a third degree consanguineous marriage and had a healthy elder sister of 10 years of age. She had received empirical antituberculous treatment for 6 months elsewhere without improvement and also had been on inhaled corticosteroids for more than a year. Fever and diarrhea were never the significant symptoms though there had been episodes of increasing breathlessness with cough intermittently.

On examination, the child weighed only 9.5 kg with a height of 85 cm indicating severe malnutrition and growth retardation. There was pan digital clubbing with marked pectus excavatum and Harrison's sulcus. There were significant chest retractions with tachypnea. Auscultation showed bilateral fine crackles all over both lung fields. Examination of other systems did not reveal any abnormalities. His oxygen saturation was 82% in room air.

X-ray chest showed diffuse bilateral air filling pattern, especially in the perihilar regions. High resolution computerized tomography showed ground glass opacities of alveolar spaces and thickening of the interlobular and intralobular septa and called crazy paving. Echocardiography showed features of mild pulmonary hypertension. Investigations for tuberculosis, immunodeficiency and cystic fibrosis were negative. Bronchoalveolar lavage aspirate showed typical findings of PAP.

The above two cases typically illustrate the clinical presentation of PAP as an ILD in two different age groups.

Q. What is the etiology and pathogenesis of pulmonary alveolar proteinosis?

Acquired, secondary, idiopathic and congenital are the types of PAP described.

Congenital

Congenital alveolar proteinosis (CAP) may be caused by inborn errors of surfactant metabolism, lysinuric protein intolerance, and mutations in the components of the granulocyte-macrophage colony-stimulating factor (GM-CSF) receptor and the histopathologic manifestations are different from the autoimmune or classic form of PAP.

- Surfactant protein B deficiency: It is a hydrophobic protein which interacts with surfactant lipids to facilitate adsorption to the air-liquid interface. If deficiency is present, infants born at term may have severe respiratory failure immediately not responding to exogenous surfactant or glucocorticoids, or aggressive respiratory support. Some may initially have a mild respiratory distress later succumbing to respiratory failure
- Surfactant protein C deficiency: This is an autosomal dominant disorder. Some may present early with respiratory failure but most have an insidious onset later in life with longer survival

- *ABCA3* mutations: *ABCA3* is an ATP binding cassette protein (transmembrane protein). Patients with *ABCA3* mutations present as fatal respiratory failure of newborns or as ILD later
- In addition to the above, the following genetic causes of PAP have been described:
  - *NKX2.1* mutations
  - lysinuric protein intolerance
  - Granulocyte-macrophage colony-stimulating factor receptor mutations.

Acquired form

This type of PAP, which is rare in childhood, is usually an autoimmune disease with antibodies to GM-CSF (anti-GM-CSF) in most cases.

Secondary form

This group can be due to:

- Infections (e.g., TB, nocardiosis, pneumocystis, atypical mycobacteria, HIV)
- Hematologic malignancies and immune deficiencies
- Exposure to inhaled chemicals and minerals.

Idiopathic form

It is possible that many of these children have defects in intracellular surfactant metabolism that has not been identified.

Q. What is the histopathology of lung in pulmonary alveolar proteinosis?

Accumulation of granular, PAS positive, and lipoproteinaceous material within the alveoli is the characteristic finding in autoimmune PAP. The alveolar septae usually display neither fibrosis nor inflammatory reaction.

Electron microscopic evaluation of the material filling the air spaces and vacuoles of the alveolar macrophages reveals lamellar bodies and tubular myelin, characteristic of surfactant. Several distinguishing features have been described in various individual congenital forms of PAP due to mutations in surfactant proteins.

Q. Are there any differences in the clinical features of pulmonary alveolar proteinosis in infancy, older children, and adults?

Signs and symptoms

In the congenital form, infants may present with severe respiratory failure in the newborn period or may show symptoms of chronic ILD in older children such as dyspnea, exercise intolerance, chronic cough, decreased activity, and failure to thrive. Hypoxemia is a prominent and characteristic feature.

In older children, the primary symptom is progressive breathlessness breath, initially with exercise. Chest pain and hemoptysis are rare. Fever is unusual in the absence of superadded infection. The physical examination may give clues to chronic pulmonary disease, including tachypnea, cyanosis, digital clubbing, and fine crackles. Characteristically, there is a significant discordance between the auscultatory findings, which appear minimal, and the radiographic findings of extensive infiltrates.

Q. What are the clues to diagnosis of pulmonary alveolar proteinosis in imaging studies?

High resolution computerized tomographty typically shows ground glass opacities of alveolar spaces and thickening of the interlobular and intralobular septa, with preservation of architecture, showing characteristic crazy paving.

Q. What is the essential diagnostic workup for pulmonary alveolar proteinosis?

Evaluation for disorders of surfactant metabolism in any child with the following clinical features:

- Severe pulmonary disease in the neonatal period without an obvious cause
- High resolution computerized tomography features suggestive of ILD

- Histopathology that demonstrates findings of CAP, desquamative interstitial pneumonia, nonspecific interstitial pneumonia, or chronic pneumonitis of infancy
- Lamellar bodies being absent or abnormal in electron microscopy.

In older children, the diagnosis is confirmed by bronchoscopy with BAL showing presence of PAS positivity or with transbronchial or open lung biopsy.

Laboratory tests

Genetic testing for mutations in the surfactant proteins and *ABCA3* genes is required to definitively diagnose an inborn error of surfactant metabolism. Some patients may require open lung biopsy. Testing for *CSF2RA* and *CSF2RB* mutations should be included, if available. Testing for *SLC7A7* mutations is necessary to detect lysinuric protein intolerance.

In the acquired forms of PAP, elevation in serum lactate dehydrogenase concentration might give a clue to the diagnosis, and anti-GM-CSF antibodies may be positive in autoimmune PAP.

Bronchoscopy

Milky effluent may be seen in noncongenital forms of PAP. Under microscopy, large amounts of amorphous, lipoproteinaceous material that stains brightly positive with PAS and large macrophages may be present. Inflammatory cells are usually absent. Open lung biopsy or transbronchial biopsy may show confirmatory findings of accumulation of PAS positive, lipoproteinaceous material in air spaces in an otherwise normal appearing lung tissue.

Q. What is the approach to management of infants and children with pulmonary alveolar proteinosis?

Neonates

It is mainly supportive and corticosteroids and surfactant therapy are ineffective. Lung transplantation is the only option that might improve the prognosis. Oral citrulline therapy and protein restriction help infants with lysinuric protein intolerance.

Infants and older children

- Anti-inflammatory therapy: In infants and older children, anti-inflammatory therapy with corticosteroids and hydroxychloroquine is tried in spite of the lack of clinical trials since it is believed that such therapy might reduce or prevent abnormal protein folding leads to protein degradation within the endoplasmic reticulum and release of toxic mediators. However, the disease progression is not reversible with such heroic measures
- Whole lung lavage: This procedure using saline has been the traditional choice of treatment for all forms of PAP and is tried for children and adults though not been universally recommended. Many authors advocate massive pulmonary lavages only for children suffering from respiratory distress or the debilitating effects of the disease (i.e., exercise intolerance, poor growth, and pulmonary hypertension). Some children and adults with PAP experience long-term resolution of the disease after one or more whole lung lavages
- Recombinant GM-CSF: Because reduced GM-CSF function is thought to play a role in some forms of PAP, some adults with secondary PAP have been treated with recombinant GM-CSF, given subcutaneously or as an aerosol, with some success.

Q. What about the prognosis of pulmonary alveolar proteinosis?

Surfactant protein B mutations in neonates with PAP with respiratory failure are usually fatal without lung transplantation. If the disease is identified in older children, it is slowly progressive and may ultimately also require lung transplantation. Few children with inborn errors of surfactant metabolism may have stable chronic lung disease and acceptable quality of life. *SFTPC* mutations have been reported as a rare cause of idiopathic pulmonary fibrosis and nonspecific interstitial pneumonia in young adults. Children with mutations in the GM-CSF receptor often have severe, progressive lung disease. Spontaneous remission or long-term resolution of symptoms after a single lavage has been reported. Some patients may require repeated lavages, as often as twice a year. Deterioration of respiratory status despite repeated lavages may occur, resulting in death. Recurrence of PAP has been reported after lung transplantation.

LEARNING POINTS

- Acquired, secondary, idiopathic, and congenital are the types of pulmonary alveolar proteinosis (PAP) described
- Diagnostic workup include high-resolution computerized tomography features suggestive of interstitial lung disease, in older children, the diagnosis is confirmed by bronchoscopy with bronchoalveolar lavage showing presence of periodic acid-Schiff positivity or with transbronchial or open lung biopsy
- Laboratory tests: Genetic testing for mutations in the surfactant proteins and *ABCA3* genes is required to definitively diagnose an inborn error of surfactant metabolism intolerance
- In the acquired forms of PAP, elevation in serum lactate dehydrogenase concentration might give a clue to the diagnosis, and anti-granulocyte macrophage colony-stimulating factor antibodies may be positive in autoimmune PAP.

SUGGESTED READINGS

1. Brody AS, Kurland G, Deterding RR, Hagood JS, Young LR, Castile RG, et al. An official American Thoracic Society clinical practice guideline: classification, evaluation, and management of childhood interstitial lung disease in infancy. American Thoracic Society Committee on Childhood Interstitial Lung Disease (chILD) and the chILD Research Network. Am J Respir Crit Care Med. 2013;188(3):376-94.
2. Coulomb A, Enaud L, Hadchouel A, Berteloot L, Lacaille F, Boccon-Gibod L, et al. Pulmonary alveolar proteinosis in children on La Réunion Island: a new inherited disorder? Orphanet J Rare Dis. 2014;9:85.
3. Luisetti M, Suzuki T, Sakagami T, Young LR, Carey BC, Wood RE, et al. Hereditary pulmonary alveolar proteinosis: pathogenesis, presentation, diagnosis, and therapy. Am J Respir Crit Care Med. 2010;182(10):1292-304.
4. Radpay B, Tabatabaei SA, Karimi A, Sedigheh RT, Jadali F, Shiva F, et al. Pulmonary alveolar proteinosis in children: a case series. J Res Med Sci. 2010;15(2):120-4.
5. Shah PL, Hansell D, Lawson PR, Reid KB, Morgan C. Pulmonary alveolar proteinosis: clinical aspects and current concepts on pathogenesis. Thorax. 2000;55(1):67-77.

CHAPTER

36

Interstitial Lung Disease

Meenu Singh, Nandini Paul, Pankaj C Vaidya

CASE 1

A 1.5 years child was admitted to hospital with complaints of recurrent fever, cough, noisy breathing, and vomiting since 1 month of age. There was a history of sudden fall in hemoglobin requiring blood transfusion. On examination, the child had fever, cough and respiratory distress. Anthropometry was normal.

Birth and family history: Not-significant

Environmental history: No history of exposure to smoke, and birds excreta.

Immunization: Complete for age.

Development: Appropriate for age.

Q. What are the differential diagnoses?

Possible differential diagnoses could be interstitial lung disease (ILD), gastroesophageal reflux disease (GERD), and Heiner's syndrome (as there was history of sudden fall in hemoglobin requiring blood transfusion).

Q. What further evaluation should be performed to make a final diagnosis?

Following investigations may be considered:

- Routine hemogram and biochemistry
- Chest X-ray and computed tomography (CT) chest
- Immunoglobulin profile
- Workup for tuberculosis
- Bronchoscopy and bronchoalveolar lavage (BAL)
- Antinuclear antibody (ANA) and anti-neutrophil cytoplasmic antibody (ANCA)
- Lung biopsy, if required.

Case Progression

Investigations of case 1 include: Mantoux test—negative; gastric aspirate for acid-fast bacilli (AFB)—negative for three times; abdominal ultrasound—normal; erythrocyte sedimentation rate—57 mm first hour; two-dimensional echocardiography—3 mm restrictive atrial septal defect with left to right shunt; human immunodeficiency virus serology—negative; immunological profile—normal; CD3, CD4, CD8, and CD4/CD8 ratio—normal; sweat chloride (19 mEq/dL) and stool for fat globules—normal; ANA/ANCA—negative. Gastroesophageal reflux (GER) scan revealed high grade reflux. Chest X-ray revealed inhomogeneous opacities in right middle and lower zone, and left middle zone (Fig. 1). Contrast-enhanced CT chest showed ground glass opacities, mediastinal and hilar lymphadenopathy with bilateral septal thickening (Fig. 2). The child required ventilation and finally died after a stormy course. Endotracheal aspirate grew *Acinetobacter*. The final diagnosis was ILD, GERD, *Acinetobacter* pneumonia, sepsis, meningitis, and multiorgan dysfunction syndrome.

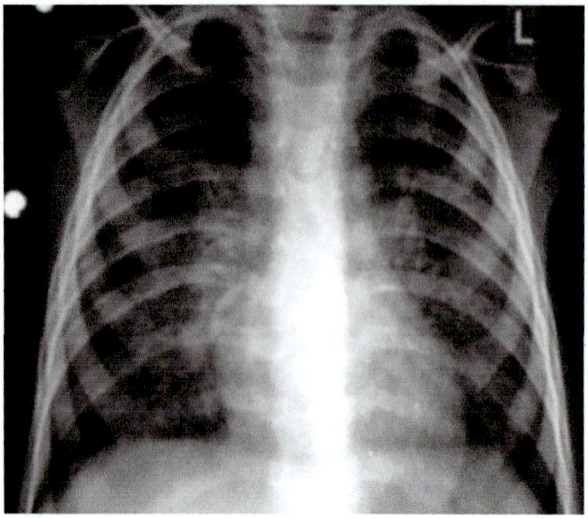

Figure 1: Chest X-ray showing inhomogeneous opacities in right middle and lower zone, and left middle zone

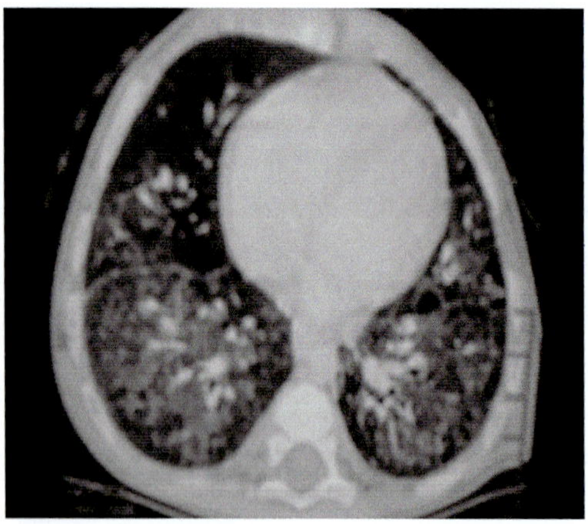

Figure 2: Computed tomography chest revealing bilateral ground glass opacities with bilateral septal thickening

Q. What is interstitial lung disease in children?

Interstitial lung disease in children are characterized by inflammatory and fibrotic changes of the alveolar walls causing reduced diffusing capacity of the lung for carbon monoxide. Interstitial lung disease is assessed by chest radiography and pulmonary function tests, and is characterized mainly by diffuse infiltrates, restrictive ventilator defect, and impaired gas exchange. There is a lack of proper pediatric guidelines for diagnosis and treatment.

Q. What is the approach to recognize interstitial lung disease disorders in children?

The recognition of ILD disorders in children is a challenging task for clinicians as a number of diagnostic measures are required. In several cases, interstitium is not involved, but airways are affected. The clinical features of ILD consist of cough in 75% of cases, tachypnea in 80% of cases, wheezing in 50% of children, failure to thrive in 30% children, and other respiratory symptoms such as impaired lung function and radiological abnormalities. As defined by interstitial lung disease in children (chILD) cooperative group, the diagnosis of chILD syndrome can be confirmed by three or four of the following criteria:

1. The presence of respiratory symptoms, i.e., cough, difficult breathing, exercise intolerance etc.
2. Hypoxemia
3. The presence of clubbing, respiratory failure, retractions, and resting tachypnea
4. Diffuse abnormality on X-ray or CT imaging.

Q. What is the classification approach of interstitial lung disease in children?

The classification approach in children differs from adults, although there may be certain overlaps. It is based on clinical findings, chest imaging, and pathological investigations. European Respiratory Society and a study conducted by Deutsch et al. have classified ILD as:

- In infancy: Abnormal development and growth, altered function of surfactant proteins, pulmonary interstitial glycogenosis, and neuroendocrine cell hyperplasia
- Primary lung diseases: Lymphatic and vascular disorders, alveolar hemorrhage etc.

- Associated systemic disorders: Malignancy, sarcoidosis and disorders of connective tissue
- Specific causes: Hypersensitivity pneumonitis, postinfectious bronchiolitis obliterans, storage disorders, and drug-induced lung disorders.

Q. What is the pathophysiology of interstitial lung disease?

The pathophysiology of ILD is poorly understood, yet it is believed that ILD is caused due to chronic inflammation by injury to alveolar epithelium. Although during the repair process reepithelialization is initiated yet the proper repair of epithelium is impaired, resulting into profound modifications of cell functions altering the production of oxidants, proteases, and mediators of immune response, i.e., cytokines and growth factors mainly transforming growth factor (TGF)-β and endothelin (ET)-1. Various pathways are involved in the disease progression including apoptosis, developmental, and endoplasmic reticulum associated pathways.

The genetic defects in surfactant proteins (*SP-B* gene, *SP-C*), *ABCA3* and *TTF-1* genes result into surfactant deficiency. Moreover, misfolded *SP-C* in alveolar epithelium stimulates the formation of aggregates and conformational defects.

Q. How is interstitial lung disease evaluated?

A careful history can help in establishing a proper diagnosis and further noninvasive testing.

Patients should be asked the following questions while making diagnosis of ILD:

- Family history of lung disease or infections
- Birth history of the child
- Environmental history of exposure to organic matter, allergens, and other hypersensitivity mediators
- Other respiratory infections.

Various related disorders resembling the signs and symptoms of chILD are cystic fibrosis, respiratory distress, acute infections, immune deficiencies, GERD, and congenital heart disease.

Imaging

Chest imaging techniques are essential in confirmation of ILD ruling in/out differential diagnosis, and localization for lung biopsy. Chest radiography is done in all patients with presenting symptoms, but this is not a very efficient way of evaluation. High-resolution computed tomography (HRCT) is a necessary technique to delineate pulmonary abnormalities such as bronchiectasis, ground-glass appearance, and cysts.

Pulmonary function testing

Despite being a nonspecific test, pulmonary function testing (PFT) is very useful in making diagnosis and managing the disease. Pulmonary function testing findings help in reflecting the lung compliance and diffusion capacity of carbon monoxide which is often reduced in chILD.

Bronchoscopy and bronchoalveolar lavage

Bronchoscopy is used for evaluation of the distal airways and in ruling out airway abnormalities and any infection in immunocompromised patients. The presence of CD4+ T-lymphocytes in BAL indicates sarcoidosis and CD8+ cells suggest hypersensitivity pneumonitis. Bronchoalveolar lavage eosinophilia indicates pulmonary infiltrates with eosinophilic syndromes.

Tissue biopsy

There is no consensus on the indications of tissue biopsy and no universal approach exists.

An early invasive tissue biopsy, via video-assisted thoracoscopic surgery or open biopsy, should be performed in immunocompromised children as diagnostic yield is high compared to immunocompetent children with chILD syndromes. The choice of procedure depends on the availability of expertise and maintaining the balance between invasiveness and tissue amount biopsied. Other methods like transbronchial lung biopsy and percutaneous needle lung biopsy in pediatric ILD are yet to be established.

Q. What are the general measures for treatment of interstitial lung disease?

Administration of oxygen for chronic hypoxemia, nutrition, proper immunization against respiratory pathogens, treatment of intercurrent infections, avoidance of air pollutants (tobacco smoke), bronchodilators, and steroids can be used as supportive care in chILD. In addition to this, the treatment of GERD, whether it is primary or secondary is important.

Q. What is the pharmacologic approach for treatment of interstitial lung disease?

The most common drug used for ILD is oral prednisolone or pulsed intravenous methylprednisolone. The recommended dose for prednisolone is 1–2 mg/kg/day and it may be given alone or in combination with hydroxychloroquine. A single daily dose of hydroxychloroquine (6–10 mg/kg/day) can be used to treat patients with fibrotic abnormalities in airways. Lung biopsy is very essential investigation to decide the therapeutic agent to be used because in cases showing a large amount of inflammation, steroids are preferred; whereas in cases with prefibrotic changes, hydroxychloroquine alone is recommended. In severe cases, both drugs are suggested and the recommended dose of pulsed methylprednisolone is 10–30 mg/kg/day for three consecutive days at 3-6 months interval. Once response is achieved, alternate day oral prednisolone is continued and response is monitored. Other immunosuppressive agents such as azathioprine, cyclophosphamide cyclosporin, or methotrexate are also recommended when steroids and hydroxychloroquine are not effective (especially in children with autoimmune disorders).

Q. Are there specific treatment strategies?

Yes, in case of patients with underlying systemic disorders, primary treatment should be specific to that disorder, e.g., chemotherapy for malignancy and immunoglobulin for hypogammaglobulinemia. For chronic respiratory infections (e.g., cytomegalovirus and Epstein-Barr virus), anti-infective treatment, interferon-α for pulmonary hemangiomatosis or recurrent whole lung lavage by bronchoscopy and subcutaneous or aerosolized administration of Granulocyte monocyte-colony stimulating factor should be considered to treat the underlying condition. In hypersensitivity pneumonitis patients, trigger factors must be avoided.

Q. What are the newer therapeutic agents rather than conventional treatment?

Immunological treatment agents, i.e., interferon-α therapy, have been associated with reduced mortality in patients with idiopathic pulmonary fibrosis (IPF). Pirfenidone, an antifibrotic and anti-inflammatory agent, which reduces the production of tumor necrosis factor-α and interferon-1β has also been studied extensively in adult patients with IPF and has been found to inhibit the decline in lung function and improved oxygenation. Tumor necrosis factor-α inhibitors like infliximab, etanercept, thalidomide, and pentoxifylline are currently tried for adult patients with pulmonary sarcoidosis as steroid sparing agents. However, none of the agents mentioned have been evaluated in infants and children.

Q. What are the treatment measures for end stage interstitial lung disease patients?

Lung transplantation can be offered to patients with end stage ILD and for the diseases caused by mutations in the surfactant protein B and *ABCA3* genes. The chances of recurrences of several ILDs in the recipient lung do remain, as indicated by some anecdotal case reports.

Q. How are patients monitored and followed up after diagnosis and treatment?

The patient should be regularly monitored at the intervals of 3–6 months or more frequently depending upon the severity of disease. Response to treatment is monitored by PFT and improvement is considered as decreased breathlessness or cough, and 2–4 % increase in arterial oxygen saturation at rest. Radiological improvement can be seen, however, it occurs over a long period of 2–4 years. Histological findings have not been found to be associated with outcomes of patients due to the variable extent of severity in different parts of the lung. A majority of cases (40–60%) with idiopathic interstitial pneumonitis respond well to corticosteroid therapy, but in infants the outcome is variable.

CASE 2

A 3-year-old boy was admitted to hospital with complaints of cough for 3 months and difficulty in breathing for 1.5 months. The child was operated for lumbar meningocele on day 15 of life. No residual neurological deficits. No history of recurrent pneumonia, recurrent illness, or infections. No history of tuberculosis and contact with. No other significant history. The child was admitted four times for these complaints, for duration 5–10 days each. He received multiple intravenous antibiotics, oxygen therapy, and was advised antitubercular therapy. On examination, the child had respiratory distress with diffuse fine inspiratory crepts with some pallor and hepatomegaly.

Q. What is the possible diagnosis in this case?

Differential diagnoses include persistent pneumonia, chronic infections (tuberculosis, *Pneumocystis jirovecii*, fungal), underlying immunodeficiency, cystic fibrosis, and ILD.

Q. How to investigate the child further?

Further investigation in form of CT chest, immunoglobulin profile, bronchoscopy and BAL, and liver and lung biopsy are required.

Case Progression

The immunological workup was negative. High resolution computed tomography chest showed bilateral consolidation, ground glass opacities, and septal thickening (Fig. 3). Computed tomography features were suggestive of infection on a possible background of ILD.

Bronchoscopy revealed normal anatomy. Milky white fluid came on lavage with pinkish hue. Culture was sterile. Fungal smear and culture—negative. Nocardia—negative. Cytology revealed macrophages polymorphs, degenerated cells, few epithelial cells, few hemosiderin laden macrophages, AFB negative, but no malignant cells.

Fine-needle aspiration cytology from lung showed consolidation with neutrophils, lymphocytes, alveolar and foamy macrophages, fibroconnective tissue fragments, and few mesothelial cells in a hemorrhagic background. Liver biopsy was suggestive of glycogen storage disease. Open lung biopsy was suggestive of ILD, not otherwise specific. The diagnosis of glycogen storage disease with ILD was made.

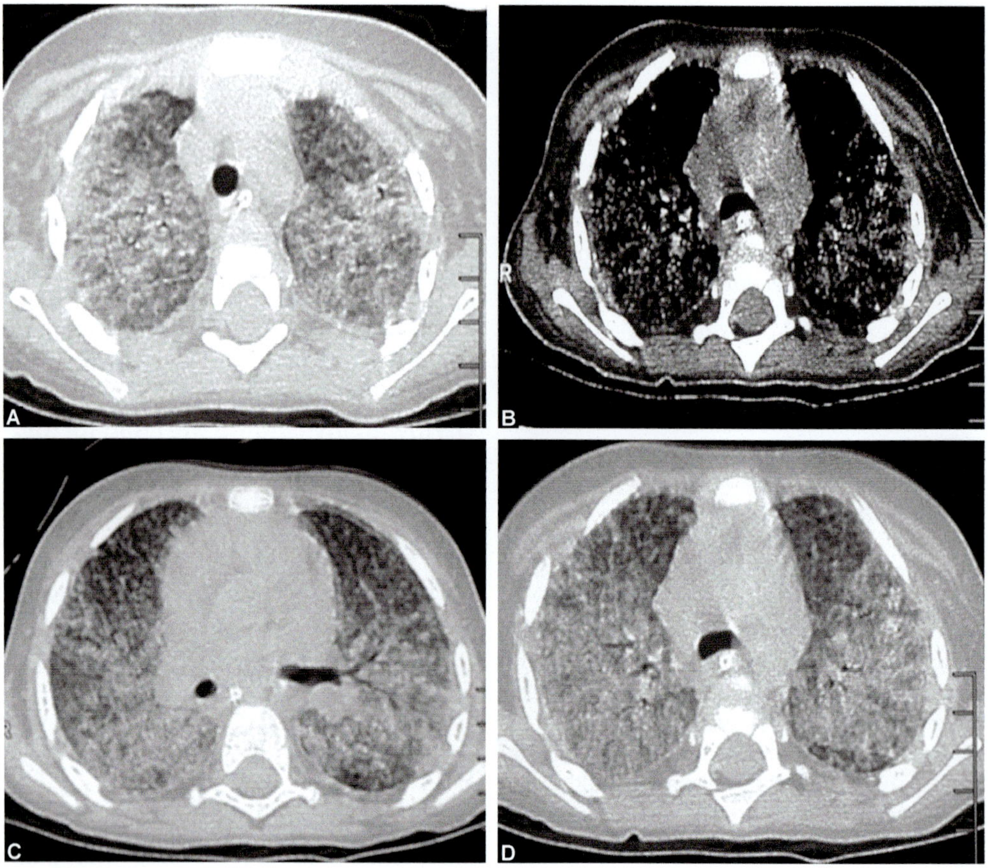

Figure 3: High-resolution computed tomography chest showing bilateral consolidation, ground glass opacities, and septal thickening

LEARNING POINTS

- Interstitial lung disease (ILD) is diagnosed by a combination of clinical, radiological, and histo-pathological findings
- Family history of respiratory illness, environmental history of allergen exposure, and birth history are important for evaluation of children with ILD
- Corticosteroids are first choice of treatment in ILD, but in case of associated disorders, primary approach is to treat the specific disorders first
- Immunological treatments such as interferon-α, tumor necrosis factor-α inhibitors like infliximab, etanercept, thalidomide, and pentoxifylline inhibitors have steroid-sparing effect.

SUGGESTED READINGS

1. Clement A, Nathan N, Epaud R, Fauroux B, Corvol H. Interstitial lung diseases in children. Orphanet J Rare Dis. 2010;22(5):1-24.
2. Deterding R. Evaluating infants and children with interstitial lung disease. Semin Respir Crit Care Med. 2007;28:333-41.
3. Deterding RR, Wagener JS. Lung biopsy in immuno-compromised children: when, how and who? J Pediatr. 2000;137:147-49.
4. Deutsch GH, Young LR, Deterding RR, Fan LL, Dell SD, Bean JA, et al. Diffuse lung disease in young children: application of a novel classification scheme. Am J Respir Crit Care Med. 2007;176(11):1120-8.
5. Dinwiddie R, Sharief N, Crawford O. Idiopathic interstitial pneumonitis in children: a national survey in the United Kingdom and Ireland. Pediatr Pulmonol. 2002;34(1):23-9.
6. Klusmann M, Owens C. HRCT in pediatric diffuse interstitial lung disease—a review for 2009. Pediatr Radiol. 39:471-81.

7 SECTION

Pleural Diseases

CHAPTER

37

Pneumothorax in Children

Ankit Parakh, Dhulika Dhingra, Pooja Abbey

CASE 1

An 8-year-old child presented with complaints of high grade fever, cough for one week, respiratory distress, and chest pain on the left side for 3 days. There were multiple boils (>1 cm) over both feet. On physical examination, left side of chest showed bulging with reduced chest movements. Percussion note was dull and air entry was reduced on the left hemithorax. The chest X-ray showed a homogenous opacity on the left side with an air fluid level with shift of mediastinum to the right suggestive of a pyopneumothorax (Fig. 1).

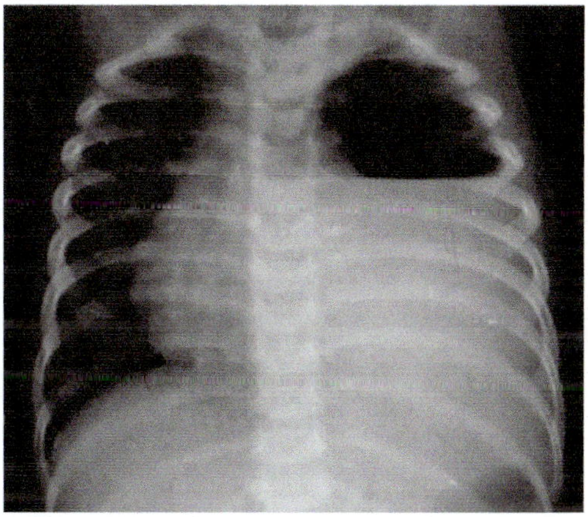

Figure 1: Frontal chest radiograph reveals a large air-fluid level within the left hemithorax, consistent with a large pyopneumothorax. There is mild mediastinal shift towards right. The left lung is not visualized

Q. What is a pneumothorax?

Pneumothorax refers to the intrapleural (between the visceral and parietal pleura) collection of air or gas. Many a times it is associated with accumulation of fluid or pus as well when it is termed as pyopneumothorax. Pneumothorax ensues when there is a communication between the pleural space and the atmosphere. This occurs usually from an alveolar rupture or uncommonly from a chest wall defect through the parietal pleura. Occasionally, infection with gas forming organisms leads to formation of a pneumothorax.

Pneumothorax can be classified in the following ways:

- Free vs. loculated pneumothorax: Air may flow freely within the chest or can be loculated by fibrous bands or other tissues
- Tension pneumothorax: It refers to a progressive build up of air in the pleural cavity with a mediastinal shift and resultant circulatory compromise

- Spontaneous or traumatic: Spontaneous pneumothorax, occurs in the absence of any identified trauma to the chest. A traumatic pneumothorax is caused either by blunt, crush, or penetrating trauma to the chest or by injury from a diagnostic or therapeutic procedure, or as a consequence of mechanical ventilation
- Primary spontaneous vs. secondary pneumothorax: Primary spontaneous pneumothorax occurs in the absence of any underlying lung disease. Secondary spontaneous pneumothorax occurs secondary to underlying lung diseases such as pneumonia, lung abscess, tuberculosis (TB), pulmonary tumors, lung infarcts, interstitial lung disease etc. Box 1 summarizes the causes of secondary pneumothorax in children.

Box 1: Causes of pneumothorax in children

Causes of pneumothorax in children

- Traumatic or iatrogenic
  - External trauma to chest wall
  - Blunt trauma to chest (bronchial transaction or rupture without any external injury)
  - During pulmonary procedure: Diagnostic thoracocentesis, pleural biopsy, percutaneous lung biopsy, transbronchial lung biopsy.
  - During other procedures: Central line insertion, nasogastric tube placement, cardiopulmonary resuscitation
- Spontaneous pneumothorax
  - Primary spontaneous pneumothorax
  - Secondary spontaneous pneumothorax
    - Necrotizing pneumonia
    - Asthma
    - Tuberculosis
    - Cystic fibrosis
    - Interstitial lung diseases associated with connective tissue diseases
    - Langerhans cell histiocytosis
    - Thoracic endometriosis and catamenial pneumothorax
    - Collagen vascular disease, including Marfan syndrome

Q. How do you assess the size of a pneumothorax on chest X-ray?

The size of the pneumothorax is determined by measuring the distance between the lung margin and the chest wall at the level of the hilum on a chest X-ray. A distance of approximately 2 cm signifies a large pneumothorax. There are formulas to calculate the size of pneumothorax in adults but not standardized for children of various ages.

Q. What is a pyopneumothorax?

Pyopnemothorax is defined as the collection of air and pus in the pleural cavity. It is the commonest cause of pneumothorax in children in India. These collections result from the spread of inflammation and infection to the pleura. Less commonly, infections in other adjacent areas, such as the retropharyngeal, vertebral, abdominal, and retroperitoneal spaces may spread to the pleura resulting in the development of pyothorax.

Q. How do you diagnose a case of pyopneumothorax?

Pneumothorax is a clinical diagnosis confirmed with X- ray chest. On examination, absent breath sounds and bulging chest are pointers towards diagnosis. Chest X-ray shows air pockets with an air fluid level. Ultrasound of the chest is a very useful modality in confirming the presence of fluid, indicating the best site for aspiration and looking for septations and loculations. A contrast computed tomography (CT) chest is warranted only in specific situations like a possibility of lung abscess, chronic empyema where surgery is planned etc. Routine use of CT chest should be avoided in view of the very high radiation associated.

Q. What can be the possible differential diagnosis?

The possible differentials are hemopneumothorax, i.e., blood in the pleural cavity (usually secondary to a chest trauma) or a peripheral lung abscess with bronchial communication. Infected cyst like hydatid can rarely rupture into a bronchus and present with a similar picture. The other mimickers of pneumothorax/pyopneumothorax are:

- Emphysema-obstructive or compensatory
- Congenital lobar emphysema
- Hyadatid cyst with communication
- Congenital cystic adenomatoid lung malformation

Q. What is the mechanism of air leaks?

Two mechanisms have been described in causation of pneumothorax especially in ventilated children. Sometimes during mechanical ventilation (invasive or noninvasive) or continuous positive airway pressure, the air can dissect along perivascular planes to the hilum. There it can rupture into the mediastinum leading to a pneumomediastinum. Air can further rupture through the visceral pleura, into the pleural space leading to a pneumothorax. Alternatively, when air is under tension in the interstitial space it leads to formation of pulmonary interstitial emphysema. Air can then rupture directly through the visceral pleura, into the pleural space leading to a pneumothorax. Uncommonly, when under sufficient pressure, air may dissect out of the thorax, along subcutaneous tissue planes causing subcutaneous emphysema, or into the peritoneal cavity causing a pneumoperitoneum or into the pericardial space causing a pneumopericardium. Figure 2 shows some illustrative chest X-rays.

Q. How would you manage a case of pyopneumothorax?

The standard management of children with a pyopneumothorax remains antibiotics and intercostal tube drainage (ICD) for removal of air and fluid. Intercostal tube drainage needs to be inserted as per standard procedure. Post ICD insertion, the air column has to be observed for air leaks on deep breathing and coughing suggesting a bronchopleural fistula. After reduction in the amount of the drainage to <25–30 mL/day and no air leak, the ICD can be safely removed.

Choice of antibiotics depends on the causative agents. In India, *Staphylococcus aureus* and *Streptococcus pneumoniae* are the common causative agents. First line antibiotics in such cases are either co-amoxiclav, cefuroxime, or a combination of third generation cephalosporin and cloxacillin. Child failing the first line drugs but having an adequate drainage can be shifted to a combination of third generation cephalosporin and vancomycin. In children presenting with hemodynamic instability or respiratory failure, vancomycin can be used upfront to cover community-acquired methicillin-resistant *S. aureus* (CA-MRSA).

CASE 2

A 5-month-girl presented to the outpatient department with cough and cold for the past 1 week. On examination, the child was comfortable, respiratory rate was 51/min with reduced air entry on the left side. Chest X-ray was sought in view of the respiratory distress and difference in air entry. The chest X-ray (Fig. 3) showed a hyperlucent left hemithorax with right mediastinal shift.

Q. What are the causes of a unilateral hyperlucent hemithorax?

Rotation is the commonest reason. The other causes are emphysema (obstructive or compensatory), pneumothorax, unilateral congenital absence of pectoral muscles, pulmonary vascular abnormalities, and Swyer-James-Macleod syndrome.

Q. What is unusual in this case?

There was a discrepancy in the clinical condition and radiological findings. The child appeared well for a pneumothorax, although the respiratory rates were high and air entry was reduced on the left side. A review of history suggested that there has been increased respiratory rate since birth. Hence, a possibility of a congenital lung malformation such as emphysema was kept.

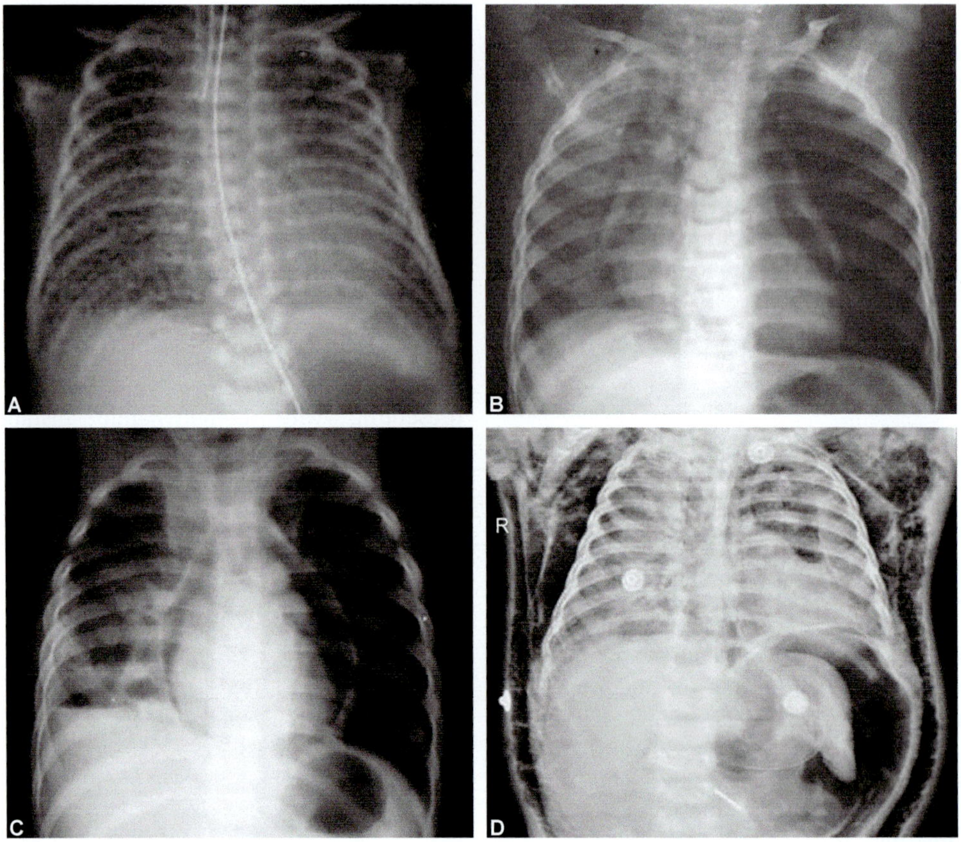

Figure 2: Frontal chest radiographs (different patients) demonstrating different radiographic presentations of air-leak phenomena. **A,** Radiograph demonstrates multiple cystic and linear lucencies radiating outward from the hila on both sides (Right > left), consistent with pulmonary interstitial emphysema, endotracheal tube is seen *in situ*; **B,** shows presence of air around the heart, great vessels and superior mediastinum-pneumomediastinum, along with a small right sided pneumothorax; **C,** shows a right pyopneumothorax, along with air seen to surround the heart on all sides (also seen to cross the midline below the heart), or pneumopericardium; **D,** shows extensive bilateral subcutaneous emphysema, along with left pyopneumothorax and air below the left hemidiaphragm, seen to outline the spleen/left lobe of liver—suggestive of pneumoperitoneum

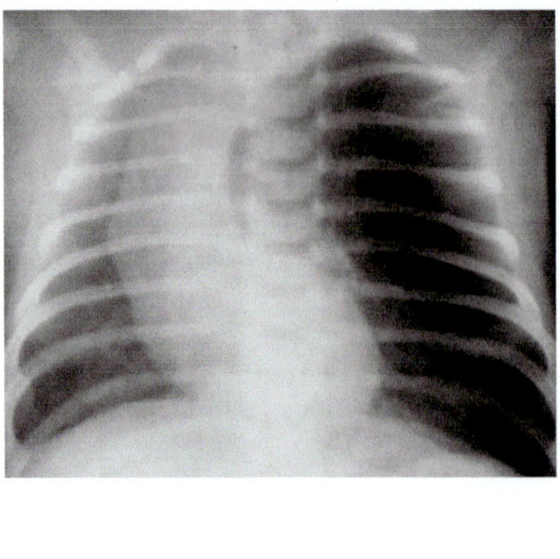

Figure 3: Frontal chest radiograph reveals a hyperlucent left hemithorax with significant mass effect and mediastinal shift towards right. There is suggestion of herniation of the left upper lung across the midline, with rotation and displacement of superior mediastinal structures. No margin of collapsed left lung is seen. Pulmonary vascular markings are visible in the left lower zone (paracardiac location). Findings suggest a hyperinflated left lung (upper lobe), rather than a pneumothorax

Q. How do we distinguish between emphysema and pneumothorax?

Two major things which need to be appreciated are presence or absence of vascular markings and lung border. Radiographs with emphysema would have vascular markings although they might be attenuated. Pneumothorax would have absent vascular markings although in cases of loculated pneumothorax it can be difficult since the other part of the lung would superimpose. In cases of pneumothorax, the collapsed lung border would usually be visible. In the current case, the left hemithorax shows obstructive emphysema. There is a right sided mediastinal shift. The X-ray in the current clinical setting is suggestive of congenital lobar emphysema of the left side with a shift to the right. Another common differential in this case is a hypoplastic lung. In case of hypoplastic lung, mediastinal shift of the normal lung to the affected side (side with volume loss) is well seen, however the shift may not be as severe as in CLE. This is evident as shown in figure 4 in CXR and CT scans.

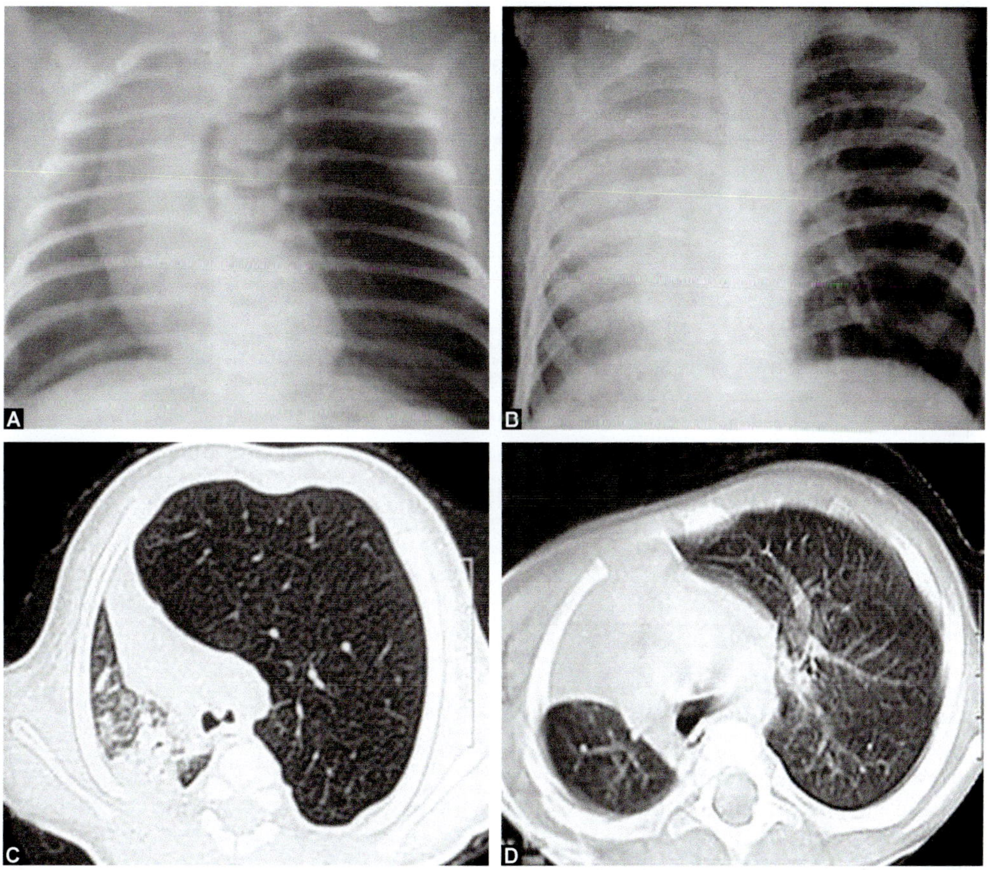

Figure 4: The frontal radiograph and computed tomography (CT) images (**A** and **C**) of a patient with left upper lobar (obstructive) hyperinflation (same patient as in case 2) compared with those of a different patient with hypoplasia of right lung (**B** and **D**) showing compensatory hyperinflation of left lung. In the case with obstructive emphysema, there is marked attenuation of pulmonary vasculature seen within the hyperinflated lung, both on radiographs and CT (**A** and **C**), when compared with the images of the patient with compensatory hyperinflation (**B** and **D**), which reveal normal vascularity

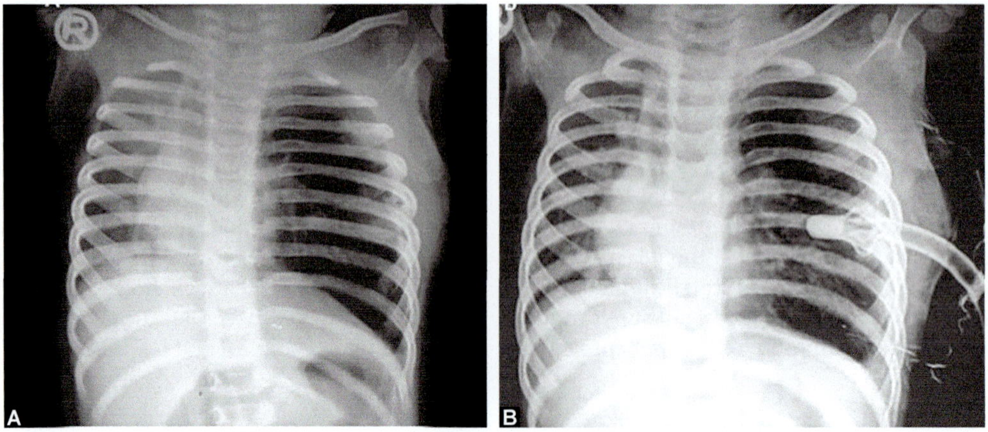

Figure 5: Frontal chest radiographs, pre- and postintercostal tube drainage (ICD) tube insertion, of a 9-month-old child with obstructive emphysema (due to foreign body) misdiagnosed as pneumothorax. The initial radiograph **A**, reveals a hyperlucent left hemithorax with mass effect, mediastinal shift towards right, and flattening of the left hemidiaphragm. However, vascular markings, though attenuated, are seen within the area of hyperlucency. The subsequent (post-ICD tube) radiograph **B**, reveals similar findings. An obstructing foreign body (peanut) was recovered from the left main bronchus on bronchoscopy

CASE 3

A 9-month-old boy presented with history of cough and respiratory distress for the past 3 weeks. Fever was present off and on. On examination, reduced air entry was revealed on the left side. Chest X-ray is shown in figure 5A. Diagnosis of tension pneumothorax was made and hence an ICD was inserted on the left side. The post ICD insertion chest X-ray is shown in figure 5B. Since there was no improvement in the symptoms, signs, and radiological findings, the child was referred.

The chest X-ray (pre ICD insertion) shows a left hyperlucent hemithorax with shift of the mediastinum to the right. The border of the collapsed lung is not identified. In such cases, the radiological differential diagnosis of either a hyperinflated lung or a lobe should be considered. The post ICD X-ray shows similar findings with no change in the radiological hyperlucency.

Q. What is different in this case compared to the previous case?

The situation is similar to the earlier case but with certain differences. The age is comparatively older and the infant was absolutely normal before. The bronchovascular marking are reduced but not absent and the lung border is not seen. Also, these findings must be correlated with the sickness of the child. A child with a tension pneumothorax would be extremely sick with circulatory compromise. The correlation sometimes can be very subjective but helpful in such situations.

CASE 4

A 5-month-old girl presented with fever, cough, nasal discharge, and respiratory distress for the past 5 days. On examination, the child was well looking and alert. The respiratory rates were 70/min with mild intercostals and subcostal recessions. Reduced air entry on the right side was noticed and wheezing was heard on the left side. The X-ray of the child is

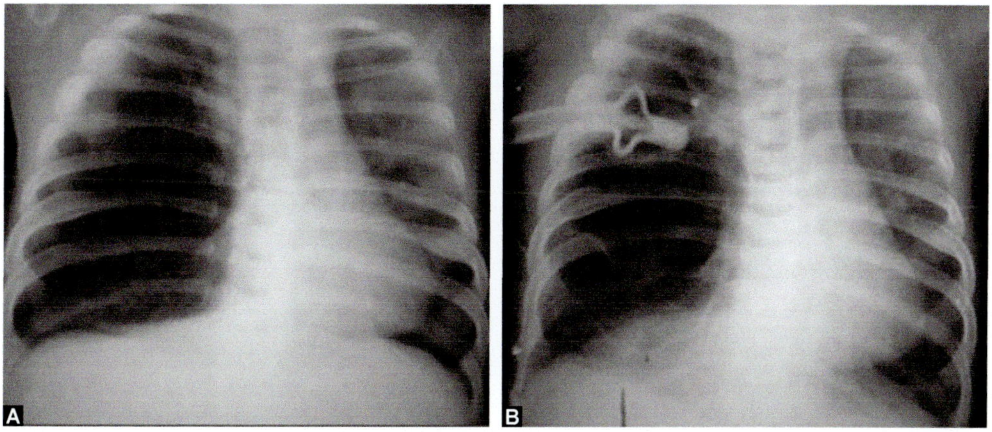

Figure 6: Frontal chest radiograph of a 5-month-old girl with respiratory distress **A,** reveals an area of hyperlucency in the right hemithorax, with mass effect, and mediastinal shift towards left. The possibility of a loculated pneumothorax was considered at a primary care center and a drainage tube was inserted. Post intercostal chest tube drainage radiograph **B,** reveals persistence of the abnormality

shown in figure 6A. The possibility of a loculated pneumothorax was considered at a primary care center and a drainage tube was inserted. Since the post ICD radiograph (Fig. 6B) reveals persistence of the abnormality, child was then referred for further workup to rule out a congenital lung malformation.

Q. How will you manage a case of foreign body inhalation?

The history may provide important clues as was in this case. The illness started suddenly with acute onset of cough and wheezing. On further asking it was realized that the child has history of choking while eating peanuts. Fever has been there but not very significant. The child underwent a flexible bronchoscopy and a cotyledon of peanut was seen obstructing the left main bronchus. In cases of any collapse or emphysema in children, possibility of a tracheobronchial foreign body should be considered and should undergo a diagnostic fiberoptic bronchoscopy. Where available rigid bronchoscopy is a safe procedure to remove the foreign body from the airways although many centers are using flexible bronchoscopy for extraction of tracheobronchial foreign bodies.

Q. What is the differential diagnosis to be considered in this case?

The differential diagnosis in such cases include a loculated pneumothorax, large post infectious pneumatoceles, and congenital lung malformations like cystic adenomatoid lung malformations.

In doubtful cases CT chest is diagnostic as in the present case (Fig. 7). Congenital cystic adenomatoid malformation would be located in a single lobe or lung without any other findings of infections. In doubtful cases follow-up would help since the post infectious pneumatoceles would reduce and disappear by up to 12 weeks.

CONCLUSION

Commonest cause of pneumothorax in children include secondary spontaneous pneumothorax. Necrotizing pneumonia, lung abscess, TB, foreign body are amongst the common causes of secondary pneumothorax. High index of suspicion, a good clinical examination, and a simple investigation like a chest X-ray may help in diagnosing the condition. Oxygen supplementation, drainage of pneumothorax (depending on the size), and monitoring of the cardiovascular system form the mainstay of management.

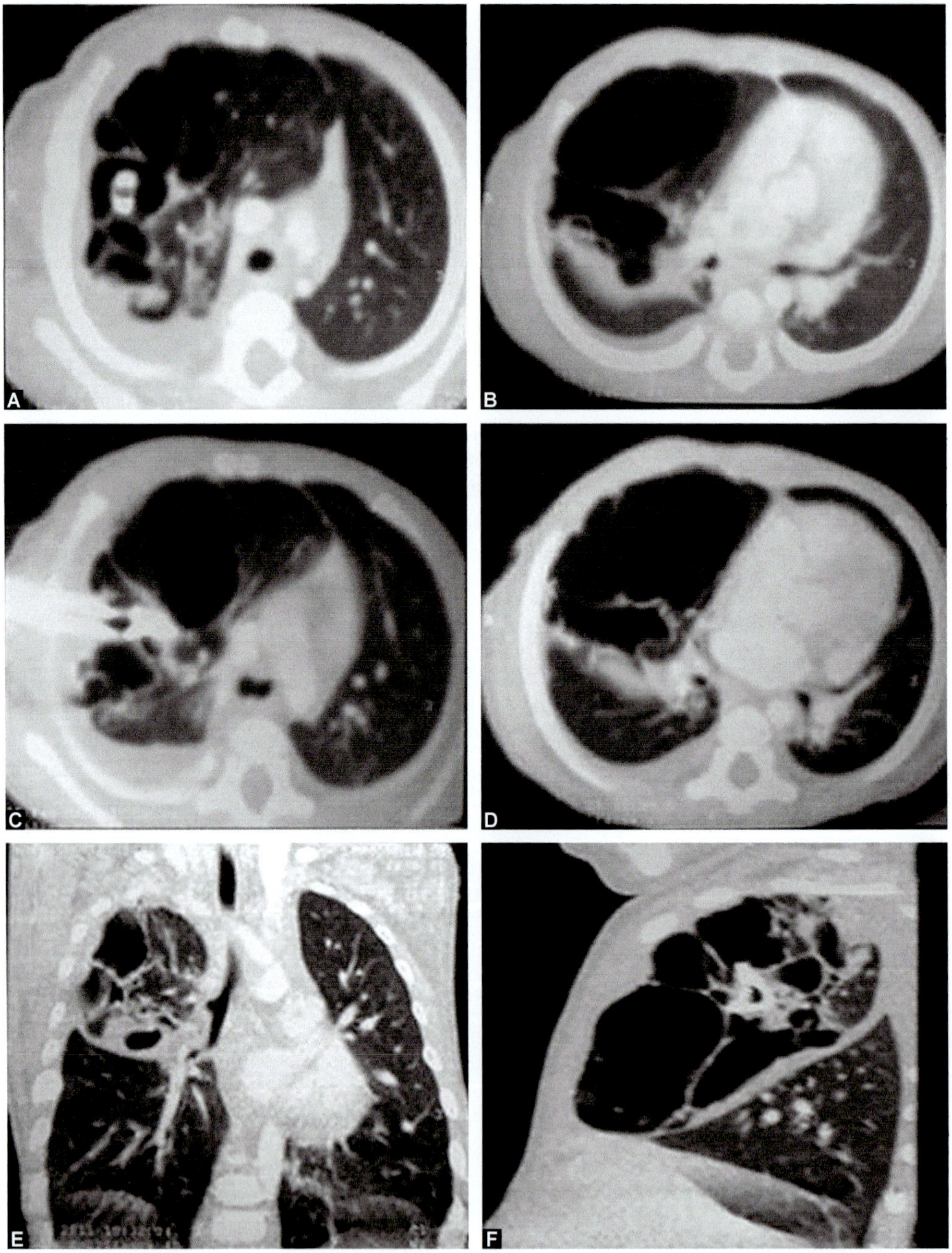

Figure 7: Cumputed tomography images of the patient, lung window settings, axial (**A** to **D**), coronal (**E**), and sagittal (**F**), reformatted images reveal a large intrapulmonary lesion in the right upper lobe, which comprises of multiple air-filled cysts, largest >2 cm in size, consistent with a type 1 congenital pulmonary airway malformation. A small right pleural effusion is noted. The intercostal tube drainage tube is seen *in situ* within the lesion. There is significant mass effect and shift of mediastinum towards left

LEARNING POINTS

- Pneumothorax is a common condition that clinicians face in clinical practice
- Differentials include emphysema due to any cause (foreign body etc), congenital lung malformations like congenital pulmonary airway malformation and congenital lobar emphysema and cystic lung lesions like hyadatid lung cysts. Congenital cystic adenomatoid malformation, tuberculosis, and hydatidosis
- A detailed history and a complete clinical examination is one of the most important pointers to definitive diagnosis
- A tension pneumothorax is a medical emergency and requires immediate attention.

SUGGESTED READINGS

1. Gupta A, Dutt N, Patel N. The different treatment modalities of pyopneumothorax-study of 50 cases. Int J M ed Sci Public Health. 2013;2: 609-12.
2. Halwai O, Bihani A, Dabholkar J. A study of clinical presentations and complications of foreign body in the bronchus-our experience. Otolaryngol Pol. 2015;69:22-9.
3. Laberge JM, Bratu I, Flageole H. The management of asymptomatic congenital lung malformations. Paediatr Respir Rev. 2004;5(Suppl A):S305-12.
4. Maconochie IK, Howell A, Walton E. Spontaneous pneumothorax in children: the pr oblem with rare presentations. Arch Dis Child. 2015;100:903-4.
5. Poenaru D, Yazbeck S, Murphy S. Primary spontaneous pneumothorax in children. J Pediatr Surg. 1994;29:1183-5.

CHAPTER

38

Pleural Effusion Including Empyema

Gautam Ghosh

CASE 1

History: A 10-year-old previously healthy boy presented with high fever for 3 days, progressive respiratory distress for 2 days, and heaviness in right chest for 1 day.

Examination: He was febrile (103°F) with tachypnea (respiratory rate 50/min) and tachycardia (heart rate 120/min) He had trachea shifted to left with diminished movement all over right chest with dull percussion note and diminished breath sound and vocal resonance below right 3rd intercostal space.

Investigation: Showed mild pallor (hemoglobin 10 g) with polymorphonuclear leucocytosis with high erythrocyte sedimentation ESR rate of 78 mm/h. Tuberculin test (TST) was positive (20 × 18 mm). Pleural fluid was clear and showed high protein (>3 g/dL), low sugar (33 mg/dL), and raised adenosine deaminase (ADA) 78% and acidic pH 7.0. Cell count was 200 cells (lymphocytes 80%) with negative Gram stain, cartridge based nucleic acid amplification test (CBNAAT), and culture. Chest X-ray and chest ultrasound are shown in figure 1. The case was diagnosed as right-sided tubercular pleural effusion and was managed with supportive therapy and the Revised National Tuberculosis Control Programme category I anti-tubercular therapy (new case). Contact tracing and CBNAAT for induced sputum was searched.

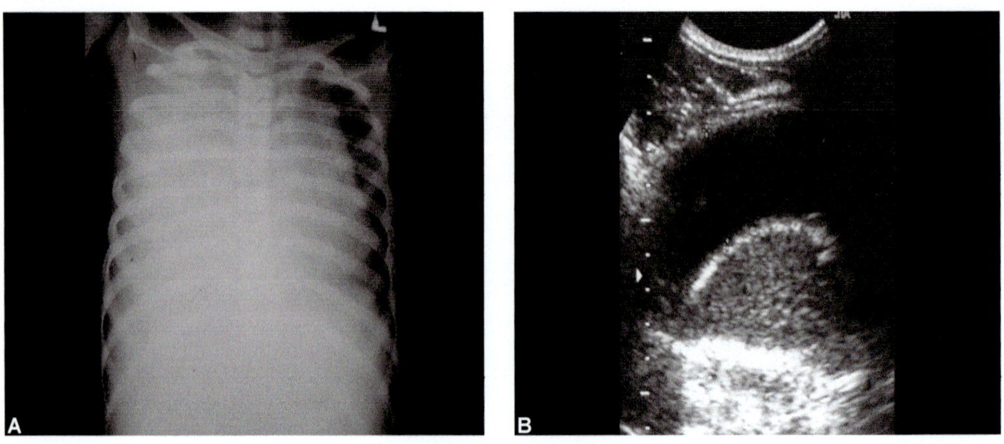

Figure 1: X-ray and ultrasound of chest showing right-sided pleural effusion

Q. What suggested tubercular pleural effusion in case 1?

History clues

Acute onset of pleural effusion in a normal child with high fever suggests tuberculosis, trauma, dengue, or collagen disease. Empyema is usually more toxic and a bit delayed. Malignancy is uncommon in a healthy child.

Supportive clues

Positive TST and exudative pleural fluid with high ADA (not confirmatory) and high ESR suggests tuberculosis pleural effusion.

Q. What is the pathophysiology of pleural effusion?

Normally, pleural fluid volume is only 0.3 mL/kg. However, there is continuous circulation of a large amount of pleural fluid through lung by arteriovenous (90%) and lymphatics (10%) flow. The pleural fluid dynamics is depicted in figure 2. A positive pressure (+6 cm of water) forces fluid in the pleural space and a negative pressure (–13 cm of water) pulls it into pulmonary circulation. Alteration of this pressure dynamics causes effusion.

Q. What is the classification or staging of pleural effusion/empyema?

Various terminologies related to pleural effusion are as follows:

- Transudates: Due to diseases that affect the filtration of pleural fluid; e.g., congestive cardiac failure (CCF) and nephritis
- Exudates: Inflammation or injury increases pleural membrane permeability to proteins and various types of cells
- Parapneumonic effusion: Pleural collection associated with infective parenchyma (pneumonia/abscess)
- Pleural effusion: Abnormal collection of fluid in pleura
- Empyema: Presence of pus in pleural fluid (usually thick but there is no strict agreement on number of cells that define empyema)
    - Exudative stage: Inflammatory process associated with pneumonia in underlying lung—fluid clear with low cell count, no infection per se in the fluid, <72 hours (simple)
    - Fibrinopurulent stage: Fibrin deposits with septae and loculations and increased white blood cells (WBC), after 4–10 days (complicated)
    - Organizational: Fibroblasts enter, membranes thicken, and lung fails to reexpand, >10 days
- Lung abscess: Parenchymal necrosis with cavitation and pus collection.

Modified light classification of pleural fluid is shown in table 1 and pleural fluid findings in various types are shown in table 2.

Pearls in Light's classification

- pH is the most early and sensitive index
- pH <7.2 needs intervention while <7.0 denotes poor outcome. pH has the advantage that it is not affected by loculations as carbon dioxide diffuses through all membranes (glucose may be affected by loculations)

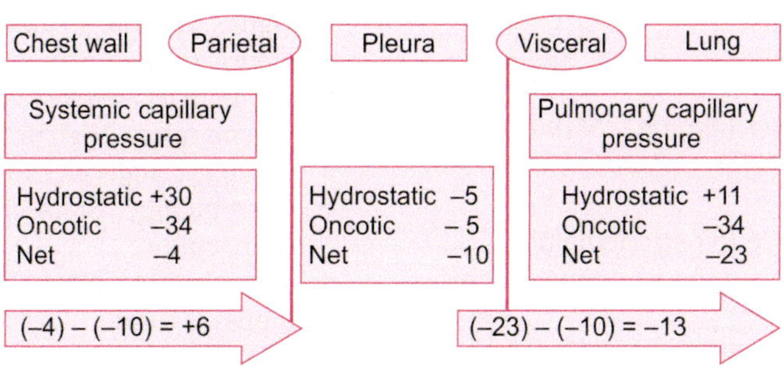

Figure 2: Pleural fluid dynamics

TABLE 1: **Modified light classification (pleural effusion)**

Type	Management
Class 1 para pneumonic effusion	
• CXR lateral decubitus view <10 mm fluid	Antibiotics only
• Chest X-ray lateral decubitus view >10 mm fluid	Antibiotics only
○ pH >7.2, glucose >40 mg, Gram stain negative	Antibiotics + thoracocentesis
○ pH <7.2, glucose <40 mg, Gram stain positive	Antibiotic + tube thoracostomy
Class 2 empyema	
No loculations	Antibiotic + tube thoracostomy
Multiple loculations/pleural peel	Antibiotics + thrombolytics (intrapleural) or debridement (VATS) or decortication

VATS, video-assisted thoracoscopic surgery.

TABLE 2: **Pleural fluid analysis**

Test	Tranudate	Exudates (tubercular)	Exudates (empyema)
Physical appearance	Clear	Straw colored	Turbid yellow
Microscopy	No cells	Predomonantly lymphocytes	Pus cells
Pleural fluid protein	<2 g/dL	>3 g/dL	>3 g/dL
Pleural fluid protein/serum protein	<0.5	>0.5	>0.5
Pleural fluid LDH/serum LDH	<0.6	>0.6	>0.6
Pleural fluid pH	>7.2	<7.3	<7.2
Pleural fluid glucose	>40 mg/dL	<40 mg/dL	<40 mg/dL

LDH, lactate dehydrogenase

- The difference of >0.3 from arterial blood pH is more significant than a single measurement
- Poor prognostic points: pH <7.0, glucose <40 mg/dL, lactate dehydrogenase (LDH) >3 times, total cells >1,000/mm3, or loculations and advanced stage.

Q. What are the common causes of pleural effusion in a child?

Common etiologies of pleural effusion in children include:

- Bacterial pneumonias (most common), e.g., *Streptococcus pneumonia, Staphylococcus aureus, Haemophilus influenzae, anaerobes,* etc.
- Tuberculosis, CCF, hypoproteinemia
- Obstruction to lymphatic drainage (chylothorax)
- Collagen vascular disease
- Malignancies, rheumatoid arthritis
- Aspiration pneumonia, traumatic
- Pulmonary embolism.

Q. What is the approach to pleural effusion?

- Step I: Confirm effusion—chest radiology/ultrasound
- Step II: Is intervention required? (>10 mm wide fluid in X-ray)
- Step III: Transudate or exudates?
  - Light's criteria: Exudate will have either pleura or serum protein >0.5, pleura or serum LDH >0.6, pH <7.2
  - Biochemistry: High protein or low sugar
  - Cytology: High cell count (types may vary)
  - Microbiology: Gram stain, Ziehl-Neelsen stain, culture
  - Special: ADA/CBNAAT, etc.
  - Biopsy: ?Tumor
- Step IV: Management. Transudate—general therapy, exudate— specific therapy.

Q. Any other imaging or scan needed in diagnosis of pleural effusion?

Decubitus film only when ultrasound not available and free fluid present (Fig. 3). It detects early collection and free flow (no loculations) of fluid in pleural space.

Q. What are indications of chest computed tomography scan in pediatric pleural effusion?

Rarely indicated, only when debridement or surgical decortication is needed in empyema. However, it is expensive and have very high radiation dose. It helps to differentiate.

- Lung consolidation versus pleural effusion
- Cystic versus solid lesions
- Peripheral lung abscess versus loculated empyema
- Aids in identification of necrotic areas
- Pleural thickening, nodules, masses
- Extent of tumor.

Q. How to manage a child with pleural effusion?

Mainstay of treatment of pleural effusion includes supportive therapy, drainage of fluid, and appropriate antibiotics.

- Supportive therapy and monitoring:
  - Admission with control of dehydration and good nutrition support and monitoring
  - Acute care with correct position (back rest) and oxygen
  - Symptomatic: Antipyretic or analgesic
  - Nursing care: Care of drainage or look for complication
- Specific: Appropriate antibiotics, antituberculosis, steroids, etc. Role of steroids: massive or bilateral effusion/severe distress after exclusion of severe sepsis
- Drainage of pus
- Expansion of lungs: Inspiratory breathing exercise
- Avoid complications.

CASE 2

History: A 12-year-old previously healthy male presented with high grade fever since 5 days and rapidly progressive breathlessness since 2 days. No past history of trauma.

Examination: He had tachycardia (heart rate 140/min) and tachypnea (respiratory rate 50/min) with respiratory distress. He showed bulging left chest with trachea shifted to right and dull note with diminished breath sound and vocal resonance on entire left chest. There was no engorged neck vein

Investigations: Pallor (hemoglobin 6 g) with polymorphonuclear leucocytosis and high ESR (rate of 120 mm/h) Tuberculin test was negative. X-ray chest showed massive pleural effusion on the left. Pleural fluid was hemorrhagic exudates with normal amylase, lipase level. Pleural biopsy showed pleural endothelioma and the child was managed with oncologic consultation and surgery.

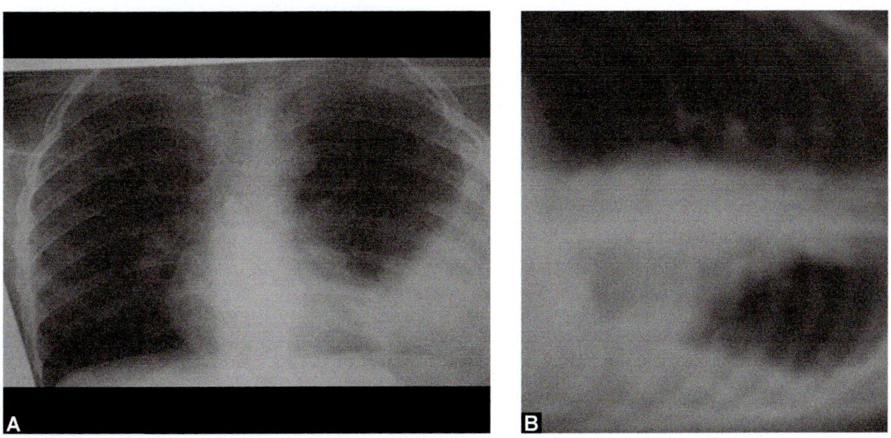

Figure 3: A decubitus film showing effusion on left side

CASE 3

History: An 8-year-old healthy girl presented with biphasic fever accompanied by drowsiness, mild cough, skin rash, and acute respiratory distress on second phase of illness.

Examination: She was in shock with facial puffiness, tachypnea with blood pressure 70/50 mmHg and had vasculitis like rash. On respiratory examination, there was diminished breath sound in bilateral lower zone and minimal ascites.

Investigation: Hemoconcentration (hemoglobin 17 g), normal WBC and thrombocytopenia (76,000). Pleural fluid was clear with 100 cells (lymphocytes 90%), with normal protein and sugar. X-ray chest showed bilateral minimal hydrothorax and ascites. The child was diagnosed with dengue (severe variety) (World Health Organization 2011) and was managed with supportive measures.

CASE 4

History: A 10-year-old boy came with high fever, cough, and respiratory distress accompanied by pain on the right chest during cough since 4 days.

Examination: He was alert but apprehensive, with fever (103°F), tachycardia (heart rate of 140/min), tachypnea (respiratory rate of 55/min), and had mild intercostal fullness with retractions and reduced breath sounds on right lower zone.

Investigations: Polymorphonuclear leucocytosis (20,500, N80), normal ESR, high C-reactive protein (CRP) was seen. Chest X-ray showed right lower zone consolidation with small pleural effusion (<10 mm) (Fig. 4)

Pleural fluid: Cell 1,200 (P70%/L30%), pH 7.2, protein 3.2 g/dL, sugar 40/90, Gram stain, and culture negative. The child was diagnosed with right-sided pleural effusion—class 1b1 (synpneumonic and uncomplicated). He was treated conservatively with antibiotics (amoxicillin-clavulanic acid). No intercostal drain given as thickness <10 mm. Blood culture grew *S. pneumonia*. He was discharged after 7 days with advice of antibiotics and other therapies.

Q. How to choose antibiotics in pyogenic effusion?

Antibiotics are chosen as per suspected organism (Table 3):

- Associated skin pustules: *Staphylococcus aureus*
- Green-colored pus: *Pseudomonas aeruginosa*
- Foul smelling pus, delayed neurodevelopment, foreign body: anaerobes
- History of contact: Tuberculosis
- Bilateral effusion: hydrothorax.

Second line of antibiotics

If no progress or deterioration within 4 days of therapy and drainage, one should consider anaerobic organisms too. Choices are vancomycin and ceftazidime or cefepime/linezolid, according to organisms.

Duration of antibiotics use

Antibiotics (preferably parenteral) to continue till child is afebrile, WBC counts normal, thoracostomy yield <50 mL/day, and X-ray chest is clearing. Subsequently, appropriate oral antibiotics (linezolid/co-amoxiclav, etc.) to be given for a total of 4–6 weeks.

CASE 5

History: A 3-year-old girl presented with fever and cough since 6 days and chest on the pain left side since 2 days.

Examination: She looked sick and preferred to lie on the left side, had tachycardia (heart rate 124/min), tachypnea (respiratory rate 45/min) and fever with left sided chest retractions. She had reduced breath sounds, tenderness on percussion, and mild intercostal edema on left lower zone

Investigation: She had mild pallor (hemoglobin 11.3), polymorphonuclear leucocytosis (23,000, N87), high CRP (98). Tuberculin skin test was negative. Chest X-ray (Fig. 5) and ultrasound chest shows effusion (>20 mm) with consolidation but no septae. Pleural fluid showed 25,000 cells [neutrophils 50%, red blood cells 1 million), sugar (38/70)], protein 4 g, LDH 1,200, pH 7.0, Gram-positive cocci in chains. The effusion was classified as class II uncomplicated (Gram-positive cocci in chains = *S. pneumonia*) as per modified Light's criteria. She was managed with appropriate antibiotics for 3 weeks and intercostal drain for 2 weeks that improved the child.

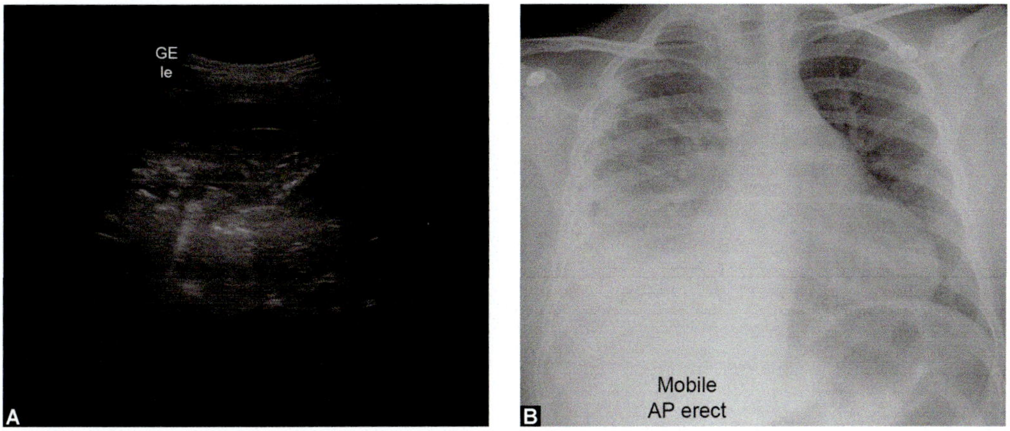

Figure 4: Ultrasound and chest X-ray showing right sided pleural effusion (thickness of effusion <10 mm only)

TABLE 3: Choice of antibiotics as per organisms for pleural effusion or empyema

Organism	Drugs (first line)	Drugs (second line)	Duration
Staphylococcus aureus	Amoxicillin + cloxacillin.	Third generation cephalosporins + cloxacillin (MSSA) Vancomycin/linezolid (MRSA)	2–4 weeks
Streptococcus pneumoniae	Penicillin G/amoxycillin	Ceftriaxone/amoxyclav	2–3 weeks
Haemophilus influenzae/ Escherichia coli/Klebsiella (Gram negative)	Cefuroxime/ceftriaxone/ cefotaxime + aminoglycosides	Cholramphenicol/amoxycillin	2–3 weeks
Pseudomonas (Immunodeficient patients)	Ceftazidime cefoperazone	Imipenem/merpenem/ticarcillin/ aztreonam	2–4 weeks
Bacteroides fragilis (anaerobic)	Penicillin/metronidazole	Clindamycin/chloramphenicol	3–6 weeks
All other anaerobes	Metronidazole	Clindamycin/chloramphenicol	3–6 weeks

MSSA, methicillin-susceptible *Staphylococcus aureus*; MRSA, methicillin-resistant *Staphylococcus aureus*.

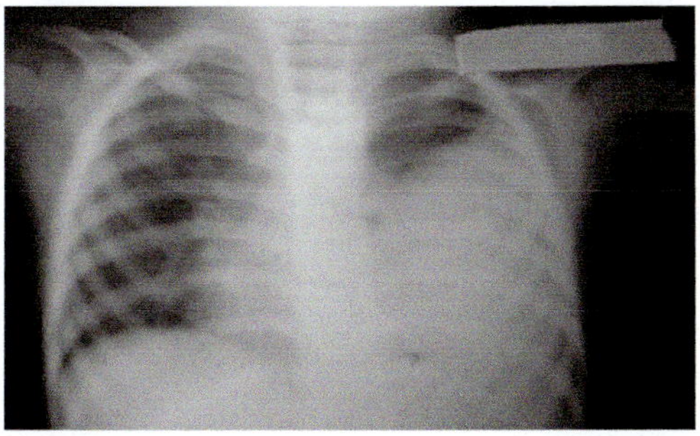

Figure 5: X-ray chest showing pleural effusion (thickness >20 mm)

Q. What are guidelines for empyema drainage intercostal drain?

Following are the guidelines for intercostal tube drainage:

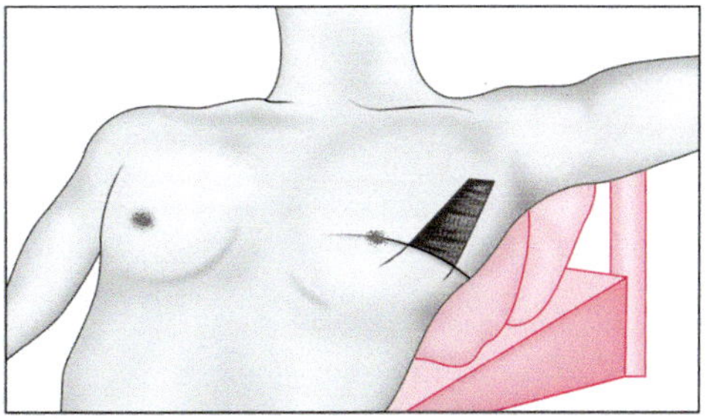

Figure 6: Safe triangle to insert intercostal drain

- It should be closed drainage, under water seal, large catheter inserted in the site of pus accumulation (ultrasound guided) in safe triangle (mid axillary line, 5th space) (Fig. 6)
- Small drains (including pigtail catheters) may be used if pus is not thick

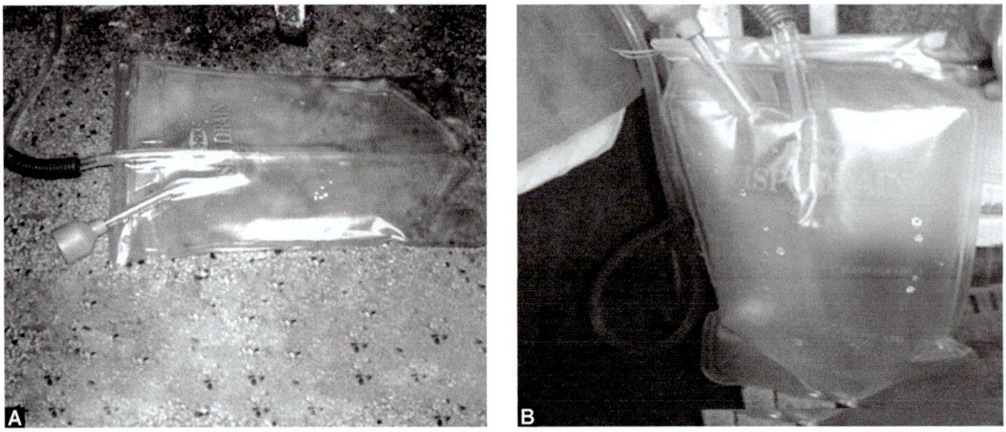

Figure 7: Pitfalls in intercostal drain management *(For color version, see Plate 3)*

- Chest tube kept till drainage is <30–50 mL/day and cavity size is <50 mL in size and no bubble in the tube on deep inspiration
- Keep the system patent and airtight, gravity dependent, avoid kinking of tube, and remove thick pus in tube if blocking drainage (Fig. 7). Maintain sterility of the system. Drain should be clamped for 1 hour once 10 mL/kg pus is initially removed. Allow as much activity as possible and encourage deep breathing and coughing
- If multiloculated, surgeon must be consulted early for his opinion on video-assisted thoracoscopic surgery (VATS) or decortications.

CASE 6

History: A 6-years-old girl, who had measles 2 week back, came with fever, cough, and respiratory distress for 8 days.

Examination: She had toxic looks, was drowsy, and in shock with tachycardia (heart rate 160/min), tachypnea (respiratory rate 50/min), and low blood pressure (74/60 mmHg). She showed signs of massive right-sided pleural effusion.

Investigations: Showed polymorphonuclear leukocytosis (32,000, N91) high ESR (of 60 mm/h,) and CRP (156).

Pleural fluid: Cells 40,000 (polymorph 70%), sugar 30, protein 4.5 g, pH 7.1, Gram-positive cocci in clusters. Chest X-ray showed massive right-sided pleural effusion (Fig. 8). Ultrasound revealed septae and loculations (Fig. 9). Computed tomography chest showed complicated empyema (Fig. 10). The child was managed with antibiotics, fluids, oxygen, fibrinolytics, chest physiotherapy, analgesics, monitoring, and nutrition initially. Later, the child also required VATS. After VATS, and with a chest drain in place, pus continues to drain for 3 days, but less in amount. On day 5, still persists up to 102–103°C. Same treatment was continued and fever subsided gradually.

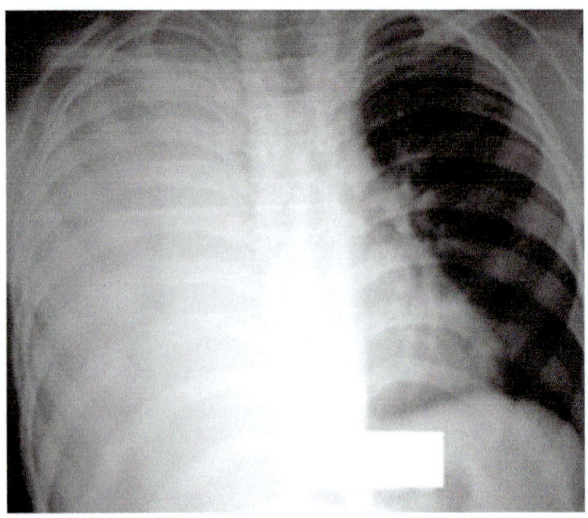

Figure 8: Massive effusion

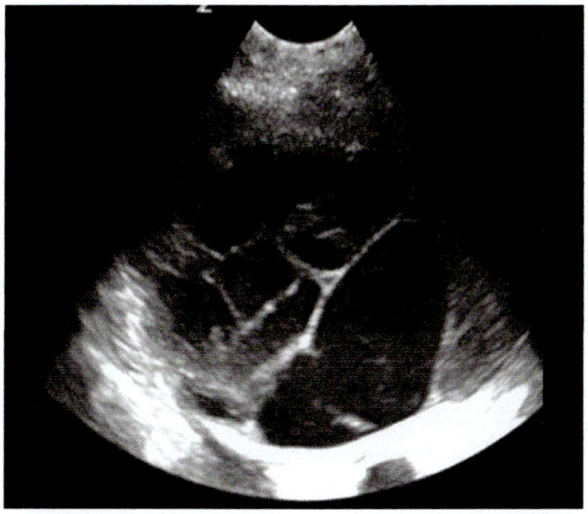

Figure 9: Septae and loculation

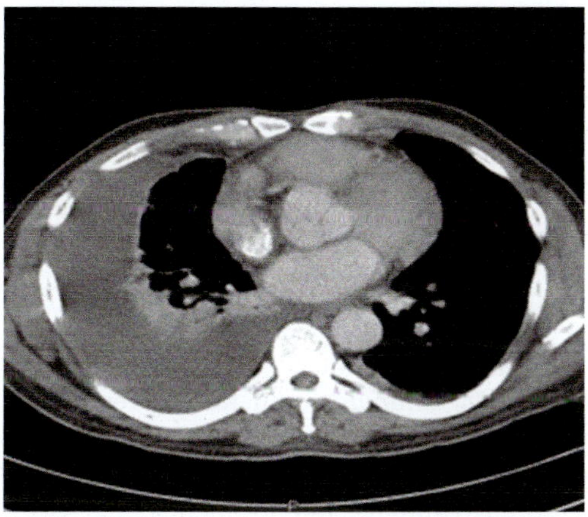

Figure 10: Computed tomography chest-complicated empyema

Q. What is the role of fibrinolytics in empyema?

There are three fibrinolytics; namely, streptokinase, urokinase, and recombinant tissue plasminogen activator. None reduce viscosity of pus. Only human recombinant deoxyribonuclease may reduce viscosity of pus.

Doses

Urokinase—40,000 IU 8 to 12 hourly with 4 hour dwell time. Available as 250,000 IU. Postreconstitution life is of 8 hours. Maximum 2 doses can be used.

Complications

Hemorrhage, fever, pleural pain, arthralgia, and adhesions (makes VATS difficult). Evidence-Cochrane review does not support its universal use.

Q. What is the role of surgery in empyema?

There are three surgical options for empyema:

1. Video assisted thoracoscopic surgery: VATS in multiloculated effusion. It may be used early with expertize/before using fibrinolytics/skill oriented
2. Minithoracotomy and debridement: It may be required in case of multiloculated and complicated nonresponding empyema after >2 weeks of drugs and intercostal drain
3. Open thoracotomy and debridement (decortication): In pleural thickening/non-expansion of lung/bronchopleural fistula.

Cochrane database review comparing medical management with fibrinolysis and VATS concluded that VATS appeared to be superior to chest tube drainage with streptokinase in terms of duration of chest tubes and hospital stay for large and loculated empyemas.

An algorithm for management of pleural effusion is shown in flowchart 1.

Q. What are the complications of empyema?

Empyema may be complicated by the followings:

- Bronchopleural fistula
- Cutaneous fistula
- Pyopneumothorax
- Purulent pericarditis
- Pulmonary abscess
- Peritonitis secondary to rupture through diaphragm
- Septic complications-meningitis, arthritis, osteomyelitis.

Q. What is prognosis of empyema?

In adequately treated cases, prognosis is excellent. Follow-up pulmonary functions suggest that residual disease is uncommon.

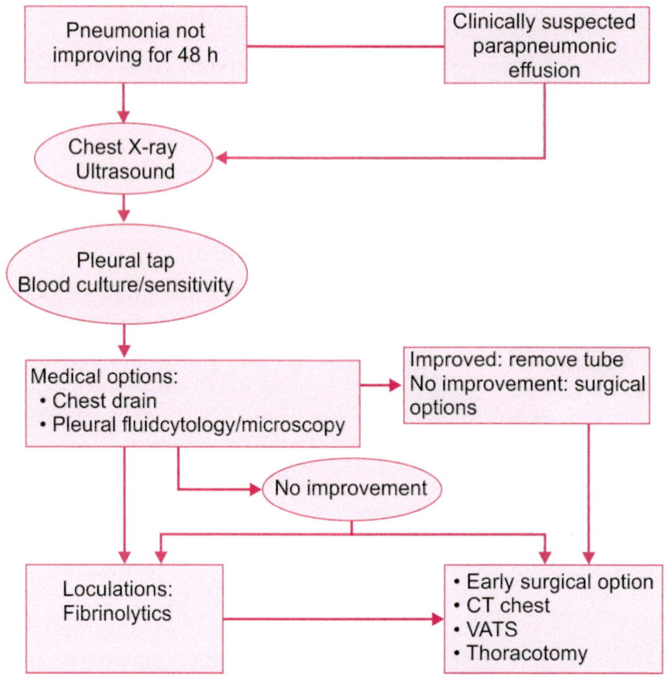

CT, computed tomography; VATS, video-assisted thoracoscopic surgery.

Flowchart 1: Algorithm for management of pleural effusion in children

Q. How can empyema be prevented?

Early diagnosis and appropriate treatment of all cases of pneumonia would reduce the incidence of complicating parapneumonic effusions and empyema. Immunization against organisms such as measles virus, *H. influenzae,* and *S. pneumoniae* could further reduce the incidence. Strong suspicion should be taken during pneumonia in immunocompromised children (human immunodeficiency virus/malnutrition/postsplenectomy, etc.).

LEARNING POINTS

- A short rapidly progressive course with severe pallor, massive effusion, and bloody exudates suggest malignancy. Pancreatitis and trauma has to be excluded in such cases
- Epidemic season, biphasic fever with worsening second peak, shock, vasculitis rash, hemoconcentration, thrombocytopenia, and bilateral hydrothorax with ascites suggest systemic disease and third space collection of fluid like dengue fever
- Intercostal edema and tenderness on percussion point to empyema. Intercostal drain is essential if pleural fluid thickness (radiological) >10 mm
- As fever may take >2 weeks to subside even after proper management of empyema, one should wait with careful observation before taking next action based on only fever. Blood or pleural fluid culture report may also help
- Multiple septae within the effusion may need early video-assisted thorascopic surgery surgery.

SUGGESTED READINGS

1. Light MJ, Blaisdell CJ, Homnick DN, Schechter MS, Weinberger MM. In: Pediatric Pulmonology (AAP). 1st ed. Jaypee Brothers Medical Publicshers (P) Ltd.2012. pp. 423-6.
2. Montogomery M. Air and Liquid in the pleural space. In: Robert W. Wilmott MD, editor. Kendig and Chernick's Disorders of the Respiratory Tract in Children. 8th ed. Philadelphia: Elsiever; 2014. pp. 976-83.
3. Shah N, Singh V, et al. The Respiratory Tract infections-Group Education Module. Respiratory Tract Infection—General Education Module for Pediatricians. Indian Academy of Pediatrics; 2012.
4. Subramanyan L, et al. Suppurative lung disease. In: Pediatric Pulmonology Foundation of India. Essentials of Pediatric Pulmonology. 3rd ed. Chennai, 2008.

8

SECTION

Pulmonary Diseases in Pediatric Intensive Care Unit

CHAPTER

39

Pulmonary Edema

Praveen Narsaria, Rakesh Lodha

CASE 1

- A 6-year-old boy presented to pediatric emergency with 2 days history of rapid breathing, cough, and decreased urine output. There was history of fever and sore throat 2 weeks back. The past medical history was insignificant.
- There was no family history of any chronic renal disease.
- On examination, the child had a respiratory rate of 64/min, with subcostal and intercostal retractions. Oxygen saturation at room air was 92%, heart rate 168/min, blood pressure 134/96 mmHg, good peripheral pulses, and capillary refill time of 3 seconds. Child had periorbital puffiness with pitting pedal edema. On chest auscultation, bilateral air entry was equal with bilateral crepitations in all lung fields, no gallop rhythm. The liver span was 6 cm. Investigations revealed hemoglobin 9.8 g/dL, total leukocyte count (TLC) 7,800/mm^3, differential count of 58% neutrophils, 30% lymphocytes, platelets 2.5 lakh/mm^3, urea 57 mg/dL, and creatinine 2.5 mg/dL. The chest radiograph showed perihilar infiltrates with prominent bronchovascular markings; there was no cardiomegaly (Fig. 1).

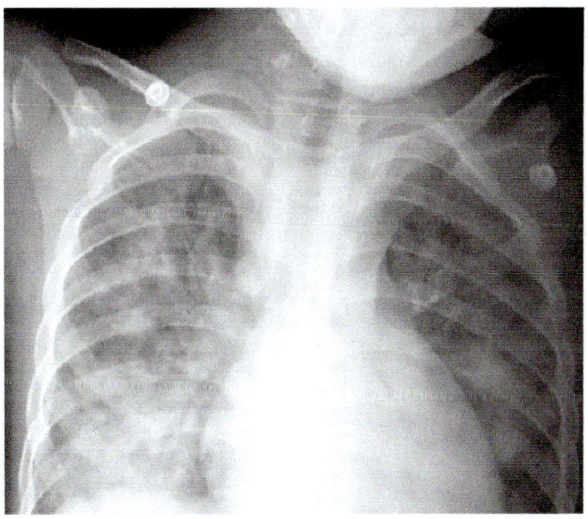

Figure 1: Chest X-ray showing perihilar infiltrates with prominent bronchovascular markings suggestive of pulmonary edema

Q. What are the possible causes for the above respiratory condition?

Various conditions may be responsible for the above respiratory manifestations. Table 1 highlights the points in favor of and against each differential diagnosis.

So, the most probable cause of respiratory condition in this child is acute pulmonary edema.

Pulmonary edema is a state of abnormal fluid accumulation in the alveoli, interfering with oxygenation and ventilation. The heart, lung, and vascular system work together to ensure adequate fluid movement through the capillary and lymphatic system of lung so that minimal fluid transudates from interstitium to

TABLE 1: **Differential diagnosis for respiratory manifestations in case 1**

	Points in favor	Points against
Pulmonary edema	• No fever, reduced urine output • Pedal edema with facial puffiness and bilateral basal crepitations • Hypertension	• No history of any comorbidity
Pneumonia	• No history of any comorbidity, presence of crepitations	• No history of fever • Bilateral basal crepitations and edema
Toxin inhalation	• No fever, short history, bilateral crepitations	• No history of toxin exposure • History of reduced urine output • Presence of edema

alveolus, thus ensuring adequate oxygenation and ventilation. In disease states, this balance is disrupted and lead to accumulation of fluid into alveolar space (both inflammatory and noninflammatory fluid).

Q. What is the pathophysiology of pulmonary edema?

Pulmonary edema occurs when there is a positive flow of fluid across the alveolar-capillary membrane. In disease states, when the alveolar epithelial barrier is breached (inflammatory edema) or the pulmonary interstitial fluid volume increases (noninflammatory edema), alveolus is filled with fluid due to increased positive net flow across the alveolar-capillary membrane. The net flow across the alveolar-capillary membrane is dependent on the oncotic and hydrostatic pressures in capillary lumen and interstitial fluid (Starling equation). In normal condition, the hydrostatic pressure of capillary lumen and interstitial fluid are approximately equal, and the capillary oncotic pressure is more than the interstitium oncotic pressure, thus allowing very less net fluid movement. In conditions of increased capillary hydrostatic pressure (such as fluid overload, hypoalbuminemia), the increased net fluid movement toward the pulmonary interstitium is handled by the lymphatic channels in interstitium. Pulmonary edema sets in these conditions when fluid movement overwhelms the clearance capacity of lymphatics. Changes in the alveolar-capillary membrane integrity can also lead to changes in its permeability (increased net flow across the alveolar-capillary membrane) and, hence, development of pulmonary edema, commonly seen in inflammatory conditions.

Q. What are the different causes of pulmonary edema?

The causes of pulmonary edema can be cardiogenic and noncardiogenic.

Cardiogenic (noninflammatory)

- Left heart failure causes, e.g., intracardiac left to right shunts, congenital arteriovenous malformation, myocarditis, arrhythmias
- Obstructive lesions, e.g., mitral stenosis, congenital obstruction to pulmonary venous drainage, pulmonary veno-occlusive disease.

Noncardiogenic (inflammatory and noninflammatory)

- Local causes:
  - Pneumonia: Infection, aspiration, drowning, toxin and smoke inhalation
  - Lymphatic insufficiency
  - Re-expansion pulmonary edema
  - Upper airway obstruction
  - Pulmonary venous fibrosis
  - Radiation
- Systemic causes:
  - Circulating toxins in sepsis
  - Uremia
  - Transfusion-related acute lung injury

- Significant increase in circulating blood volume, e.g., acute renal failure, overzealous fluid administration, syndrome of inappropriate antidiuretic hormone secretion
- Hypoalbuminemia: Renal and hepatic causes, malnutrition
- Neurogenic pulmonary edema
- Pancreatitis.

Q. How to differentiate between cardiogenic and noncardiogenic pulmonary edema?

Table 2 shows the features that may help to differentiate between cardiogenic and noncardiogenic pulmonary edema.

Q. What type of pulmonary edema is likely to be present in the index case and what is the cause for it?

This child had features of increased circulating blood volume (suggested by reduced urine output due to acute renal failure, edema, and hypertension) which led to increased capillary hydrostatic pressure and more seepage of fluid into the alveolus and pulmonary interstitium. This increased net flow of fluid led to development of pulmonary edema with no features of left heart failure.

So, pulmonary edema in this child is noncardiogenic, noninflammatory, and secondary to fluid overload due to acute renal failure. Acute renal failure in this child is due to post streptococcal glomerulonephritis, as child had history of throat infection followed by oliguria. Management strategy in such cases should focus on correction of fluid balance. A positive fluid balance with features of pulmonary edema is an indication for urgent dialysis to remove excess body fluid. Dialysis can be hemodialysis or peritoneal dialysis depending on feasibility and hemodynamic stability of patient. In small children, peritoneal dialysis is preferred due to difficulty in placement of hemodialysis catheter, availability of appropriate size hemodialysis catheter, and smaller blood volumes. Amongst hemodynamically unstable patients, peritoneal dialysis or continuous renal replacement therapy can be used. Till pulmonary edema resolves, other supportive measures should be provided, e.g., ventilation (invasive or noninvasive) if required, nursing in propped-up position, correction of anemia, etc.

TABLE 2: Differentiation between cardiogenic and noncardiogenic pulmonary edema

Clinical	Cardiogenic	Noncardiogenic
Crepitations	Generally basal or whole of lung field	May be present in nondependent parts of lung
Gallop	Mostly present	Absent
Hepatomegaly	Usually present	Usually not present
Radiographic		
Heart size	Normal or increased	Usually normal
Vascular distribution	Balanced or inverted	Normal or balanced
Distribution of edema	Central or even	Peripheral or patchy
Pleural effusion	Present	Absent
Peribronchial cuffing	Present	Usually not present
Septal lines	Present	Usually not present
Air bronchogram	Usually not present	Usually present

CASE 2

A 1-year-old child with a known case of ventricular septal defect, presented to pediatric emergency with complaints of increased difficulty in breathing and excessive cry for a day. Child had an upper respiratory tract infection (URTI) like illness since 2 days. On examination, the child had a respiratory rate of 78/min with subcostal and intercostals retractions, oxygen saturation on room air was 94%, heart rate was 182/min, peripheral pulses were feeble and capillary refill time of 3 seconds. On auscultation, there were bilateral basal crepitations, had gallop, with liver of 4 cm below the right costal margin.

Investigations revealed hemoglobin 6.3 g/dL, TLC 10,000/mm^3 (Neutrophils$_{56}$ lymphocytes$_{33}$), and platelet count 2.5 lakh/mm^3. Chest X-ray revealed cardiomegaly with increased perihilar infiltrates and mild bilateral pleural effusion (Fig. 2).

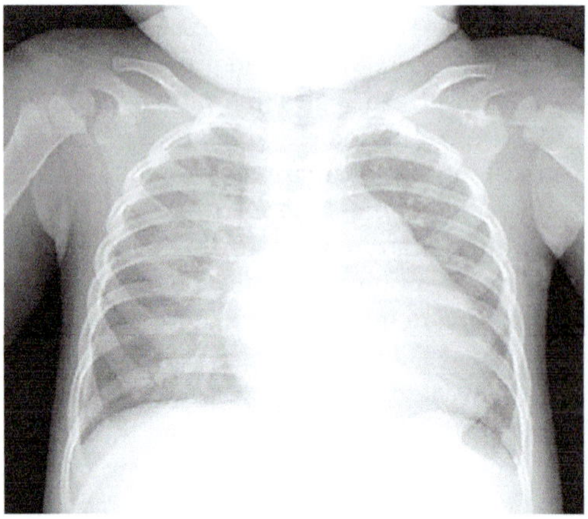

Figure 2: Chest X-ray of infant showing cardiomegaly with increased perihilar infiltrates and mild bilateral pleural effusion suggestive of pulmonary edema

Q. What is the cause of the above respiratory condition?

Differentiation between pulmonary edema and respiratory tract infection (as in present case) sometimes becomes difficult in children with congenital heart disease, as clinical features in either conditions overlap and cardiomegaly can be present due to underlying heart disease, but some points help us to differentiate between these two. In children with pulmonary edema, generally there is short history of viral illness followed by onset of respiratory distress (viral illness may point toward onset of viral myocarditis and short history toward development of pulmonary edema rather than pneumonia), whereas in pneumonia, children generally have high grade fever with lack of URTI symptoms and a slower course. Also, on examination, findings suggestive of lung parenchyma pathology are localized in pneumonia and more diffuse and evenly distributed in pulmonary edema which is confirmed by chest X-ray. Further, total counts are elevated with neutrophilic response in pneumonia, whereas counts are normal in pulmonary edema. So, in our present case, child has a short URTI like illness, followed by onset of symptoms. On examination, child has diffuse findings (bilateral crepitations with gallop rhythm) with chest X-ray showing bilateral perihilar infiltrates. Also, total counts are normal, so this child is having acute pulmonary edema of cardiogenic cause.

Q. What are the possible causes for congestive heart failure in this child?

The child has congenital heart disease and features of pulmonary edema which may be due to:

- Acute viral myocarditis
- Anemia
- Pneumonia with congestive cardiac failure (CCF) without myocarditis in such an underlying cardiac condition.

The presentation of viral myocarditis in an infant can be very dramatic with severe heart ventilation, leading to a requirement for mechanical support early in the course of treatment. The most common viruses causing myocarditis are enterovirus/coxsackie virus, adenovirus, and parvovirus. The possibility of viral myocarditis should be kept in child presenting with acute heart failure, with viral prodrome, and elevated troponin I. Other supportive evidence comes from echocardiography and magnetic resonance imaging (MRI), but definitive diagnosis requires myocardial biopsy. Management of viral myocarditis is supportive (as most of the cases in children and adults are self-limiting), with use of diuretics, inotropes (preferably milrinone—to be used with caution, can precipitate arrhythmias), and mechanical ventilation if required.

Anemia causes increased stress on myocardium due to tachycardia and increased stroke volume. In severe anemia, the glomerular filtration rate also decreases, leading to electrolyte and fluid retention along with reduced oxygen delivery to myocardium. This causes additional burden on myocardium and thus, can precipitate heart failure. In underlying congenital heart disease with left to right shunts, the myocardium is already stressed and any extra burden (anemia, fever, infection) on it can easily topple over the balance toward failure.

Children with congenital heart disease are anemic due to poor nutritional intake, recurrent episodes of pneumonia, and higher metabolic demand, so they are more prone to develop heart failure. In our case, child had a history of short viral prodrome followed by heart failure.

Possibility of pneumonia is less likely as TLC is normal, precipitation of CCF is shortly after a viral prodrome, and there are bilateral lung findings.

Q. Why is it important to differentiate between cardiogenic vs. noncardiogenic pulmonary edema?

It has therapeutic implications. In cardiogenic causes, mainstay of treatment is inotropes (after myocarditis has been ruled out) and fluid restriction, whereas in noncardiogenic causes management depends on underlying etiology. It may include fluid restriction, dialysis, antibiotics, and mechanical ventilation.

Q. What is the probable cause of CCF in this child and how to manage?

As discussed above, the probable cause seems to be viral myocarditis or anemia. Further workup of this child showed normal troponin I and echocardiography showed an ejection fraction of 45% with normal chamber size. These findings keep the possibility of anemia leading to CCF more likely, as troponin I was normal and echocardiography was not suggestive of myocarditis. Anemia can cause fluid retention as described above and fever in such a condition can lead to compromised cardiac output. The already overloaded pulmonary vasculature (increased capillary hydrostatic pressure) will lead to net positive flow of fluid into alveolus, due to increased hydrostatic pulmonary capillary pressure generated due to failing myocardium.

Management of such case is supportive and includes correction of anemia with blood component therapy, decongestive measures, control of fever, and if required inotropes. After acute phase is over, child should be put on oral loop diuretics, iron supplements, adequate diet, and planned for corrective surgery.

Q. How to manage a child with pulmonary edema?

Any patient presenting with respiratory distress, first step is to assess patency of airway and steps should be taken accordingly. After this, supplemental oxygen should be started and adequacy of breathing should be assessed. If patient has increased work of breathing or has signs of respiratory failure, adequate corrective measures should be taken. Similarly, circulation should be assessed and taken care of. Now, after ABC (airway, breathing, and circulation) stabilization, a focused and rapid history and clinical examination should be done to localize the cause for respiratory distress. In our case 2, cause of respiratory distress is pulmonary edema of cardiogenic origin as discussed above. In cardiogenic cause of pulmonary edema, focus is on improvement of myocardial oxygen demand-supply balance by reducing its workload, improving oxygen delivery, and improving cardiac inotropy. These are achieved by correction of anemia (better oxygen supply) and reduction in afterload (by use of vasodilators and maintaining a negative fluid balance). Inotropes should be used cautiously as presence of myocarditis can worsen condition. In cardiogenic causes of pulmonary edema, conditions with fluid overload (e.g., renal failure with oliguria), dialysis should be used upfront and in other causes, antibiotics are used with general supportive measures. All patients with pulmonary edema should be nursed in propped-up position, if hemodynamically stable. Ventilation strategy should be planned to minimize ventilator-associated lung injury and a negative overall fluid balance should be maintained (Flowchart 1).

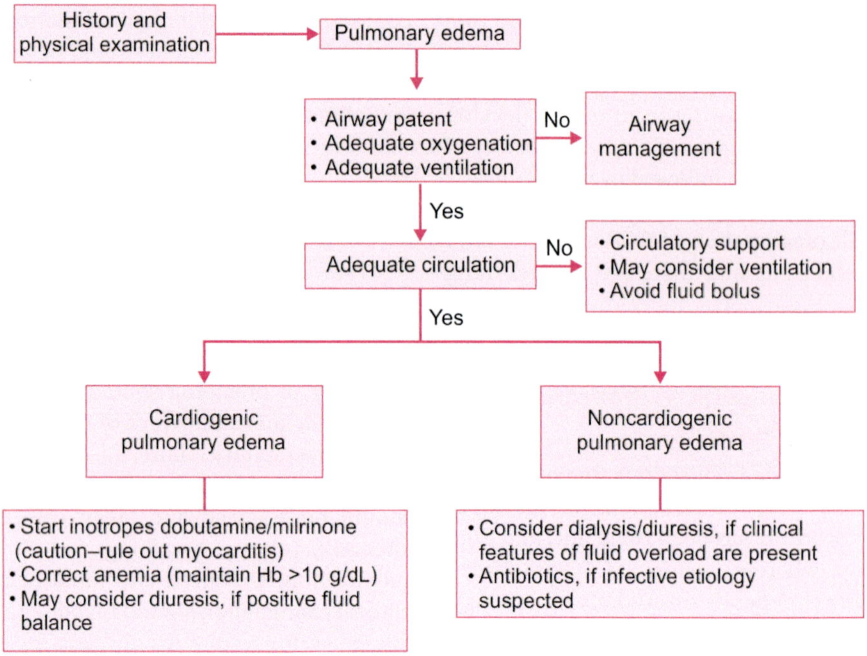

Flowchart 1: Management of pulmonary edema

LEARNING POINTS

- Presence of respiratory distress, bilateral basal crepitations, and hepatomegaly with chest X-ray showing bilateral perihilar infiltrates with or without cardiomegaly are pointers toward pulmonary edema
- Pulmonary edema can be due to cardiogenic and noncardiogenic causes and differentiation between these two has therapeutic implications
- Amongst patients with underlying congenital heart disease presenting with respiratory distress, pulmonary edema and pneumonia are common causes for respiratory distress and should be differentiated
- Amongst cardiac causes of pulmonary edema, myocarditis should also be considered as an important cause
- Management of pulmonary edema is removal of extravascular lung water through dialysis, cardiac inotropy and other supportive measures determined by the causes
- Protective lung strategy of ventilation should be used if ventilator support is required.

SUGGESTED READINGS

1. Mazor RL, Green TP. Pulmonary edema In: Kliegman RM, Stanton BM, Geme JS, Schor NF, editors. Nelson Textbook of Pediatrics, 20th ed. Elsevier: Philadelphia; 2016. pp. 2061-63.
2. O'Brodovich H. Pulmonary edema. In: Wilmott RW, Boat TF, Bush A, Chernick V, Deterding RR, Ratjen F, editors. Disorders of Respiratory Tract in Children, 8th ed. Elsevier: Philadelphia; 2012. pp. 570-85.
3. Ware LB, Matthay MA. Acute pulmonary edema. N Engl J Med. 2005;353(26):2788-96.

CHAPTER

40

Acute Respiratory Distress Syndrome

Krishan Chugh, Vikas Taneja

CASE 1

A 4-month-old boy was admitted with complaints of cough and coryza for 8 days, and fever and fast breathing for 1 day. On admission, the child had increased work of breathing with significant oxygen requirement, tachycardia, poor perfusion, and drowsiness. Examination of the chest revealed only few crepitations. The child was intubated and mechanically ventilated in view of signs of respiratory failure (SpO_2 84%, PaO_2 45 mmHg on FiO_2 100%). Chest X-ray showed bilateral fluffy infiltrates. The respiratory secretions were positive for swine flu influenza (H1N1) on reverse transcriptase polymerase chain reaction. The child required very high ventilatory settings with 100% FiO_2. Positive end expiratory pressure (PEEP) was stepped up in small increments and best titration was achieved at a PEEP of 15 cmH_2O.

The child had a stormy course in the pediatric intensive care unit (PICU) with very high ventilatory requirements for almost 7 days. Seventy two hours into ventilation, when the hemodynamic stability was achieved, prone positioning was tried for 24 hours. It did not show much change in the oxygenation. By day 8, the child started showing improvement by decreasing in the ventilatory requirements and inotropes. He was gradually weaned off the ventilatory support and extubated by day 16.

Q. What is acute respiratory distress syndrome and how is it defined?

Acute respiratory distress syndrome (ARDS) was first defined by Ashbaug et al. in 1967, as a clinical entity marked by profound hypoxemia and bilateral chest infiltrates. The initial name was adult respiratory distress syndrome, as it occurred in adults and pathologically was similar to respiratory distress syndrome in neonates. Later it was replaced by ARDS as it was reported in children as well. A lot of work has been done since then on defining the syndrome.

The American-European Consensus Conference, in 1994, came up with standard definition of acute lung injury (ALI) and ARDS (Table 1). This definition was extrapolated to

TABLE 1: American-European Consensus Conference Definition of acute respiratory distress syndrome

Timing	Acute onset	
	ALI	ARDS
Oxygenation (PaO_2/FiO_2)—regardless of PEEP level	<300	<200
Chest radiograph	Bilateral infiltrates	Bilateral infiltrates
Pulmonary artery wedge pressure	<18 or no clinical evidence of left atrial hypertension	<18 or no clinical evidence of left atrial hypertension

ALI, acute lung injury; ARDS, acute respiratory distress syndrome; PEEP, positive end-expiratory pressure; FiO_2, fraction of inspired oxygen; PaO_2, partial pressure of arterial oxygen.

TABLE 2: The Berlin definition of acute respiratory distress syndrome

Timing	Chest imaging*	Origin of edema	Oxygenation#		
			Mild	Moderate	Severe
Within 7 days of a known clinical insult Or New or worsening respiratory symptoms	• Bilateral opacities • Not fully explained by effusions, lobar lung collapse or nodules	• Need echocardiography to exclude hydrostatic edema if no risk factors present	• 200 mmHg $<PaO_2/FiO_2$ >300 • With PEEP or CPAP ≥5 cmH_2O‡	• 100 mmHg $<PaO_2/FiO_2$ >200 • With PEEP >5 cmH_2O	• PaO_2/FiO_2 ≤100 • With PEEP ≥5 cmH_2O

*Chest radiograph or computed tomography scan chest.
#If altitude is higher than 1,000 m, the correction factor should be calculated as follows [PaO_2/FiO_2 (760 barometric pressure)].
‡This may be delivered noninvasively in the mild acute respiratory distress syndrome group.
PEEP, positive end-expiratory pressure; ARDS, acute respiratory distress syndrome; CPAP, continuous positive airway pressure; FiO_2, fraction of inspired oxygen; PaO_2, partial pressure of arterial oxygen.

children, and for years, have been used by pediatric intensivists for management and prognostication. However, this definition had a lot of limitations in terms of diagnosis and management of ARDS patients. To address some of the limitations of this definition, new criteria named as the Berlin definition was put forward in 2011 by an international expert panel comprising members from European Society of Intensive Care Medicine, American Thoracic Society, and Society of Critical Care Medicine (Table 2). However, the Berlin definition did not address pediatric specific considerations. This led the pediatric intensive care societies across the world to convene a consensus conference to define pediatric ARDS (PARDS) in 2015 (Table 3). The recommendations of this consensus conference have been published, which focus on every aspect of PARDS including definition, pathophysiology, management, research, and prognostication. The authors' case met the criteria of severe PARDS.

Q. What is the etiopathology of pediatric acute respiratory distress syndrome?

The injury to the lung and subsequent ARDS can result from direct insult to the lung (pneumonia, aspiration, inhalational injury, transfusions, and ventilator induced lung injury) or a systemic insult like sepsis and septic shock. The basic pathology is injury to the alveolar capillary unit, leading to the accumulation of proteinacious exudate in the alveoli and microvascular thrombi in the capillary bed, thereby affecting the gas exchange. This fluid accumulation in the alveoli in the setting of dysregulated inflammation, cytokine release, and deranged coagulation leads to marked hypoxemia, radiographic opacities, decreased functional residual capacity, and decreased lung compliance. Acute respiratory distress syndrome is a heterogenous disease with different units of the lung having varying degrees of inflammation, thus leading to V/Q mismatch. The pathological features of ARDS involve three overlapping phases:

1. Inflammatory or exudative phase (0–7 days)
2. Proliferative phase (7–21 days)
3. Fibrotic phase (after 21 days).

In the authors' case, the cause of ARDS was H1N1 pneumonia. Overall prognosis of ARDS is bad and the one caused due to H1N1 has even worse prognosis.

Q. What is the clinical presentation of pediatric acute respiratory distress syndrome?

History at the time of presentation gives clues not only to the primary diagnosis like pneumonia or sepsis but also points to the

TABLE 3: The Pediatric Acute Lung Injury Consensus Conference definition of acute respiratory distress syndrome

Age	Exclude patients with perinatal lung disease			
Timing	Within 7 days of a known clinical insult			
Origin of edema	Respiratory failure not fully explained by cardiac failure or fluid overload			
Chest imaging	Findings of new infiltrates consistent with acute pulmonary parenchymal disease			
Oxygenation	Noninvasive mechanical ventilation	Invasive mechanical ventilation		
	PARDS (no severity stratification)	Mild	Moderate	Severe
	• Full face mask bilevel ventilation or CPAP >5 cmH_2O# • P/F ratio ≤300 • S/F ratio ≤264*	4 ≤OI <8 5 ≤OSI <7.5*	8 ≤OI <16 7.5 ≤OSI <12.3*	OI ≥16 OSI ≥12.3*
Special population				
Cyanotic heart disease	Standard criteria above for age, timing, origin of edema, and chest imaging with an acute deterioration in oxygenation not explained by underlying cardiac disease*			
Chronic lung disease	Standard criteria above for age, timing, and origin of edema with chest imaging consistent with new infiltrate and an acute deterioration in oxygenation from baseline which meets oxygenation criteria above‡			
Left ventricular dysfunction	Standard criteria above for age, timing, and origin of edema with chest imaging changes consistent with new infiltrate and an acute deterioration in oxygenation from baseline which meets criteria above not explained by left ventricular dysfunction			

OI = (FIO_2 × mean airway pressure × 100)/PaO_2

OSI = (FIO_2 × mean airway pressure × 100)/SpO_2

*Use PaO_2 based metric when available. If PaO_2 is not available, wean FIO_2 to maintain SpO_2 ≤97% to calculate OSI or SF ratio.

#For non-intubated patients treat with supplemental oxygen or nasal modes of non-invasive ventilation.

‡Acute respiratory distress syndrome severity groups stratified by OI or OSI should not be applied to children with chronic lung disease who normally receive invasive mechanical ventilation or children with cyanotic congenital heart disease.

PARDS, pediatric acute respiratory distress syndrome; OI, oxygenation index; OSI, oxygen saturation index; CPAP, continuous positive airway pressure; FiO_2, fraction of inspired oxygen; PaO_2, partial pressure of arterial oxygen. PF ratio, PaO_2:FiO_2; SF ratio, SpO_2:FiO_2.

presence of risk factors for developing acute lung injury or ARDS. Tachypnea followed by respiratory distress may progress fast indicating reducing lung compliance. Most of the time, ARDS develops within 24–72 hours after the onset of the primary disease process.

On clinical examination, the child may have significant work of breathing with subcostal and intercostal retractions. Chest auscultation may be normal or reveal fine crepitations all over. Over time, the patient develops hypoxia which is out of proportion to the clinical signs. As the disease progresses, the hypoxia worsens and the patient may have worsening of the respiratory distress requiring mechanical ventilation. Acute respiratory distress syndrome patients may have associated hemodynamic instability as part of the sepsis if it is the underlying cause, or as a result of the high ventilatory pressures required to maintain oxygenation. Severe hypoxia, hypercarbia, and metabolic acidosis may cause elevated pulmonary artery pressures resulting in increased right ventricular workload.

Q. What are the investigations required to establish the diagnosis of pediatric acute respiratory distress syndrome?

As per the definition of PARDS, one needs only a chest radiograph and a blood gas analysis along with the clinical presentation to define PARDS. Wherever blood gas analysis is not available, SpO_2 can be used in the place of pO_2 to calculate oxygen saturation index and PaO_2:FiO_2 ratio.

All other investigations as done in any critical patient like sepsis work-up, kidney function test, liver function test, electrolytes, lactates, and coagulation parameters help in establishing the cause of ARDS as well as in the management of such patient. Hypoalbuminemia is predictive of ARDS, weight gain, and death in patients with severe sepsis.

Echocardiography will help in evaluating cardiac contractility, intravascular volume status, pulmonary hypertension, and any other congenital cardiac defects. Computed tomography of the chest, although not routinely ordered, may be helpful in differentiating between atelectasis and consolidation.

Q. How do we differentiate cardiogenic from noncardiogenic pulmonary edema?

By definition of PARDS, we need to rule out any cardiac cause leading to fluid accumulation in the lungs. Assessment of left ventricular function can be done by bedside echocardiography, which is a good predictor of cardiac symptoms in children with left ventricular failure. Assessment includes cardiac output (aortic Doppler flow velocities), systolic function (shortening fraction and ejection fraction), and diastolic function (mitral valve inflow techniques).

Consolidated or fluid filled lung on ultrasonography would reveal absence of the sliding sign and presence of B lines. Pleural effusion is detected as a hypoechoic and homogeneous structure with no gas inside, free from echoes.

Q. How is pediatric acute respiratory distress syndrome managed?

The management of pediatric ARDS is mainly supportive. Critical aspects of management are treating the primary cause (sepsis/pneumonia/aspiration) and minimizing the risk of complications. Strategies proposed for an effective management of PARDS are lung protective ventilation, conservative fluid management, adequate sedation, analgesia and paralysis, and adequate nutrition. Still, PARDS carries very high mortality due to the nature of the disease itself and the early development of multi-organ failure. The stepwise management of PARDS is given in flowchart 1.

Q. What is the ventilation strategy in pediatric acute respiratory distress syndrome managed?

The goal of mechanical ventilation in ARDS is to maintain adequate oxygenation. However,

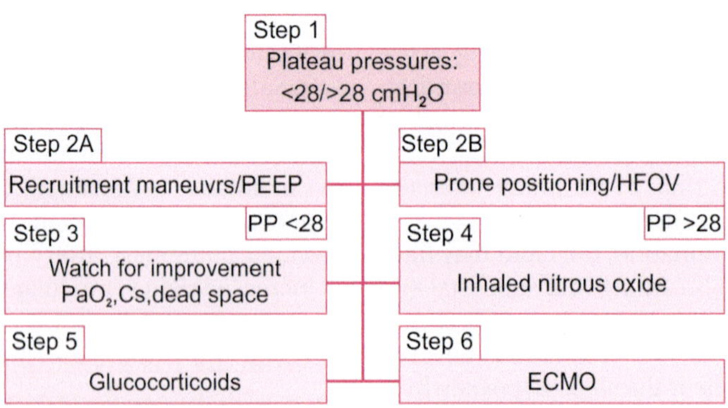

PEEP, positive end-expiratory pressure; HFOV, high frequency oscillatory ventilation; ECMO, extracorporeal membrane oxygenation; PaO_2, partial pressure of arterial oxygen; Cs, compliance, PP, plateau pressure.

Flowchart 1: Algorithm showing stepwise approach to management of acute respiratory distress syndrome.

because of the nonuniform nature of the disease in ARDS, mechanical ventilation has the potential to aggravate lung injury.

Endotracheal tubes

The recent PARDS guidelines recommend the use of cuffed endotracheal tubes in ventilating children with ARDS.

Ventilation modes

Besides conventional modes of ventilation, newer modes like airway pressure release ventilation (APRV) have shown promise in adult population in terms of lower inspiratory pressures and better patient ventilator synchrony. However, in pediatric ARDS, none of the modes have been shown to improve outcome.

Tidal volume

The ARDS Network (ARDSNet) study has been the landmark study after which a number of lung protective ventilation strategies have been proposed. The ARDSNet study demonstrated that the low tidal volume strategy (6 mL/kg) compared to traditional ventilatory methods (tidal volumes 12 mL/kg) decreased mortality (31 vs. 39.8%), increased ventilator free days, and decreased plasma interleukin concentrations in adult patients with ARDS. Similar ventilatory strategy of low tidal volumes and high PEEP has become the standard of care in pediatric population as well. As per the recent PARDS guidelines, it is recommended to use patient specific tidal volumes according to disease severity. Tidal volumes should be 3–6 mL/kg for patients with poor lung compliance and 5–8 mL/kg for patients with better preserved lung compliance (Table 4).

Inspiratory pressures

In the absence of transpulmonary pressure measurements, the PARDS guidelines recommend a lower inspiratory plateau pressure limit of 28 cmH_2O and a slightly higher plateau pressures (28–32 cmH_2O) for patients with reduced chest wall compliance.

TABLE 4: Acute Respiratory Distress Syndrome Network lung protective (6 mL/kg predicted body weight) strategy

Mode	Time cycled, pressure regulated, volume controlled ventilation
Tidal volume	• Set at 8 mL/kg predicted IBW and titrate to 6 mL/kg over 6 h • May titrate up to 8 mL/kg IBW if plateau pressure <30 cmH_2O and evidence for breath stacking (>3/min) or airway pressure < PEEP • Titrate down to 4 mL/kg IBW if plateau pressure >30 cmH_2O
Plateau pressure	• The goal is to keep the plateau pressures <30 cmH_2O
I:E ratio or inspiratory flow	• Target—I:E ratio at 1:3 to 1:1 • I:E ratio can be reduced to 1:1 if inadequate oxygenation. This would mean a longer inspiratory times which would help in recruitment of alveolar units and improve oxygenation
Arterial pH	• Target—7.30 <pH <7.45 (if possible)
Arterial pH (goal)	• Increase ventilator rate to 35 to maintain pH ≥7.30 • If ventilator rate = 35 and pH <7.30, bicarbonate may be given • If ventilator rate = 35, bicarbonate has been considered, and pH <7.15, tidal volume may be increased (plateau pressure may rise >30 cmH_2O) • This concept is called permissive hypercapnia and minimizes ventilator induced lung injury
PEEP and FiO_2	• Target: PaO_2 = 55–80 mmHg or SaO_2 = 88–95%

Continued

Continued

Mode	Time cycled, pressure regulated, volume controlled ventilation
PEEP and FiO_2	• PEEP 5 5 8 8 10 10 10 12 14 14 14 16 18 18 20–24 • FiO_2 0.3 0.4 0.4 0.5 0.5 0.6 0.7 0.7 0.7 0.8 0.9 0.9 0.9 1.0 1.0 • Increase PEEP to recruit alveoli and maintain adequate PaO_2. Titrate PEEP (8–20 cm) to reduce FiO_2 ≤0.6. This concept is known as permissive hypoxemia and helps to minimize oxygen toxicity
Sedation, analgesia and paralysis	• Adequate sedation and analgesia in order to avoid patient ventilator asynchrony. Intermittent paralysis rather than a continuous infusion should be preferred. This would also help in weaning off the ventilator faster

IBW, ideal body weight; PEEP, positive end-expiratory pressure; I:E, inspiratory expiratory ratio; PaO_2, partial pressure of arterial oxygen; SaO_2, oxyhemoglobin saturation; FiO_2, fraction of inspired oxygen.

Positive end expiratory pressure

Pediatric ARDS guidelines recommend PEEP levels of 10–15 cmH_2O titrated to oxygenation and hemodynamic response in severe PARDS. Positive end expiratory pressure levels greater than 15 cmH_2O may be needed in severe PARDS, but attention should be paid to limiting the plateau pressures. However, oxygen saturation/oxygen saturation index, respiratory system compliance, resistance, and hemodynamics should be closely monitored as PEEP is increased.

Lung recruitment maneuvers

It is believed that providing high inspiratory pressures (e.g., 40 mmHg) sustained for prolonged period (e.g., 40 s) can open many of the collapsed alveoli (recruitment) and improve the oxygenation and ventilation. However, the risk of air leaks has limited the use of this strategy in children. Instead most centers practice incremental PEEP application to find the optimum level of PEEP where oxygenation and lung compliance are best and the hemodynamic parameters are not compromised. Higher levels of PEEP lead to a breaking effect on the pressure volume loop. Thus ventilatory settings should be such that the patient is ventilated in the safe zone (Fig. 1). Constant monitoring of the patient including ventilator graphics helps to ensure safe zone ventilation. However, no pediatric data exists on the effect of recruitment maneuvers on morbidity, mortality, length of stay, or duration of mechanical ventilation.

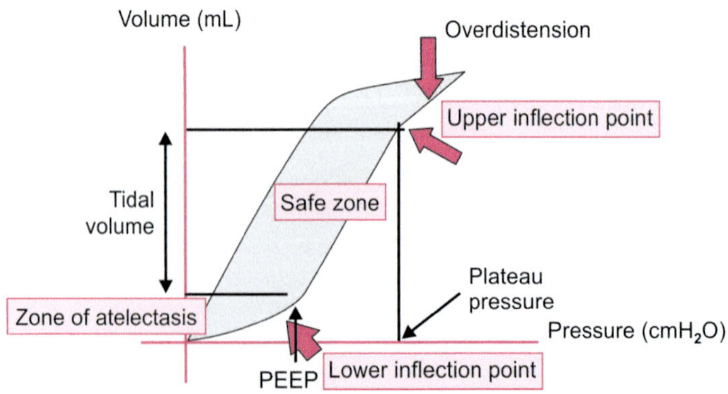

Figure 1: Safe zone for ventilation as seen on the pressure-volume curve

Q. What is permissive hypoxemia and permissive hypercarbia?

The concept of permissive hypoxemia and hypercarbia has come as part of the lung protective ventilation strategies to achieve the best oxygenation with minimal ventilator induced lung injury (Table 4).

Oxygenation

For mild PARDS with PEEP requirement less than 10 cmH_2O, maintain SpO_2 between 92–97%. For severe PARDS requiring PEEP >10 cmH_2O, maintain SpO_2 in the 88–92% range. When SpO_2 is less than 92%, monitoring of central venous saturation and markers of oxygen delivery is strongly recommended.

Ventilation

For moderate to severe PARDS, permissive hypercapnia should be considered to minimize lung injury. It is recommended to maintain pH between 7.15-7.30. Use of soda bicarbonate is not recommended. Exceptions to permissive hypercapnia include intracranial hypertension, severe pulmonary hypertension, select congenital heart disease lesions, hemodynamic instability, and ventricular dysfunction.

Q. What is the role of noninvasive ventilation in pediatric acute respiratory distress syndrome?

Noninvasive ventilation (NIV) should be tried in "early" ARDS (ALI) that is not responding to high flow oxygen. There should be very low threshold for intubation if the patient shows worsening hypoxemia or increasing work of breathing because the window of opportunity is small. Hence, very strict vigil is required. Very few studies on use of NIV in PARDS have been done and the outcome is also conflicting.

There is relatively little published data to support the routine use of NIV in PARDS. However, in mild PARDS, the addition of NIV to standard medical therapy may prevent intubation and mechanical ventilation. Noninvasive ventilation is not recommended in children with severe disease. Humidified high flow nasal cannula (HHFNC) has been tried but its efficacy has not been demonstrated to be equivalent to NIV. There have been very few studies that demonstrate the use of HHFNC in children with PARDS.

Q. How should fluids be manage in a child with acute respiratory distress syndrome?

Fluid management in ARDS is of utmost importance and over time has shown to affect the outcome in terms of oxygenation index, number of ventilator free days and ICU length of stay. Compared to the liberal fluid strategy, the conservative fluid strategy has shown to improve the outcome though has not had any significant effect on the mortality. Similar results have also been reproduced in pediatric studies. Once the hemodynamics have been stabilized in the initial period, fluid boluses should be avoided and in later stages albumin-furosemide infusion may be used to remove excess fluid out of the body.

As per PARDS guidelines, pediatric patients with PARDS should receive fluids adequate enough to maintain sufficient intravascular volume, end-organ perfusion, and optimal delivery of oxygen. After initial fluid resuscitation and stabilization, fluid therapy should be titrated based on a goal directed protocol that includes total intake, output, and fluid balance. However, further studies are needed to determine the optimal fluid management strategy in PARDS.

Q. What is the role of prone positioning in pediatric acute respiratory distress syndrome?

There is increasing evidence of beneficial effects of prone positioning on outcomes (significant reduction in 28- and 90-day mortality). Risks of prone positioning are mainly logistical, e.g., dislodgement of endotracheal tube or vascular lines, increased intra-abdominal pressure, feeding intolerance, and edema (facial). The greatest effects are achieved when patients are maintained prone for 12 hours or longer and oxygenation improves in 60–70% of patients.

In PARDS, prone positioning has been associated with improved oxygenation in children with hypoxemic respiratory failure. However, it is not a routine therapy in PARDS. It may be considered as an option in therapy for severe PARDS.

Q. What is the current status of high frequency oscillatory ventilation in acute respiratory distress syndrome?

High frequency oscillatory ventilation (HFOV) has been in use since the 1970s. Though it has a proven role in neonatal RDS, role in pediatric ARDS was never clearly established. Recent PARDS guidelines recommend using HFOV as an alternate mode of ventilation in hypoxic respiratory failure where plateau pressure requirements are exceeding 28 cmH_2O (moderate to severe PARDS). In HFOV, optimal lung volume should be achieved by stepwise increase or decrease in the mean airway pressure. The recent PARDS guidelines do not recommend the use of high frequency jet ventilation, high frequency percussive ventilation, or liquid ventilation in children with severe ARDS.

Recent studies in adults have not shown any survival benefit with HFOV compared to the conventional ventilatory strategies (OSCAR and OSCILLATE trials).

Q. Do steroids have any role in the management of acute respiratory distress syndrome?

While a study performed about 2 decades back suggested benefits of administration of steroids in later (fibroproliferative) stages of PARDS, including significant reduction in mortality, the findings were not confirmed in later large trials.

Similarly, the anti-inflammatory actions of steroids have not been shown to be beneficial in the early course of PARDS.

At this stage, neither high doses nor medium doses of corticosteroids can be recommended in PARDS. Low dose steroids are recommended in children with refractory septic shock.

Majority of studies on role of steroids were done before the era of lung protective strategy became the norm. It remains to be seen what would be the effect of steroids when this less injurious and less inflammation ventilation practice is being followed.

Currently, steroids are not recommended for the management of PARDS.

Q. Are there any newer therapies for pediatric acute respiratory distress syndrome?

Newer modes of ventilation

A number of new ventilation modes are being used in the management of ARDS such as APRV, adaptive support ventilation, and neurally adjusted ventilatory assist. However, studies have not conclusively shown mortality benefit or reduction in the number of ventilator days.

Surfactant

Acute respiratory distress syndrome leads to significant surfactant depletion and theoretically replacing surfactant should help in improving lung mechanics and oxygenation. However, pediatric studies showing benefit from surfactant replacement are not convincing to give any clear recommendations for the use of surfactant in severe PARDS.

Inhaled nitrous oxide

Inhaled nitrous oxide (iNO) is a selective pulmonary vasodilator with no significant systemic hemodynamic effects. Inhaled nitric oxide improves V/Q mismatch by improving the pulmonary blood flow and thus would help in improving oxygenation. Pulmonary pressures are also reduced which in turn reduces right ventricular afterload. So there may be an early improvement in oxygenation but the effects are not sustained beyond 1–2 days. Also use of iNO has not shown any mortality benefit.

Presently, the use of inhaled nitric oxide is not recommended for routine use in PARDS. However, it may be considered in patients with documented pulmonary hypertension or severe right ventricular dysfunction.

Q. What is the role of extracorporeal membrane oxygenation in the management of pediatric acute respiratory distress syndrome?

Extracorporeal membrane oxygenation (ECMO) is used to support oxygenation and perfusion to the organs of the body for the time till the lungs heal. The initial studies on ECMO with successful outcomes came from neonatal RDS and have been extrapolated to adults and children. Despite limitations (including very high costs) and high rate of complications, ECMO is being used in children with mixed outcomes. According to the Surviving Sepsis Guidelines 2013, ECMO is reserved for patients with refractory septic shock with respiratory failure, refractory hypoxemia due to severe ARDS and H1N1 pneumonia with respiratory failure.

As per the PARDS guidelines, ECMO should be considered to support children with severe PARDS, where the cause of respiratory failure is believed to be reversible or child is likely to be suitable for lung transplant. It is not possible to apply strict criteria for selection of children for ECMO, so it is recommended that children with severe PARDS should be considered for ECMO when lung protective strategies are not showing much benefit.

Q. What is the guidance for nutrition in pediatric acute respiratory distress syndrome?

Critically ill children in the PICU are in the hypercatabolic state and nutrition usually gets neglected while more aggressive therapy is being instituted for shock, sepsis, ARDS, renal failure, etc. Studies have shown significant malnutrition in such critically ill patients which has a significant impact on the clinical outcomes in terms of morbidity and mortality. Early institution of nutritional support has been shown to contribute to improved outcomes in critically ill children. Enteral rather than the parenteral is the preferred route.

LEARNING POINTS

- Lung protective ventilatory strategies (low tidal volume ventilation with the maintenance of plateau pressures, optimal positive end-expiratory pressure, high inspiratory-time) whenever possible remains the standard of care as it is the only method that has been proven to reduce the mortality rate
- The other therapeutic approach that has improved clinical outcomes in pediatric acute respiratory distress syndrome (ARDS) is the use of a fluid conservative strategy once shock has been resolved
- Good supportive care, early nutrition, early recognition, and management of various complications have resulted in better outcomes in pediatric ARDS
- Advances in extracorporeal membrane oxygenation therapy have regenerated interest as better outcomes with severe ARDS are being shown in recent studies.

SUGGESTED READINGS

1. ARDS Definition Task Force, Ranieri VM, Rubenfeld GD, Thompson BT, et al. Acute respiratory distress syndrome: the Berlin Definition. JAMA. 2012;307:2526-33.
2. Bernard GR, Artigas A, Brigham KL, et al. The American-European Consensus Conference on ARDS. Definitions, mechanisms, relevant outcomes, and clinical trial coordination. Am J Respir Crit Care Med. 1994;149:818-24.
3. Ferguson ND, Cook DJ, Guyatt GH, et al.; OSCILLATE Trial Investigators; Canadian Critical Care Trials Group. High-Frequency oscillation in early acute respiratory distress syndrome. N Engl J Med. 2013;368:795-805.
4. Guérin C, Reignier J, Richard JC, et al.; PROSEVA Study Group. Prone positioning in severe acute respiratory distress syndrome. N Engl J Med. 2013;368:2159-68.
5. Khemani RG, Conti D, Alonzo TA, Bart RD 3rd, Newth CJ. Effect of tidal volume in children with acute hypoxemic respiratory failure. Intensive Care Med. 2009;35:1428-37.
6. Khemani RG, Smith LS, Zimmerman JJ, Erickson S; Pediatric Acute Lung Injury Consensus Conference Group. Pediatric acute respiratory distress syndrome: definition, incidence, and epidemiology: proceedings from the Pediatric Acute Lung Injury Consensus Conference. Pediatr Crit Care Med. 2015;16(5):S23-40.
7. Ventilation with lower tidal volumes as compared with traditional tidal volumes for acute lung injury and the acute respiratory distress syndrome. The Acute Respiratory Distress Syndrome Network. N Engl J Med. 2000;342:1301-8.
8. Young D, Lamb SE, Shah S, et al.; OSCAR Study Group. High-frequency oscillation for acute respiratory distress syndrome. N Engl J Med. 2013;368;806-13.

CHAPTER

41

Nosocomial Pneumonia

Tanu Singhal

CASE 1

An 8-year-old boy presented to the emergency department of a tertiary care hospital during an ongoing influenza outbreak with history of fever and cough of 2 days duration followed by breathlessness. At admission, the child had fever with tachypnea, respiratory rate of 50/min, severe recessions, distress, and oxygen saturation of 80% on room air. Over the next couple of hours, the child needed intubation and mechanical ventilation. The chest X-ray showed extensive bilateral infiltrates with normal blood counts. Empiric therapy with ceftriaxone, azithromycin, and oseltamivir was initiated. The child soon met the criteria for acute respiratory distress syndrome needed increasing ventilator settings over the next 2 days. The nasopharyngeal swab was positive for influenza A. He then started improving. By day 5, the child was on weaning settings and extubation was planned. On day 6, the child had one spike of fever of 102°F and increase in tracheal secretions. The secretions were now thick and yellow. The white blood cell count increased from 10,000 to 16,000 with 80% polymorphs. The ventilator settings increased significantly. The chest X-ray which was previously almost a complete white out did not show any further changes.

Q. What is the differential diagnosis?

Ventilator-associated pneumonia (VAP) appears to be the most likely diagnosis. Ventilator-associated pneumonia is defined as pneumonia occurring in a mechanically ventilated patient at or 48 hours after ventilation. Other ventilator-associated events (VAE) that may cause worsening in a mechanically ventilated child include lobar atelectasis, pulmonary edema, pneumothorax, and rarely acute pulmonary embolism. However, these will not be associated with fever. Conversely, ventilator-associated tracheobronchitis is a close differential of VAP except that there may not be significant clinical respiratory deterioration or radiologic changes.

Q. How will you diagnose VAP?

Early diagnosis is important to achieve good outcomes while over diagnosis leads to excess antibiotic use. However, the diagnosis of VAP is challenging and fraught with debate since the gold standard of lung histology or lung cultures is usually not available. In usual clinical practice, the diagnosis is based on a combination of clinical, radiologic, and microbiologic features. Recently, the Centers for Disease Control proposed new surveillance definitions for VAE, infection-related ventilator-associated complications, possible VAP, and probable VAP. These are mainly surveillance definitions for reporting in adults. Clinical criteria for diagnosis of VAP in children <1 year and those between 1 year and 12 years are detailed in table 1.

TABLE 1: Clinical criteria for diagnosing VAP in children

Children 1–12 years (at least three of the following criteria)	• Fever (>38.4°C or 101.1°F) or hypothermia (<37°C or 97.7°F) with no other apparent cause • Leukopenia (<4,000 WBC/mm^3) or leukocytosis (>15,000 WBC/mm^3) • New onset of purulent sputum, change in character of sputum, increased respiratory secretions, or increased suctioning requirements • Rales or bronchial breath sounds • Worsening gas exchange [O_2 desaturations (pulse oximetry of <94%), increased oxygen requirements, or increased ventilation demand]
Children <1 year: Worsening gas exchange (as defined above) with at least three of the following criteria	• Temperature instability with no other recognized cause • New onset of purulent sputum, change in character of sputum, Increased respiratory secretions, or increased suctioning requirements • Apnea, tachypnea, nasal flaring with retraction of chest wall or grunting, wheezing, rales or rhonchi, cough • Bradycardia (<100 beats/min) or tachycardia (>170 beats/min)

VAP, ventilator-associated pneumonia; WBC, white blood cells.

These criteria have good sensitivity (around 100%), but very poor specificity (15%) for diagnosing VAP. Radiologic criteria also have limitations including poor specificity and interobserver variation. Hence, microbiologic criteria involving culture of respiratory secretions are essential. The lower respiratory tract can be sampled by a variety of methods. Table 2 compares the accuracy of these methods in diagnosis of VAP.

The use of nonbronchoscopic broncho-alveolar lavage (BAL) wherein a suction catheter is inserted till resistance is felt and then a small quantity of saline instilled and withdrawn [presence of bubbles (surfactant) indicating that the lower respiratory tract has been sampled] combines ease with accuracy.

The clinical pulmonary infection score (CPIS) is based on a combination of six criteria (Table 3).

When compared to histopathology, two adult studies reported the sensitivity of CPIS score as 72 and 77%, with a specificity of 85 and 42% respectively. Recently, a simplified CPIS score of 8 (based on clinical, oxygenation, and radiologic criteria) reported a sensitivity of 80%, specificity 80%, positive predictive value 86.9%, and negative predictive value 70.5% in diagnosing VAP in children in an Indian intensive care unit (ICU) when the gold standard was a positive BAL culture of >10^4/mL.

TABLE 2: Comparison of various sampling methods for diagnosis of VAP in children

Technique	Criteria	Sensitivity and specificity
Endotracheal aspirates	105 CFU/mL	Sensitivity 90%, specificity 40%
Bronchoalveolar lavage (BAL)/ nonbronchoscopic BAL	104 CFU/mL	Sensitivity 70–82%, specificity 80–88%
	Bacterial index >5 (sum of log of all species grown)	Sensitivity 78%, specificity 86%, PPV of 70%, and NPV of 90%
	Intracellular bacteria and Gram stain	Sensitivity (30 and 50%), specificity (95% and 81%)
PSB	10^3 CFU/mL	Sensitivity 70%, specificity 90%
PSB and BAL	Quantitative cultures and intracellular bacteria	Sensitivity 88%, specificity 90%

CFU, colony forming units; PSB, protected specimen brush; PPV, positive predictive value; NPV, negative predictive value.

TABLE 3: Clinical pulmonary infection score calculation

Parameter	Score
Temperature (°C)	
36.5–38.4	0
38.5–38.9	1
≥39.0 and ≤36.0	2
Blood leukocyte level, leukocytes/mm^3	
4,000–11,000	0
<4,000 or >11,000	1
Plus band forms ≥500	2
Tracheal secretions	
<14+	0
≥14 +	1
Plus purulence 2	2
Oxygenation PaO_2:FiO_2	
>240 or ARDS	0
≤240 or no ARDS	2
Pulmonary radiograph finding	
No infiltrate	0
Diffuse or patchy infiltrate	1
Localized infiltrate	2
Culture of tracheal aspirate specimen (semiquantitative: 0–1, –2, or 3+)	
Pathogenic bacteria cultured ≤1 or no growth	0
Pathogenic bacteria cultured >1+	1
Plus same pathogenic bacteria on Gram stain >1+	2

ARDS, acute respiratory distress syndrome; PaO_2:FiO_2, ratio of partial pressure of arterial oxygen to the fraction of inspired oxygen.

Diagnostic algorithm for VAP is suggested in flowchart 1.

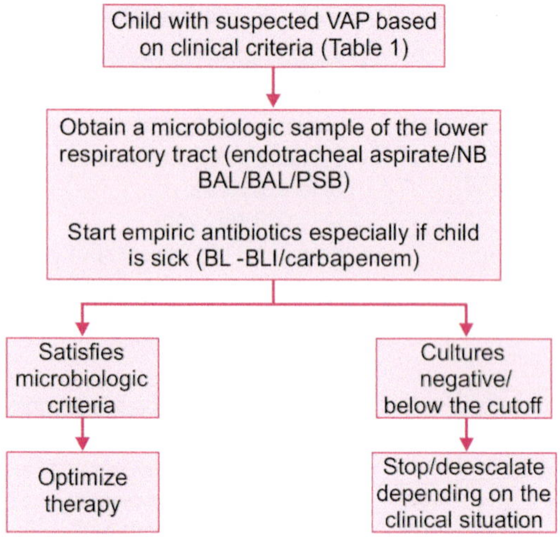

VAP, ventilator-associated pneumonia; NB BAL, nonbronchoscopic bronchoalveolar lavage; BAL, bronchoalveolar lavage; PSB, protected specimen brush; BL-BLI, β-lactam-β-lactamase inhibitor.

Flowchart 1: Diagnostic and management algorithm for ventilator-associated pneumonia

Q. How common is VAP and which are the causative organisms?

Ventilator-associated pneumonia is the second commonest hospital-associated infection in critically ill children and neonates and develops in 3–10% of pediatric intensive care unit patients (as against 15–30% in adults). Neonatal intensive care unit VAP rates vary from 1.4–3.5/1,000 ventilator days National (Nosocomial Infection Surveillance system of the US). Indian studies have reported higher rates varying from 17.5% to 32.5%.

The etiology of VAP in children is generally independent of the duration of ventilation (unlike adults). Most studies from India in both adults and children have incriminated multidrug resistant Gram-negative pathogens including *Acinetobacter*, *Pseudomonas*, *Klebsiella*, *Escherichia coli*, *Enterobacter* as causative agents; Gram-positive organisms including methicillin-resistant *Staphylococcus aureus* (MRSA) have been infrequently reported.

Q. What empirical therapy will you start?

Empirical antibiotic cover for hospital-acquired pneumonia is determined by prior antibiotic use, local pathogens and their susceptibilities, data from surveillance cultures if available, Gram stain of the pulmonary secretions, degree of sickness, host comorbidities and finally pharmacokinetics, and pulmonary penetration of various antibiotics.

In view of the etiologic and resistance profile in Indian ICUs, use of agents active against extended-spectrum β-lactamase producing Gram-negative pathogens such as piperacillin tazobactam/cefoperazone sulbactam with or without an aminoglycoside should be chosen. In a sick patient with severe sepsis, a carbapenem such as meropenem or imipenem is preferred. In some units where carbapenem resistance is high, empirical use of colistin in very sick patients is sometimes necessary. A MRSA cover should be given if the MRSA rates in the ICU (>20%) are high or if the Gram stain of endotracheal aspirate shows Gram-positive cocci; there is some data to suggest that linezolid may be superior to vancomycin for pneumonia. There is no data to support routine use of inhalational antibiotics in VAP.

Q. How will you modify therapy and what should be the duration?

Therapy should be optimized (either escalation/deescalation) once the culture results are available. If the cultures are negative or below the cutoff, antibiotics may be stopped depending on the clinical condition and if an alternative explanation has emerged. This may not always be possible since the sensitivity of these methods is not 100%, especially if the patient has been on antibiotics. If an anti MRSA drug was started empirically, it should be stopped if no MRSA is isolated. Combination therapy can be deescalated to monotherapy if possible.

There are no clear recommendations regarding duration of therapy in both adult and childhood VAP. A multicentric randomized trial in adults, however, demonstrated that 8 days therapy was noninferior to 15 days therapy in VAP due to organisms other than nonfermenting Gram-negative bacilli (*Pseudomonas* and *Acinetobacter*).

Q. What is the likely prognosis?

Ventilator-associated pneumonia is known to significantly increase mortality, antibiotic use, duration of mechanical ventilation, hospital stay, and treatment costs. The difference in mortality rates in critically ill children with and without VAP was reported as 13% in one international study.

Q. What can be done to prevent nosocomial pneumonia?

The preventive measures target prevention of either colonization/aspiration or inhalation of pathogenic bacteria. In nonventilated patients especially following surgery, early mobilization, adequate pain control, and breathing exercises lower the risk of postoperative atelectasis and pneumonia. Strict asepsis should be maintained during intubation and suctioning. Only sterile water should be used in humidifiers and the nebulizer sets should be dry before use.

Evidence-based recommendations from the Society for Healthcare Epidemiology of America recommend the following strategies as most effective in reducing risk of VAP in children: use noninvasive positive pressure ventilation for selected populations, assessing readiness to extubate daily using spontaneous breathing trials in patients without contraindications, avoiding unplanned extubations, providing regular oral care (i.e., tooth brushing or gauze if no teeth), elevating the head of the bed to 30–45°, changing of ventilator circuits only if visibly soiled or malfunctioning, preventing gastric overdistension, and in older children using cuffed endotracheal tubes and endotracheal tubes with subglottic suction ports. The superiority of closed inline suctioning over open suction is still debated. Strategies of no clear benefit include use of systemic antibiotics to treat tracheobronchitis, stress ulcer prophylaxis, and selective oral and gut decontamination.

LEARNING POINTS

- Ventilator-associated pneumonia (VAP) should be suspected in a mechanically ventilated child with symptoms of fever, leukocytosis/leukopenia, purulent/excessive tracheal secretions, new infiltrates on chest X-ray and increased ventilatory requirements
- The microbiologic confirmation of VAP is by quantitative cultures of endotracheal aspirates/ bronchoscopic lavage
- Empirical therapy for VAP in the Indian setting usually comprises of a β–lactam–β–lactam inhibitor combination or carbapenems
- Antibiotic therapy for only positive tracheal cultures should be avoided
- Each critical care unit should implement a comprehensive VAP prevention bundle.

SUGGESTED READINGS

1. Branson R, Klompas M, Eichenwald EC, Greene LR, Howell MD, Lee G, et al. Strategies to prevent ventilator-associated pneumonia in acute care hospitals: 2014 update. Infect Control Hosp Epidemiol. 2014;35 Suppl 2:S133-54.
2. Foglia E, Meier MD, Elward A. Ventilator-associated pneumonia in neonatal and pediatric intensive care unit patients. Clin Microbiol Rev. 2007;20:409-25.
3. Lodha R, Kabra SK. Diagnosis of ventilator-associated pneumonia: is there a simple solution? Indian Pediatr. 2011;48:939-40.
4. Proulx F, Gauvin F, Dassa C, Chaïbou M, Farrell CA, Lacroix J. Ventilator-associated pneumonia in intubated children: comparison of different diagnostic methods. Pediatr Crit Care Med. 2003;4:437-43.
5. Tullu MS, Balasubramanian P. Study of ventilator-associated pneumonia in a pediatric intensive care unit. Indian J Pediatr. 2014;81:1182-6.
6. Zilberberg MD, Shorr AF. Ventilator-associated pneumonia: the clinical pulmonary infection score as a surrogate for diagnostics and outcome. Clin Infect Dis. 2010;51 Suppl 1:S131-5.

9

SECTION

Miscellaneous Respiratory Disorders

CHAPTER

42

Foreign Body Aspiration

Jagdish P Goyal

CASE 1

An 8-year-old male child presented with complaint of fever, cough and respiratory difficulty for 7 days.

Past medical history: Recurrent respiratory tract infection.

Physical examination: Tachypnea and decreased air entry on left side with crepitation. No wheeze.

Family history: No family history of asthma and allergy.

Investigations: Hemoglobin 10.3 g/dL, total leukocyte count (TLC) 18.5 × 10^3/μL, differential leukocyte count showed 88% neutrophils, 8% lymphocytes, 2% monocytes, and 2% eosinophils. Chest X-ray showed left side pleural effusion with underlying collapse (Fig. 1).

Ultrasonography (USG) thorax revealed very minimal free fluid with underlying consolidation at left costophrenic angle. USG showed few enlarged sub-centric lymph node in para-aortic region. Mantoux test with 5 tuberculin units was negative. Sputum for acid-fast bacillus was also negative for three occasions. Blood culture was sterile. Pleural tapping was done and antibiotics were started. On 5th day of admission at hospital patient had sudden respiratory arrest. Relatives provided history that child was trying to cough out. Patient had been intubated and kept on ventilator. Patient's Glasgow coma scale (GCS) was 8 and on next day neurological status further deteriorated with GCS of 4. Deep tendon and superficial reflexes were absent (probably due to excessive dose of sedative). Patient was investigated considering that he had acute central nervous system infection. His investigation suggested normal blood sugar and electrolytes, malaria parasite—negative, cerebrospinal fluid—normal, and magnetic resonance imaging of brain was normal. Patient was continued with ventilator support and gradually improved (GCS improved to 15) and weaned from ventilator in 2 days. Patient had similar X-ray pictures. Total leukocyte count was 11.5 × 10^3/μL and C-reactive protein (CRP) was 60 mg/dL, so antibiotics were changed. Again after 4 days, patient had similar episode. He had sudden respiratory arrest while coughing and again intubated and kept on ventilator.

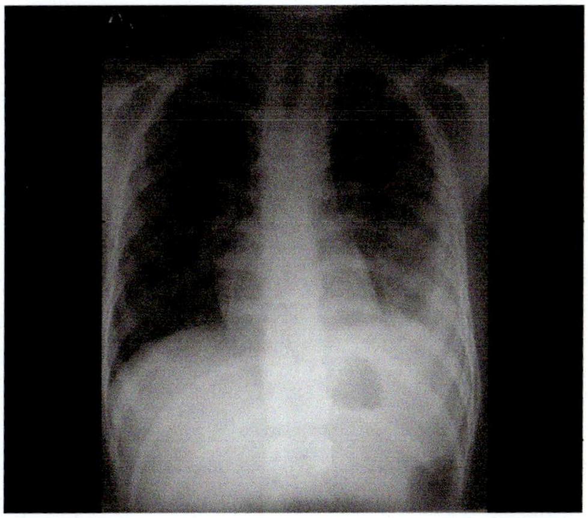

Figure 1: Left-side pleural effusion with underlying collapse

Q. What are the differential diagnoses in this case?

The differentials in this case could be:

- Airway abnormalities: Usual presenting symptom in congenital airway abnormalities is noisy breathing. However, respiratory symptoms are sometimes evident only with comorbid conditions and upper respiratory tract infections. Though child had history of recurrent respiratory tract infections with decreased air entry on left side so bronchomalacia of left side was kept as diagnostic possibility, but child had no history of noisy breathing or wheeze which pointed against airway abnormalities. Bronchoscopy helps in delineating airway abnormalities
- Foreign body aspiration: As child had history of recurrent respiratory tract infections with decreased air entry on left side. Along with, the recurrent sudden respiratory arrests that improved rapidly, strongly suggest foreign body aspiration (FBA)
- Congenital lung abnormities: Recurrent pneumonia on same side of lung is a feature of congenital lung malformation. This child had history of recurrent respiratory infections and decrease air entry on left side. So, possibility of congenital lung malformation should be kept in mind which may be ruled out by computed tomography (CT) scan of chest if indicated.

Q. When one should suspect a FBA?

A FBA should be suspected in following conditions:

- When child presents with history of sudden onset cough, choking, and respiratory distress with no previous history of asthma
- Unilateral chest examination findings (may be decreased air entry, wheezing, dull on percussion or hyper-resonant depending on complete obstruction or ball-valve mechanism by foreign body)
- Repeated sudden worsening of respiratory symptoms (may be due to mobile foreign body)
- Persistent unilateral findings on chest X-ray (collapse or hyperinflation) with no alternative explanation. History of FBA may not be there.

Q. What is epidemiology of FBA in children?

Foreign body aspiration most commonly occurs in children <4 years. Foreign body aspiration is potentially a life-threatening event and sixth most common cause of accidental death in children in United States. Serious complication due to FBA occurs in 10–20% of case. Organic (peanuts, grams, or nuts) FBA is far more common than inorganic.

Q. What are clinical features of FBA in children?

Clinical features may be divided as per location of foreign body, e.g., laryngeal, tracheal, and bronchial. Laryngeal FBA may lead to hoarseness of voice, barking cough mimicking croup, inspiratory stridor, odynophagia, and acute airway obstruction with cyanosis. Tracheal FBA may present as stridor, wheezing and dyspnea. Bronchial FBA is most common and may present as classical triad of cough, wheezing, and unilaterally decreased breath sound. Obstructive emphysema (ball valve like), atelectasis and recurrent pneumonia or non-resolving pneumonia also indicate possibility of bronchial FBA.

Q. How do we confirm a diagnosis of FBA?

Bronchoscopy is the next step in confirming diagnosis as well as ruling out other causes such as airway abnormalities. It will also help in removal of the foreign body.

Case Progression

On further questioning, parents revealed a history of sudden chocking 5 years back which almost confirms FBA. Bronchoscopy was done and foreign body in left lower lobe bronchus was found which was removed with rigid bronchoscope. Later on, child improved rapidly.

CASE 2

An 18-month-old female child presented to pediatric emergency with history of cough and respiratory difficulty for 2 days.

Past medical history: Episodic wheeze.

Physical examination: Afebrile, tachypneic, and decreased air entry on right side with bilateral wheeze.

Family history: Family history of asthma in grandmother.

Investigations: Hemogram was normal, and chest X-ray showed left lung hyperinflation and a collapsed right lung with mediastinal shift (Fig. 2)

Q. What is your assessment of the case?

This child presented with history of cough and respiratory difficulty for 2 days. Child was an episodic wheezer. She was tachypneic having bilateral wheeze with air entry reduced on right side. Based on clinical features and X-ray findings FBA was suspected.

Q. What are the differential diagnoses in this case?

The differentials in this case could be:

- Obstruction of right bronchus with thick mucus plus
- Airway abnormalities
- Acute exacerbation of asthma
- Left-side emphysema.

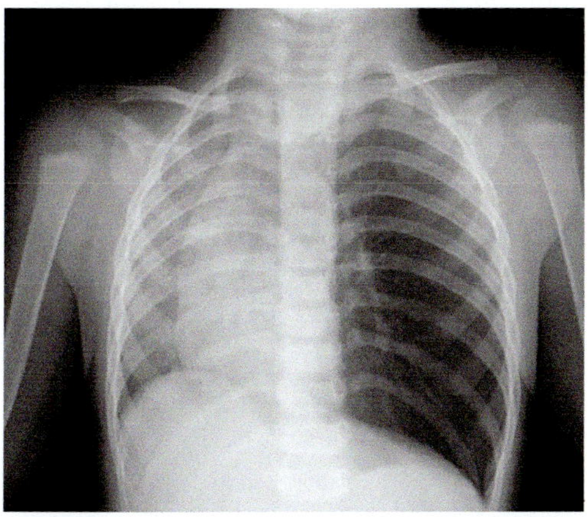

Figure 2: X-ray showing collapse of right lung with hyperinflation of left lung and mediastinal shifting toward right side

Q. What is the most appropriate next step?

Most appropriate next step would be bronchoscopy which was done and peanut was found in left main bronchus. Peanut was causing "ball-valve" like effect leading to emphysema. It was removed and child became asymptomatic. She was discharged on antibiotics and chest physiotherapy. Her pre discharge X-ray chest was normal.

Q. What are the learning points from this case?

This case suggests that FBA should be suspected in a patient who has presented with sudden onset of respiratory difficulty with X-ray showing atelectasis and hyperinflation even if no history of FBA.

CASE 3

Three-year-old male child presented to pediatric emergency with history of sudden onset of respiratory distress for 2 hours while he was eating with his elder sibling. History of choking and cyanosis was also present. There was no history of fever.

Past medical history: None.

Physical examination: Afebrile, tachypneic and decrease air entry on right side.

Family history: No family history of asthma and allergy.

Investigations: Complete blood count and X-ray chest was normal.

Q. How will you analyze this case?

This child had presented with sudden onset of respiratory distress with no significant past history. Breath sounds were diminished on right side. Even though X-ray was normal, child was suspected to have FBA.

Q. What are the differential diagnoses in this case?

- Aspiration or foreign body
- Airway anomaly
- Gastroesophageal reflux disease
- Congenital heart disease
- Dysrhythmia
- Seizure.

Q. What are the important points in history?

- History of sudden choking and cyanosis
- History of noisy breathing since birth
- History of underlying cardiac disorder
- History of feeding difficulty
- History of loss of consciousness.

Q. What is the most likely diagnosis?

Based on history and clinical examination most likely diagnosis is FBA.

Q. How FBA can be diagnosed?

Chest radiograph is initial modality for diagnosis. Fluoroscopy being a dynamic modality may be very useful when chest skiagram in inspiratory phase is inconclusive. In children, low-dose multidetector CT (MDCT) scan and virtual bronchoscopy are noninvasive tools for diagnosis of FBA and can be used where facilities are available. MRI with T1 image is helpful in diagnosis of peanut fragments in lower airway. Bronchoscopy can be used as diagnostic as well as therapeutic tool.

Q. What is management of FBA in children?

Initial management of FBA is airway support. Ensure open airway before proceeding to any diagnostic or therapeutic intervention.

In a witnessed foreign body aspiration with acute symptoms in outside hospital settings

If child is active or coughing, he or she should encourage coughing so that foreign body can be expelled. In case child is not able to cough, Heimlich's maneuver can be used to try to expel the foreign body. In infants alternate five chest thrusts or five back blows should be used instead of Heimlich's maneuver because of risk of injury to abdomen viscera in Heimlich's maneuver.

In hospital settings

If there is history of FBA or diagnosis almost certain, we can go directly for rigid bronchoscopy for diagnosis and removal of foreign body. If diagnosis of FBA is uncertain and there are other differential diagnoses, flexible bronchoscopy can be first performed and then rigid bronchoscopy may be used to remove foreign body if it is found. Only very few centers in world remove foreign body by flexible bronchoscope.

Q. What is most appropriate next step?

Most appropriate next step would be bronchoscopy in this case. Bronchoscopy was done and vegetative foreign body was found in right main bronchus which was removed.

Q. What are the learning points in this case?

Foreign body aspiration should always be considered as a differential diagnosis in any child with history of choking and sudden onset of respiratory distress along with normal chest X-ray. Because chest X-ray inspiratory film may be normal in a case of FBA.

LEARNING POINTS

- Foreign body aspiration (FBA) has variable clinical presentation in children
- Foreign body aspiration should be considered in a patient who has presented with sudden onset of respiratory difficulty with X-ray showing unilateral atelectasis and hyperinflation even if no history of FBA
- Foreign body aspiration should always be kept in differential diagnosis in a child with history of choking and sudden onset of respiratory distress despite normal chest X-ray.

SUGGESTED READINGS

1. Bertelli L, Gentili A, Modolon C, Corsini I, Cazzato S. A foreign body aspiration in a preschool child mimicking a multitrigger wheezing: a case report and review of the literature. Pediatr Emerg Care. 2012;28:1382-4.
2. Boufersaoui A, Smati L, Benhalla KN, Boukari R, Smail S, Anik K, et al. Foreign body aspiration in children: experience from 2,624 patients. Int J Pediatr Otorhinolaryngol. 2013;77:1683-8.
3. Chung PH, Wong KK, Lan LC, Tam PK. Peanut aspiration: an avoidable life-threatening condition. Hong Kong Med J. 2012;18:340-2.
4. Holinger LD. Foreign bodies of airways. In: Kliegman RE, Stanton BF, Schor NF, St Geme EW, Behrman RE (Eds). Nelson Textbook of Pediatrics, 19th edition. Philadelphia: Saunders, an imprint of Elsevier Inc; 2011. pp. 1453-4.
5. Yadav SP, Singh J, Aggarwal N, Goel A. Airway foreign bodies in children: experience of 132 cases. Singapore Med J. 2007;48:850-3.

CHAPTER 43

Hydrocarbon Aspiration

Rakesh K Dogra

CASE 1

Urmilla, a 3-year-old female child was brought to the pediatric emergency department with history of ingestion of kerosene oil stored in a polyethylene terephthalate (PET) bottle 1 hour back. She was conscious, oriented, afebrile and was interested in her surroundings. Her clothes smelt of kerosene. Her respiratory rate was 30/min and pulse rate was 92/min. On chest examination, air entry was equal on both sides and there were no added sounds.

Q. To which group of compounds does kerosene oil belong? What are the commonest modes of presentation? What are other members of the group?

Liquid hydrocarbons are by-products of petroleum and are widely used for industrial and household purpose. Kerosene, petrol, lubricating oils or motor oils, lighter fluid, diesel, lamp oil, etc. are examples of commonly used liquid hydrocarbons. Kerosene is commonly used as cooking fuel in several households in developing countries. Accidental aspiration is the most common cause of human exposure, especially in young children. Kerosene oil aspiration is the most common hydrocarbon aspiration seen in children. Hydrocarbon ingestion leading to pneumonitis is relatively rare and occurs in approximately 2% of cases. Aspiration of hydrocarbons by young children typically is an unintentional occurrence and ingestion of large quantities of hydrocarbons by children is unusual because of its foul taste. In contrast, hydrocarbon aspiration in teenagers usually occurs intentionally (e.g., suicidal attempt, recreational use, or siphoning of gasoline).

There are four structural classes of hydrocarbons. The classes with their common examples and uses are provided in table 1.

Q. What are the determinants of aspiration and toxicity of hydrocarbons?

Determinants of aspiration: The aspiration potential of the hydrocarbons is determined by three properties:

1. Volatility: The ability to vaporize or to exist in a gaseous form
2. Surface tension: The adherence or cohesiveness of molecules along a liquid surface; lower surface tension allows compounds to spread over a large area
3. Viscosity: The resistance to flow through an orifice or the tendency of a compound to resist stirring. Lower viscosity facilitates deeper penetration into the tracheobronchial tree

The aspiration hazard of hydrocarbons is inversely related to viscosity and surface tension and directly related to volatility. Thus, hydrocarbons with decreased viscosity, low

TABLE 1: Classification of hydrocarbons

S. No.	Group	Examples	Use
1.	• Aromatic hydrocarbons ○ Cyclic compounds containing a benzene ring	• Benzene • Toluene • Xylene	• Used primarily in solvents, glues, nail polish, paints, and paint removers. • Huffable
2.	• Halogenated hydrocarbons ○ They are fluorinated, chlorinated, or brominated	• Methylene chloride chloroform • Carbon tetrachloride • Trichloroethylene • Tetrachloroethylene	• Solvent, paint stripper, spot remover, white out
3.	• Terpene hydrocarbons	• Turpentine oil • Pine oil	• Solvent, paint thinner • Cleaner, disinfectant
4.	• Aliphatic hydrocarbons	• Petroleum distillates	• Cooking fuel, furniture polish, lamp oil • Lighter fluid

surface tension, and high volatility are more likely to be aspirated and cause pulmonary injury. The low viscosity permits greater penetration into the distal airways while the low surface tension facilitates spread over a greater area. As an example, simple petroleum distillates (kerosene, gasoline, liquid furniture polish) are chiefly aspiration hazards. They have high potential to cause aspiration pneumonitis, but rarely cause systemic symptoms. Chemical properties of various petroleum substances are shown in box 1

Box 1: Chemical properties of petroleum compounds

- Viscosity ↓
- Volatility ↑
- Compound
  - Gasoline
  - Naptha
  - Mineral spirits
  - Kerosene
  - Mineral seal oils
  - Mineral oil
  - Motor oil
  - Petroleum jelly
  - Paraffin

- Determinants of toxicity: with the exception of aromatic and halogenated compounds, most hydrocarbons cause clinical toxicity only when aspirated or inhaled because they are poorly absorbed through the gastrointestinal tract. The systemic toxicity of hydrocarbons is determined by their volatility.

CASE 2

Sunny, a 4-year-old male child was brought to pediatric emergency department with history of ingestion of some unknown liquid while playing at his neighbor's house which was being painted. On detailed questioning, it was found that he had consumed the liquid that was being used to polish the furniture and contained mixture of few chemicals. He had vomited the liquid immediately after consuming it. On examination, he was restless, irritable with respiratory rate of 60/min and heart rate of 130/min and signs of respiratory distress with SpO_2 of 88% in room air. He had bilateral coarse crepitations on chest examination.

Q. What is the immediate management of this case?

Immediate attention to airways, breathing, and circulation (ABC) is of utmost importance. Stabilize vitals and maintain oxygen saturations at ≥92%. Ascertain the exact contents of the container by asking a detailed history, as many a time they are mixed with agents having systemic toxicity such as camphor, aniline dyes, heavy metals, and pesticides. Immediate decontamination of the patient by removing clothes, cleaning of skin, and flushing eyes with plenty of water if any redness, swelling, or lacrimation is present is important to prevent further exposure. Initial management should comprise of history, physical examination, and chest radiograph.

Q. What are indications for gastric lavage in hydrocarbon poisoning?

Because hydrocarbons do less damage when swallowed than when aspirated into the lungs, it is important to avoid emetics or gastric lavage because of increased risk of aspiration after such procedures. However, lavage is indicated in ingestion of certain hydrocarbons and under certain circumstances such as:

- Ingestion of compounds with systemic toxic effects, e.g., halogenated and aromatic hydrocarbons
- Petroleum distillates containing toxic additives like heavy metals or insecticides
- Large volume ingestion as in suicidal attempt.

Pneumonic CHAMP is frequently used for such situations and stands for Camphor containing compounds, Halogenated hydrocarbons, Aromatic hydrocarbons, heavy Metal containing hydrocarbons, Pesticide containing hydrocarbons.

Q. What is the clinical course of hydrocarbon aspiration?

Immediate aspiration manifests in the form of coughing, choking sensation, gagging, and vomiting.

- Aspiration usually follows vomiting which might be spontaneous or induced
- Cough usually appears within 30 minutes of aspiration
- 30–60% of patients with hydrocarbon aspiration have fever at the time of presentation (38–40°C)
- Any amount of aspiration could lead to pulmonary manifestations, with a lag of 12–24 hours in some cases
- Respiratory findings include—tachypnea, dyspnea, cyanosis, diminished resonance on percussion, suppressed or tubular breath sounds, and crackles in any combination
- Severe injury manifests in the form of hemoptysis, pulmonary edema, and respiratory failure developing within 24 hours. In 88% of cases, radiographic signs develop within 2 hours and majority will develop signs within 6–12 hours
- Blood gases might reveal hypoxemia without hypercapnia suggestive of V/Q mismatch or diffusion block. Destruction of airway epithelium and bronchospasm adds to V/Q abnormalities. Displacement of alveolar gas by hydrocarbon vapors adds to hypoxemia.

Q. What are the common radiographic findings in cases of hydrocarbon aspiration?

The radiographic findings include—punctate mottled densities, fine perihilar infiltrates, features of pneumonia, air trapping atelectasis, pleural effusion, pulmonary edema, and white out. Pneumatoceles are seen as late manifestation. These findings are predominantly found in dependent portion of the lungs.

Q. What are the indications for admission and discharge of patients of hydrocarbon aspiration?

If patient is asymptomatic in the emergency room with a normal chest radiograph, observation for 6–8 hours is important and if no symptoms develop, the patient can be discharged. Arterial blood gas analysis should be performed in case of any abnormality in history, examination, or chest radiograph. In case of abnormal examination, chest radiograph, or blood gas, admit the child and start symptomatic management and assess need for ventilator support. Consider transfer to pediatric intensive care unit (PICU) under such circumstances. If patient is asymptomatic and results of examination and chest radiograph are normal after 24 hours, patient can be discharged after providing education regarding prevention of future recurrence to the family.

Q. How will you manage a case of hydrocarbon aspiration?

Supplemental oxygen must be given if the patient is hypoxemic. Adequate hydration should be maintained carefully as fluid overload can be counterproductive as pulmonary pathology evolves. Trial of bronchodilators can be given in case of progression of respiratory symptoms. Hypoxemic respiratory failure should be treated with mechanical ventilation and positive end-expiratory pressure. Extracorporeal membrane oxygenation and high-frequency jet ventilation are other modalities helpful in improving oxygenation where conventional ventilation fails. An approach to manage hydrocarbon is shown in flowchart 1.

Q. What is role of antibiotics in cases of hydrocarbon aspiration? Is there any role of corticosteroids in the management of these cases?

Superimposed bacterial infection is difficult to detect because leukocytosis and fever are common after hydrocarbon aspiration; however, superimposed bacterial infection is not a common occurrence. Antibiotics are indicated in selected circumstances such as:

- Presence of organism on Gram staining from endotracheal tube
- Positive cultures of endotracheal tube
- Patients severely compromised by malnutrition, debilitation, or underlying chronic disease
- Severe pneumonia.

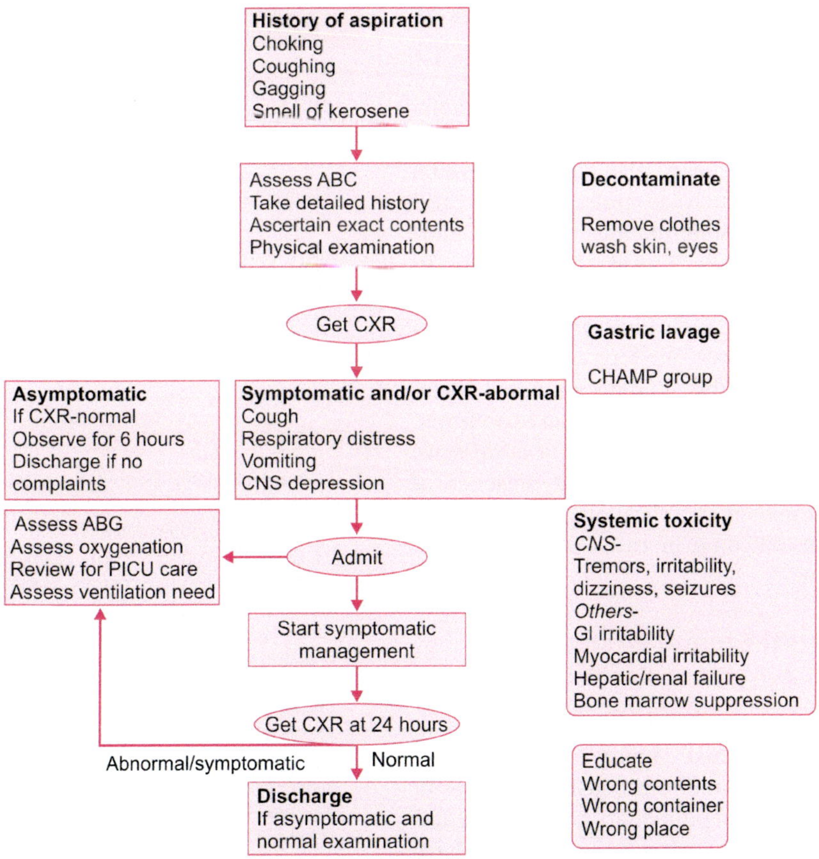

CXR, chest X-ray; CNS, central nervous system; PICU, pediatric intensive care unit; GI, gastrointestinal; ABC, airways, breathing and circulation; ABG, arterial blood gas.

Flowchart 1: Algorithm for management of hydrocarbon aspiration

There is no therapeutic or prophylactic role for corticosteroids in hydrocarbon aspiration.

Q. What are the complications of hydrocarbon aspiration? What are predictors of poor outcome?

The major pulmonary complications of hydrocarbon aspiration include:

- Asphyxia, necrotizing chemical pneumonitis, lipoid pneumonia, and hemorrhagic pulmonary edema, progressing to shock and respiratory arrest
- Pneumothorax, subcutaneous emphysema of the chest wall, and pleural effusion, including empyema, may also occur
- Secondary infection with bacteria or viruses, although rare, may occur
- Pneumatoceles may develop in areas of extensive consolidation during the recovery period.

High-resolution computed tomography (CT) scan is helpful in the diagnosis of lipoid pneumonia and can also detect possible complications, such as pneumatoceles and pneumothorax. Abnormalities on chest radiographs usually take 2 weeks to 8 months to clear with no or minimal scarring. Pulmonary function studies indicate residual injury to peripheral airways in long-term; however, significance of this finding is not known. History of prior lavage, presence of hypoxemia, secondary bacterial pneumonia at admission, need for ventilator support and presence of ventilator-related complications are associated with poor outcome in cases of hydrocarbon aspiration.

Q. What is the role of exogenous surfactant in management of hydrocarbon aspiration?

Lung parenchymal injury in cases of hydrocarbon aspiration is considered as result of direct toxicity to pulmonary parenchyma and disruption of the surfactant layer. There have been few recent case reports of use of exogenous surfactant successfully in patients developing acute respiratory distress syndrome (ARDS) following hydrocarbon aspiration. However, there is no definitive role of administration of exogenous surfactant at present in cases of hydrocarbon aspiration.

Q. What preventive steps can be taken to avoid hydrocarbon aspiration or poisoning?

Educating the family to keep the potential toxic material out of reach of children and to avoid storage of such liquids in containers, like polyethylene terephthalate (PET) bottles, which children associate with commonly used drinks in the household. Immediate decontamination of the child as explained earlier prevents further exposure.

LEARNING POINTS

- All petroleum distillates are hydrocarbons, but not all hydrocarbons are petroleum distillates. They are often mixed with dyes, heavy metals, and pesticides resulting in systemic toxicity
- The aspiration hazard of hydrocarbons is inversely related to viscosity and surface tension and directly related to volatility
- Symptomatic treatment is the mainstay of management
- There is no role of prophylactic antibiotics and corticosteroids.

SUGGESTED READINGS

1. Horoz OO, Yildizdas D, Yilmaz HL. Surfactant therapy in acute respiratory distress syndrome due to hydrocarbon aspiration. Singapore Med J. 2009;50(4):e130.
2. Jayashree M, Singhi S, Gupta A. Predictors of outcome in children with hydrocarbon poisoning receiving intensive care. Indian Pediatr. 2006;43(8):715-9.
3. Lee A, Bye MR, Mellins RB. Lung injury from hydrocarbon aspiration and smoke inhalation. In: Robert W, Bush A, Boat TF, Deterding RR, Ratjen F, Chernick V (Eds). Kendig and Chernick's Disorders of the Respiratory Tract in Children, 8th edition. Philadelphia: Elsevier; 2012.
4. Mastropietro CW, Valentine K. Early administration of intratracheal surfactant (calfactant) after hydrocarbon aspiration. Pediatrics. 2011;127(6):e1600-4.
5. Osterhoudt KC, Burns Ewald M, Shannon M, Henretig FM. Toxicologic emergencies. In: Fleisher, GR, Ludwig, S, Henretig, FM (Eds). Textbook of Pediatric Emergency Medicine, 5th ed. Philadelphia: Lippincott, Williams & Wilkins;, 2006. p. 951.

CHAPTER

44

Tumors of Lung and Chest Wall

Latha M Sneha, Julius X Scott, Sivabalan X Somu

CASE 1

A 12-year-old boy presented with complaints of fever and cough for 1 week and progressive breathlessness for 5 days. He was treated empirically with oral antibiotics and oral bronchodilators by his private practitioner at his native place. In view of persistence of symptoms after 10 days, he was referred to a private hospital. On examination he was found to be afebrile, tachypneic, and had decreased air entry in the right side. X ray chest revealed opacity in the right upper and middle lobe with right-sided pleural effusion (Fig. 1). A chest drain was inserted and he was started on intravenous antibiotics. With no resolution of symptoms after a week, a computed tomography chest was done which showed homogenous soft tissue component in the right upper and midzone with right-sided pleural effusion (Fig. 2).

Q. What is likely diagnosis in this patient?

This 12-year-old boy presented with fever and cough and his X-ray film of chest shows opacities involving right upper and middle zone and computed tomography (CT) chest showing soft tissue mass causing collapse of right upper lobe and lower lobe with ill-defined expansile lytic lesion in the posterior aspect of 5th rib. Overall clinical picture suggests a mass lesion that is arising from ribs and going inside thoracic cavity. More likely to be primitive neuroectodermal tumor.

Q. How to proceed to confirm diagnosis of this tumor?

Diagnosis can be established by biopsy of the tumor. In this child initially pleural fluid cytology attempted but was negative for malignant cells. Biopsy of the mass revealed primitive neuroectodermal tumor. He was started on chemotherapy and there was a complete resolution of the lung mass after two cycles and undergoing treatment now.

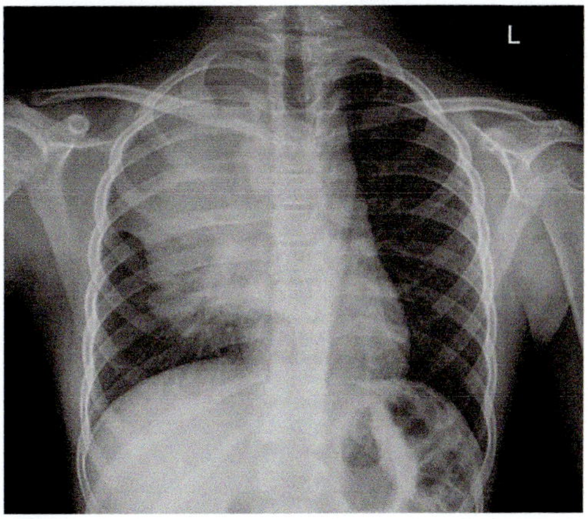

Figure 1: X-ray chest showing homogenous opacity in right upper and midzone

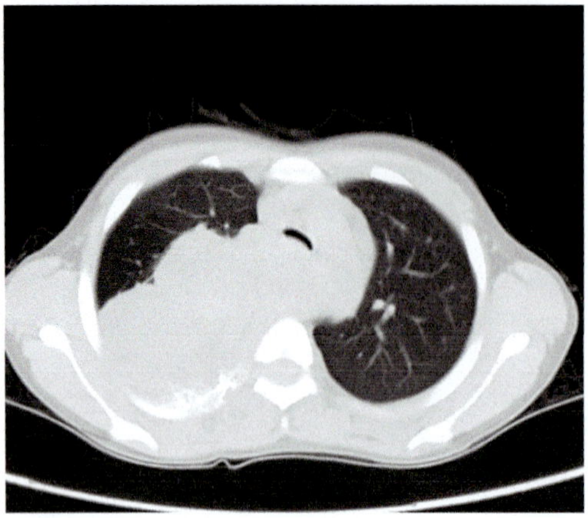

Figure 2: Computed tomography chest showing soft tissue mass causing collapse of right upper lobe and lower lobe with ill-defined expansile lytic lesion in the posterior aspect of 5th rib

CASE 2

A 3-year-old boy presented to his primary physician with cough and wheeze of 2 weeks duration. X-ray chest revealed bilateral patchy consolidation (Fig. 3). He was started on antibiotics and there was no symptomatic resolution after 1 month. Hence, child was referred to a higher center for persistent cough and wheeze with abnormal X-ray chest.

Q. What are diagnostic possibilities?

This 3-year-old child has cough and wheeze with X-ray showing multiple well-defined circumscribed opacities in all the lung fields. The differential diagnosis for such opacities includes tumor metastasis or multiple cysts like hydatid cysts.

Detailed history suggests that child was treated for Wilms' tumor; therefore, it is likely to be recurrence of Wilms' tumor.

Q. How to confirm diagnosis of recurrence of Wilms' tumor with metastasis in lungs?

Initial workup may include imaging of chest in form of positron emission tomography (PET) CT and biopsy of the lesion if possible.

In this child, a detailed history taking revealed that he had completed chemotherapy for stage II Wilms' tumor 2 years ago. Considering this history of malignancy in the past, a CT chest was done which showed coin-shaped shadows suggesting metastasis of tumor (Fig. 4). Positron emission tomography scan revealed increased uptake in the lungs and biopsy of the lung lesion was confirmatory of relapsed Wilms' tumor. Initial X-ray chest reported as pneumonia, was in fact a metastatic lesion.

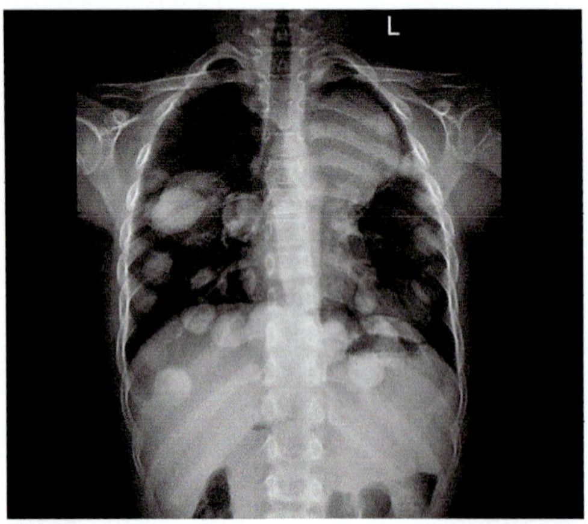

Figure 3: X-ray chest showing multiple bilateral nodular opacities

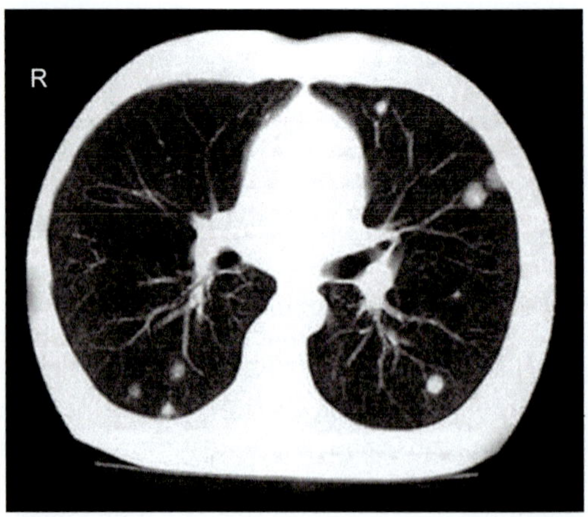

Figure 4: Computed tomography (CT) chest showing multiple nodules in the upper region of both lung parenchyma and left pleura, suggestive of pulmonary metastasis

Q. What are common lung tumors in children?

Primary lung tumors are rare in children. Lung masses in children are 10 times more likely to represent a benign developmental or a reactive lesion than a neoplasm. Common malformations forming solid and cystic masses are bronchogenic cyst, segmental bronchial atresia, intralobar and extralobar pulmonary sequestration, congenital pulmonary airway malformation, and congenital lobar over inflation.

Majority of the pulmonary neoplasms in children are due to metastatic disease, with a ratio of primary malignant tumors to metastatic disease being 1:5. The most common malignant primary tumors of the lung are bronchial tumors, pleuropulmonary blastoma, and pleural tumors (malignant mesothelioma).

Bronchial tumors

Primary endobronchial lesions are of three histologic types—carcinoid, being the most frequent, followed by mucoepidermoid and adenoid cystic types. Mucoepidermoid carcinoma accounts for 10% of malignant lung tumors in children.

The child may present clinically with recurrent atelectasis or pneumonitis, hemoptysis, cough and wheeze. The tumor presents as a painless, slow-growing mass blocking bronchial tubes and causing obstruction. Though the tumor is not encapsulated, it has a very low malignant potential, and bronchial tumors are associated with excellent prognosis even in the presence of local invasion.

Though the lesions are visible endoscopically, biopsy may be hazardous due to hemorrhage and endoscopic resection is not recommended. Bronchography or CT scan helps in determining the degree of bronchiectasis distal to the obstruction.

Resection, removal of the involved lymphatics if feasible, is the treatment of choice. Neither chemotherapy nor radiation therapy is indicated unless there is metastasis.

Pleuropulmonary blastoma

A rare and highly aggressive embryonal mesenchymal tumor, exclusively seen in children and rare beyond 12 years of age. It accounts for 15% of all primary pediatric pulmonary tumors and 25 % of them occur in familial settings. The siblings and first-degree relatives should be screened for pulmonary and extrapulmonary benign and malignant conditions, which is a significant point to be noted by the pediatrician and the pulmonologist.

Cough, dyspnea, hemoptysis, fever, chest pain, upper abdominal pain, anorexia, malaise, or neurological symptoms from brain metastasis can be the presenting features. Cases with predominant pleural involvement often present with pleuritis and empyema refractory to medical treatment. Symptomatic presentation also results from spontaneous pneumothorax in the cystic lesions.

Three types have been described based on morphology. The tumor types form a continuum with progression over time from type I to type III. The long-term survival of type I is >80% and <50% for type II and type III. The commonest site for metastasis is brain. It is associated with high risk of fatal embolic complications.

Imaging studies show varied appearance depending on the tumor type; unilocular cysts, multicystic structure, cyst containing polypoid mass, and solid-cystic mass. The entire thorax should be screened for asymptomatic cysts, which could be forerunner of type I tumors.

Fine needle aspiration cytology or a solitary needle biopsy core might sample a single tissue type can conceal the true nature of the disease, hence complete tumor resection and histological examination should be the standard procedure as it decides the appropriate therapy. Total resection is associated with improved prognosis. Recurrence or metastasis does occur in spite of primary resection.

Malignant mesothelioma

Primary pleural neoplasms in the pediatric population are quite rare. Diffuse malignant mesothelioma is extremely rare in children;

there is no clear causal relationship with asbestos exposure in children. They also occur as a secondary malignancy following radiation therapy. Mortality rate ranges from 50% to 70%.

Secondary involvement of lung in systemic disease

Langerhans cell histiocytosis

In children, lung involvement in Langerhans cell histiocytosis reflects systemic involvement rather than an isolated lung lesion. Most often occurs in infants and young children, and skeletal survey may reveal punched-out lytic lesions of skull and other long bones. Lung involvement shows a reticulonodular pattern, larger cavitary nodules, pneumatoceles, bilateral cystic disease, and pneumothorax.

Leukemia and lymphoma

Pulmonary infiltrates in leukemic patients are primarily considered as infectious, but leukemic infiltration of lung may cause a similar picture. They may manifest as patchy interstitial, septal, pleural infiltrates in contrast to Hodgkin's and non-Hodgkin's lymphoma which tend to form a larger, well-circumscribed nodules obscuring the background parenchyma. Arthi et al. has reported 3-year-old girl child who presented with fever, cough and wheeze for 6 months, X-ray chest showed military mottling and was started on antitubercular treatment for 6 months; the worsening of respiratory symptoms and increase in the pulmonary infiltrates prompted a thoracoscopic lung biopsy which revealed a non-Hodgkin's lymphoma.

Metastatic solid tumors of childhood

They account for 80% of all lung tumors in children. Wilms' tumor and osteosarcoma are the most common tumors that produce lung metastases. They appear as single or multiple circumscribed nodules, often peripherally and in the lower lobes in hematogenous spread and reticular or miliary pattern in lymphangitic spread.

LEARNING POINTS

- In pediatrics, respiratory symptoms are not always of infectious or inflammatory etiology
- Consolidation and pleural effusion can be the presenting feature of chest wall tumors and malignancy has to be ruled out, if an underlying mass is seen
- Miliary mottling, after ruling out other common etiologies, rarely can be a sign of pulmonary metastasis
- If malignancy is considered, kindly refer the child upfront to pediatric oncologist for complete evaluation as incomplete investigations prior to referral may cause resentment among the caretakers and lead to abandonment or delay in seeking intervention.

SUGGESTED READINGS

1. Cohen MC, Kaschula ROC. Primary pulmonary tumors in childhood: a review of 31 years' experience and the literature. Pediatr Pulmonol. 1992;140:222-32.
2. Fauroux B, Aynie V, Larroquet M, Boccon-Gibod L, Ducou le Pointe H, Tamalet A, et al. Carcinoid and mucoepidermoid bronchial tumours in children. Eur J Pediatr. 2005;164: 748-52.
3. Priest JR, Andic D, Arbuckle S, Gonzalez-Gomez I, Hill DA, Williams G., et al. Great vessel/cardiac extension and tumor embolism in pleuropulmonary blastoma: a report from the International Pleuropulmonary Blastoma Registry. Pediatr Blood Cancer .2011;56:604-9.
4. Srinivasan A, Ravikumar T, Andal A, Scott JX. Primary pulmonary diffuse large B-cell non-Hodgkin's lymphoma in a child. Indian J Chest Dis Allied Sci. 2013;55:225-7.
5. Weldon CB, Shamberger RC. Pediatric pulmonary tumors: primary and metastatic. Semin Pediatr Surg. 2008;17:17-29.

CHAPTER

45

Pulmonary Artery Hypertension and Cor Pulmonale

Ramesh P Menon, Arindam Choudhury

CASE 1

A 5-year-old girl, otherwise normal, was brought by her parents with complaints of panting excessively, even while doing daily activities, of recent onset. On examination her heart rate was 100/minute and blood pressure in right upper limb while sitting was 88/56 mmHg with a normal temperature. On cardiovascular system examination, the only abnormal finding was a loud P2 felt prominently in the second intercostal space, besides a left parasternal heave. There was no variation in the second heart sound with respiratory maneuvers. There was no organomegaly and rest of the systemic examination was within normal limits. On enquiry, she had the habit of snoring while sleeping and had some daytime somnolence also.

Q. What is likely diagnosis in this child?

This young girl without any comorbid condition has developed features of obstructive sleep apnea (with snoring, daytime somnolence) complicated by features of pulmonary artery hypertension (easy fatigability, normotensive with palpable and loud P2 and parasternal heave). The respiratory maneuvers and variability in P2 indicate a functional reserve of the pulmonary circulation capacitance. There is no variation in P2 with respiratory maneuvers indicating a pulmonary hypertension.

Q. How pulmonary hypertension is defined and what are the characteristic presenting feature(s) of pulmonary hypertension in children?

Pulmonary hypertension (increased blood pressure in the pulmonary circulation) is more common in children than in adults. It could be pulmonary venous or arterial hypertension.

Definition

After 3 months of age, in term babies at sea level, pulmonary hypertension is present when the mean pulmonary artery pressure (PAP_{mean}) exceeds 25 mmHg at rest, in the presence of an equal distribution of blood flow to all segments of both lungs, with normal pulmonary capillary wedge pressure. This is irrespective of the presence or absence of pulmonary hypertensive vascular disease (PHVD). In particular, pulmonary vascular reactivity (PVR) is important in the diagnosis and management of PHVD in children with heart disease.

Exercise hemodynamic abnormalities is important in the pediatric population; therefore, a PAP_{mean} >30 mmHg with exercise is an abnormal response and also defines (idiopathic) pulmonary artery hypertension.

A clinical suspicion is aroused by history of child who is unduly short of breath, tires easily or is syncopal when there is no evidence of heart or lung disease. There may be progressive exertional dyspnoea (unexplained and increasing), easy fatigability, lightheadedness, and presyncope when associated with other conditions. Children only occasionally complain of chest pain. The physical signs of pulmonary hypertension include a left parasternal, right ventricular lift, an accentuated pulmonary component of the S_2, and sometimes cool extremities. A systolic murmur of tricuspid regurgitation or a diastolic murmur of pulmonary regurgitation may be present. Increased vasoconstriction or obliteration of the vascular bed especially associated with congenital heart disease in children leads to pulmonary hypertension (PH). Childhood PH is usually related to acyanotic as well as cyanotic heart disease. In conditions like adenotonsillar hypertrophy, commonly, the young child has periodic upper airway obstruction with episodes of hypoxia and develops pulmonary arterial hypertension . A modest elevation in pulmonary arterial pressure (PAP) is tolerable, but a high pressure is associated with obstructive pulmonary vascular disease leading to right heart failure and death. Pulmonary arterial hypertension is much more common than venous hypertension, particularly in childhood, and the new therapies target arterial disease.

Q. In the above case, resting SpO_2 is 89% off O_2. What should be the approach to a child with PAH?

As given in flowchart 1, history and clinical examination would lead us to a suspicion of pulmonary hypertension. Functional capacity

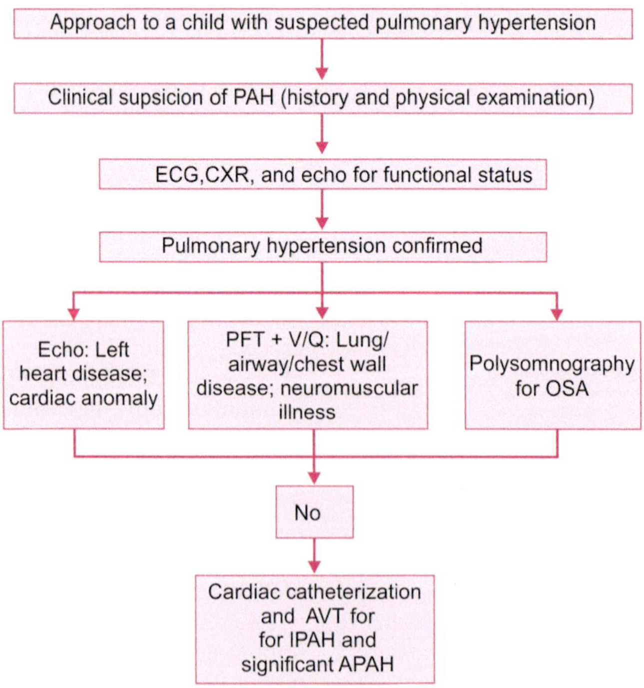

CXR, chest X-ray; ECG, electrocardiogram; echo, echocardiography; IPAH, idiopathic pulmonary arterial hypertension; APAH, associated pulmonary arterial hypertension; AVT, acute vasodilator testing; PFT, pulmonary function tests; V/Q, ventilation/ perfusion.

Flowchart 1: Approach to pediatric pulmonary hypertension

is graded according to the New York Heart Association (NYHA)/World Health Organization (WHO) classification, from the asymptomatic patient in class I to the severely disabled in class IV. Shortness of breath is a common complaint and an objective assessment of exercise capacity is helpful. In a cooperative child aged 6 years or more, the results of a 6 minutes walk test can be compared with those in normal children of the same age and sex.

The chest X-ray (CXR) may show prominent (central) pulmonary vessel markings with peripheral pruning. ECG may show P pulmonale, right ventricular hypertrophy with dilatation. Echocardiogram with Doppler interrogation may confirm the same, in addition to estimating the pulmonary artery systolic and diastolic pressures. A contrast-enhanced spiral CT, in addition to a CXR, in older children may show evidence of thrombus in the central pulmonary arteries and chronic thromboembolic disease. It may also distinguish idiopathic pulmonary arterial hypertension (IPAH) from pulmonary veno-occlusive disease (PVOD). Ventilation/perfusion (VQ) scans may be normal or show small peripheral nonsegmental perfusion defects. Magnetic resonance imaging helps in assessing right ventricular function but is resource intensive. The echocardiogram generally reveals dilated right heart chambers, right ventricular hypertrophy with posterior bowing of the ventricular and, in the absence of an atrial communication, the atrial septum. The left ventricle may be severely compressed (banana-shaped). Right atrial size and left ventricular eccentricity index are predictive of outcome in adults and are routinely assessed in children. Lung function testing can sometimes demonstrate small airways obstruction.

In addition to routine hematology and biochemistry (blood tests may show hyperuricemia, particularly in Eisenmenger's syndrome and elevation of brain natriuretic peptide, although less reliably than in adults), thyroid function tests, a thrombophilia screen including antiphospholipid antibodies (lupus anticoagulant, anticardiolipin antibodies) and an autoimmune screen are carried out. Children may seroconvert when they are older. Some children have an immunoglobulin deficiency. They may have a low level of antithrombin III, protein S, or protein C, which may be genetic in origin or result from a consumption coagulopathy. Screening of other siblings for the familial form of the disease is necessary. Angiography is the gold standard for the diagnosis and follow-up of pulmonary hypertension. Lung biopsy is rarely justified in pulmonary hypertension. The exceptions are suspicion of PVOD or pulmonary capillary hemangiomatosis (PCH), alveolar hypoplasia or dysplasia in persistent pulmonary hypertension of the newborn (PPHN), and very rarely in children with complex congenital heart disease (CHD) in whom it might still be possible to operate.

Q. What are the causes of PAH in children? How is pediatric pulmonary hypertension classified?

The etiology of PAH is more diverse in pediatric patients (Box 1). Childhood pulmonary hypertension could be IPAH, formerly known as primary pulmonary hypertension, and/or secondary-associated pulmonary arterial hypertension (APAH) when associated with other disorders such as CHD, connective tissue or lung disease.

Q. How to manage this patient?

Management of APAH (secondary PAH)

Successful treatment of the pulmonary hypertension depends on early screening for pulmonary hypertension as a major complicating factor. Presentation and the investigation of children with APAH are determined by the underlying disease process. The principal etiologies are as above [chronic hypoxia associated with obstructive sleep apnea (OSA), as in this example]. In children with APAH, treatment of the primary cause, if not of long-standing nature, would reverse the pulmonary artery hypertension also. However, if cor

Box 1: Classification of pulmonary hypertension

- Pulmonary arterial hypertension (PAH)
  - Idiopathic PAH (IPAH)
  - Familial IPAH (FIPAH) [*BMPR2, ALK1*, endoglin (+/- HHT gene)]
  - Associated with PAH (APAH)
    - Connective tissue disease
    - Congenital systemic to pulmonary shunts
    - Portal hypertension
    - Human immunodeficiency virus
    - Drugs and toxins
    - Other (hemolytic anemia, Schistosomiasis)
  - Associated with significant venous or capillary involvement
    - Pulmonary veno-occlusive disease (PVOD)
    - Pulmonary capillary hemangiomatosis
  - Persistent pulmonary hypertension of the newborn
- Pulmonary hypertension associated with left heart diseases
- Pulmonary hypertension associated with respiratory disease and/or hypoxia
  - Chronic obstructive pulmonary disease
  - Interstitial lung disease
  - Sleep disordered breathing
  - Alveolar hypoventilation disorders
  - High altitude
  - Developmental abnormalities
- Pulmonary hypertension due to chronic thrombotic/embolic disease
- Miscellaneous
  - Tumor and others (glycogen storage disease, Gaucher's disease, sarcoidosis, pulmonary Langerhans cell histiocytosis, thyroid disorders, lymphangioleiomyomatosis)

pulmonale has developed, then it would need therapeutic intervention of its own.

Treatment of PAH

It is understood as supportive therapy, pharmacotherapy, and supplementary therapy. Immunization schedules should be maintained, and young children may need respiratory syncytial virus prophylaxis. Anesthesia for any procedure requires particular care. The aim of medical treatment is to dilate the pulmonary vasculature and reverse the abnormal remodeling characteristic of pulmonary vascular disease. The practical difficulties in treating children influence management and include their age, level of understanding, size, and in some the presence of other anomalies. Three signaling pathways are targeted in pharmacotherapy—(1) prostacyclin, (2) endothelin, and (3) nitric oxide pathways.

Prostacyclin and its analogues

The most effective therapy is a continuous intravenous infusion of epoprostenol, the sodium salt of prostacyclin. It has a $t_{1/2}$ = 3–5 minutes, is unstable and the infusion has to be prepared every 24 hours. The principal side effects are jaw pain and diarrhea. Iloprost is a prostacyclin analogue which can be given by inhalation, but small, tired children find it difficult to inhale an effective dose. The drug is effective for <2 hours.

Endothelin receptor antagonists

The dual endothelin (ET) receptor antagonist (ERA) bosentan was the first oral drug shown to be efficacious in IPAH in children and has been used extensively in this and other types of pulmonary hypertension since its introduction in 2002. Its principal side effect is elevation of liver enzymes which necessitates a monthly blood test. The newer selective ET-A receptor antagonists, sitaxentan and ambrisentan, have not yet been studied in children.

Phosphodiesterase inhibitors

Sildenafil was the first drug of this class and is still the most commonly used, particularly in young children with APAH. The principal side effects include erections and systemic hypotension when high doses are used. The dose is 0.5–1 mg/kg/dose, given three to four times a day, rarely more. In 2012, after the STARTS trial (Sildenafil monotherapy) the FDA placed a safety warning on prescription of sildenafil in pediatric PAH patients. The ruling, now part of the package insert , states that sildenafil should not be started in patients 1–17 years of age. Children with APAH-CHD and those weighing <20 kg did not appear at an increased risk with high-dose sildenafil. Abruptly stopping sildenafil, may be associated with severe worsening or death.

Supplementary therapy

Patients with pulmonary vascular disease are prone to develop thrombosis in situ. Older children are given warfarin and younger ones usually receive aspirin. The international normalized ratio must be monitored particularly closely in those on ERA.

Oxygen

Oxygen is a potent pulmonary vasodilator. Nocturnal supplemental oxygen is indicated if there is nocturnal systemic arterial oxygen desaturation .

Atrial septostomy

This procedure is indicated in children with IPAH and postoperative pulmonary hypertension suffering from syncope and/or severe right heart failure. It reduces the effect of a sudden increase in pulmonary arterial and right heart pressures and maintains a left ventricular output.

Lung and heart-lung transplantation

Refer children on intravenous epoprostenol for assessment by the transplantation service when they are established on treatment and are still well.

> **CASE 2**
>
> A 25-day-old newborn infant with an acyanotic congenital heart disease (supravalvular mitral ring and atrial septal defect) with some cyanosis, which is evident on crying.

Q. Is this baby suffering from Eisenmenger's disease?

This baby is "at risk" of Eisenmenger's disease. Classical Eisenmenger's syndrome occurs in the patient who initially had a large left to right shunt and then slowly developed pulmonary vascular disease with shunt reversal. Central cyanosis and clubbing is not usually a problem in neonates or young infants. Most patients begin to deteriorate in their teenage years. A small group of children who have a high pulmonary vascular resistance (PVR) when first seen in such children, the resistance probably remains high from birth. They frequently become symptomatic in childhood and may benefit from medical therapy. Sleep studies may be indicated in those with trisomy 21. Complex, surgically naive as well as postoperative cases for which surgery is not feasible frequently need re-appraisal, including cardiac catheterization with a view to palliation by medical therapy

Q. What is acute vasodilator testing (AVT)? What is the clinical implication of vasoreactivity testing?

Acute Vasodilator testing is critical for determining the following:

- Calcium channel blockers (CCBs) utility in IPAH
- Operability in children with CHD
- Long-term prognosis.

The usual practice is: inhaled nitric oxide (iNO) (dose range 20–80 ppm) if available. Barst criteria (modified) is defined as a 20% decrease in mean pulmonary artery pressure (PAPm) with normal or sustained cardiac output and no change or decrease in the ratio of pulmonary to systemic vascular resistance (PVR/SVR). Evaluation of the Sitbon criteria (e.g., a decrease in PAPm by 10 mmHg to a value <40 mmHg with sustained cardiac output) has been done in adults primarily, with regard to long-term response . The Barst and Sitbon criteria predict IPAH in children and adults.

In the child with IPAH, a robust positive response during AVT may predict sustained response with CCBs. In assessing operability in CHD, or long-term outcomes, AVT is still nebulous, conceptually. Cardiac catheterisation remains to confirm the diagnosis, assess disease severity, and guide therapeutic management and the role of lung biopsy.

Only patients with a positive AVT can be treated with a CCB. This applies to <10% of those with IPAH. Children who improve and are stable on a CCB, need repeat cardiac catheterisation in a year to optimize or escalate therapy before they deteriorate. The majority of negative responders present in NYHA/WHO class III–IV frequently need to be started on intravenous epoprostenol. In a minority it is feasible to initiate therapy with an ERA. Most children however, in this situation, require dual therapy. Sildenafil monotherapy has not been proven to be efficacious in children. Syncopal children need an urgent atrial septostomy. After discharge from hospital, echocardiography is mandatory, since urgent intensification of therapy is frequently necessary.

Q. What are the developmental lung diseases associated with PAH in neonates? How is PPHN in a newborn treated?

Developmental lung diseases associated with pulmonary hypertension are:

- Congenital diaphragmatic hernia
- Bronchopulmonary dysplasia
- Alveolar capillary dysplasia (ACD)
- Alveolar capillary dysplasia with misalignment of veins
- Lung hypoplasia ("primary" or "secondary")
- Surfactant protein abnormalities
- Surfactant protein B (SPB) deficiency
- Surfactant protein C (SPC) deficiency
- ATP-binding cassette A3 mutation
- Thyroid transcription factor 1/Nkx2.1 homeobox mutation
- Pulmonary interstitial glycogenosis
- Pulmonary alveolar proteinosis

Persistent pulmonary hypertension of the newborn

It is usually a self-limiting condition, indicated by persistent failure to wean off the ventilator. It may signal alveolar dysplasia, especially in babies born at high altitude. Persistent pulmonary hypertension of the newborn may also be the first indication of chronic lung disease of prematurity or future IPAH. Children with a modest increase in PAP are treated with sildenafil unless it is apparent that irreversible changes have set in. In both chronic lung disease and PPHN, the aim is to encourage normalization of the pulmonary vasculature and so be able to stop treatment with relatively new, powerful drugs whose long-term effects on children are under evaluation.

Q. What are the new and emerging therapies?

Newer agents target remodelling of the pulmonary vasculature, the restoration of endothelial function, and growth of new peripheral pulmonary arteries. New modes of administration, new formulations, and new analogues of existing drugs; new ERA and new phosphodiesterase (PDE) 1/5/6 plus PDE-3 phosphodiesterase and PDE-1 inhibitors are emerging. Statins, RhoA inhibitors, antigrowth factor drugs, metalloproteinase inhibitors, K-channel openers, stem cell and gene therapy, and vasoactive intestinal peptide are being developed which may reverse (pulmonary) plexiform angiopathy. At present we can stabilize patients for many years; precision medicine(s) used in combination offer the hope of cure and greater promise to the individual child.

LEARNING POINTS

- History and examination followed by chest X-ray, electrocardiogram and transthoracic echocardiogram are required to diagnose pulmonary hypertension
- The etiology of pulmonary hypertension is diverse in pediatric patients. In the majority, pulmonary hypertension is idiopathic or associated with congenital heart disease, and rarely is associated with other conditions such as connective tissue or thromboembolic disease
- Three signaling pathways are targeted in pharmacotherapy for pulmonary hypertension—(1) prostacyclin, (2) endothelin, and (3) nitric oxide pathways
- New modes of administration, new formulations and new analogues of existing drugs, new endothelin receptor antagonists and new phosphodiesterase (PDE) 1/5/6 plus PDE-3 and PDE-1 inhibitors are emerging now for pulmonary artery hypertension.

SUGGESTED READINGS

1. Barst RJ, McGoon MD, Elliott CG, Foreman AJ, Miller DP, Ivy DD. Survival in childhood pulmonary arterial hypertension: insights from the registry to evaluate early and long-term pulmonary arterial hypertension disease management. Circulation. 2012;125(1):113-22.
2. Berger RM, Beghetti M, Humpl T, Raskob GE, Ivy DD, Bonnet D, et al. Clinical features of paediatric pulmonary hypertension: a registry study. The Lancet. 2012;379:537-46.
3. Cerro MJ, Abman S, Diaz G, Freudenthal AH, Freudenthal F, Harikrishnan S, et al. A consensus approach to the classification of pediatric pulmonary hypertensive vascular disease: report from the PVRI Pediatric Taskforce, Panama 2011. Pulm Circ. 2011;1(2):286-98.
4. Ivy DD, Abman SH, Barst RJ, Berger RM, Bonnet D, Fleming TR, et al. Pediatric pulmonary hypertension. J Am Coll Cardiol. 2013;62(25 Suppl):D117-26.
5. Moledina S, Hislop AA, Foster H, Schulze-Neick I, Haworth SG. Childhood idiopathic pulmonary arterial hypertension: a national cohort study. Heart. 2010;96(17):1401-6.
6. Simonneau G, Robbins IM, Beghetti M, Channick RN, Delcroix M, Denton CP, et al. Updated clinical classification of pulmonary hypertension. J Am Coll Cardiol. 2009;54(1 Suppl):S43-54.
7. Haworth SG. The Management of pulmonary hypertension in children. Arch Dis Child. 2008;93(7):620-5.
8. Vorhies, Erika E, Ivy DD. Drug treatment of pulmonary hypertension in children. Pediatric Drugs. 2014;16(1):43-65.

Index

Page numbers followed by *f* refer to figure, *t* refer to table, *b* refer to box, and *fc* refer to flowchart.

R

S

T

U

V

W

Y

Z